Coaching Families for Resilience

How Pediatricians Can Support Caregivers and Prevent Burnout

Gretchen A. Pianka, MD, MPH, FAAP

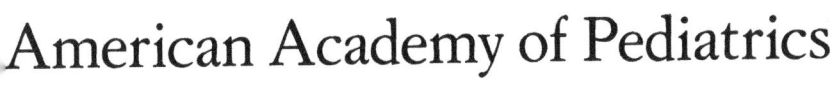

American Academy of Pediatrics

DEDICATED TO THE HEALTH OF ALL CHILDREN®

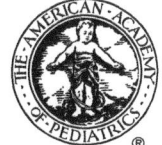

American Academy of Pediatrics Publishing Staff

Mark Grimes, *Vice President, Publishing*
Jeff Mahony, *Senior Director, Professional and Consumer Publishing*
Chris Wiberg, *Senior Editor, Professional/Clinical Publishing*
Theresa Wiener, *Production Manager, Clinical and Professional Publications*
Amanda Helmholz, *Medical Copy Editor*
Soraya Alem, *Digital Production Specialist*
Sara Hoerdeman, *Marketing and Acquisitions Manager, Consumer Products*

Published by the American Academy of Pediatrics
345 Park Blvd
Itasca, IL 60143
Telephone: 630/626-6000
Facsimile: 847/434-8000
www.aap.org

The American Academy of Pediatrics is an organization of 67,000 primary care pediatricians, pediatric medical subspecialists, and pediatric surgical specialists dedicated to the health, safety, and well-being of all infants, children, adolescents, and young adults.

The recommendations in this publication do not indicate an exclusive course of treatment or serve as a standard of medical care. Variations, taking into account individual circumstances, may be appropriate.

Statements and opinions expressed are those of the author and not necessarily those of the American Academy of Pediatrics.

Any websites, brand names, products, or manufacturers are mentioned for informational and identification purposes only and do not imply an endorsement by the American Academy of Pediatrics (AAP). The AAP is not responsible for the content of external resources. Information was current at the time of publication.

The publishers have made every effort to trace the copyright holders for borrowed materials. If they have inadvertently overlooked any, they will be pleased to make the necessary arrangements at the first opportunity.

This publication has been developed by the American Academy of Pediatrics. The contributors are expert authorities in the field of pediatrics. No commercial involvement of any kind has been solicited or accepted in the development of the content of this publication.

Every effort is made to keep *Coaching Families for Resilience* consistent with the most recent advice and information available from the American Academy of Pediatrics.

Please visit www.aap.org/errata for an up-to-date list of any applicable errata for this publication.

Special discounts are available for bulk purchases of this publication. Email Special Sales at nationalaccounts@aap.org for more information.

Printed in the United States of America

9-519/0325   1 2 3 4 5 6 7 8 9 10

MA1175

ISBN: 978-1-61002-788-5

eBook: 978-1-61002-789-2

Cover and publication design by Peg Mulcahy

Library of Congress Control Number: 2024942980

Author

Gretchen A. Pianka, MD, MPH, FAAP

Primary Care Pediatrician

Greater Portland Health

Portland, ME

Pediatrician

Pediatric Rapid Evaluation Program (PREP)

Edmund N. Ervin Pediatric Center

Augusta, ME

American Academy of Pediatrics Reviewers

Committee on Psychosocial Aspects of Child and Family Health

Council on Child Abuse and Neglect

Council on Foster Care, Adoption, and Kinship Care

Department of Healthy Resilient Children

Section on LGBT Health and Wellness

Dedication

To my high school principal, who told me I would never amount to anything.
Thank you for showing me how not to talk to struggling kids.

Equity, Diversity, and Inclusion Statement

The American Academy of Pediatrics is committed to principles of equity, diversity, and inclusion in its publishing program. Editorial boards, author selections, and author transitions (publication succession plans) are designed to include diverse voices that reflect society as a whole. Editor and author teams are encouraged to actively seek out diverse authors and reviewers at all stages of the editorial process. Publishing staff are committed to promoting equity, diversity, and inclusion in all aspects of publication writing, review, and production.

Contents

Acknowledgments xi

Introduction 1

Chapter 1. Offsetting Adversity With Resilience 5

Chapter 2. Overview of Resilience University 33

Chapter 3. Essential Toolkit 53

Chapter 4. Process for Stepwise Change 91

Chapter 5. A Structured Approach to Resilience Coaching 117

Chapter 6. Using Relationship-Based and Trauma-Informed Anticipatory
Guidance 149

Chapter 7. Examples of Tailored Anticipatory Guidance: Vignettes 175

Chapter 8. Universal Integration in Practice 209

Conclusion 231

Appendix. Handouts and Tools 235

Appendix A. Using 5 Big Deep Breaths to Calm the Nervous System 236

Appendix B. Box Breathing 237

Appendix C. Relaxation Breathing 238

Appendix D. Use Your Breath 239

Appendix E. Glitter Jar Meditation 240

Appendix F. Emotional Awareness 241

Appendix G. Loving-Kindness Meditation for Parents and Caregivers 242

Appendix H. Loving-Kindness Meditation for Older Children and Teens 243

Appendix I. Walking Meditation 244

Appendix J. Mindfulness Using 5-4-3-2-1 245

Appendix K. Mindfulness Using Toes-to-Nose 246

Appendix L. Applied Mindfulness: The Fire-Truck Brain Analogy 247

Appendix M. Building Block Worksheets Using the HOPE (Healthy Outcomes
from Positive Childhood Experiences) Framework 248

Appendix N. Conversation Topics to Support the HOPE (Healthy Outcomes
from Positive Childhood Experiences) Building Blocks 250

Appendix O. Stress Reduction Plan for Teens 251

Appendix P. 9-5-2-1-0 Checklist 252

Appendix Q. Plan-Do-Study-Act Approach in Resilience University 253

Appendix R. Blank "Back the Bus Up" Timeline 254

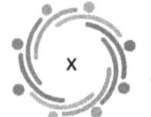

Appendix S. Feelings Sticker Chart 255

Appendix T. Family Feelings Chart.................................... 256

Appendix U. "10 Things I Can Do When I Feel Yucky" List 257

Appendix V. Validate, Validate, Validate 258

Appendix W. NICER Parenting 259

Appendix X. SUNBEAM: A Stress-Lowering, Trauma-Informed Parenting
Practice 260

Appendix Y. Emotion Coaching for Parents and Caregivers 261

Appendix Z. Resilience University Enrollment Form 262

Appendix AA. Resilience University Certificate of Completion 263

Appendix BB. Other Feeling Chart Templates 264

Appendix CC. Self-Care Nook 269

Appendix DD. Printable Glitter Jar Labels 270

Appendix EE. 6 Steps to Connect 271

Index 273

Acknowledgments

From the bottom of my heart, I would like to thank the young man at Zavala Elementary School who never spoke to me but showed up over and over to silently stand between me and those peers who were bullying me.

I am eternally grateful to my thesis adviser, Patricia O'Hara, for recognizing that I was having a trauma response in the middle of my bachelor thesis defense and supporting me through it. I didn't know what was happening. Thank you for knowing what to do.

I would probably have given up on medicine and never become a doctor if it hadn't been for Dr Mary Wilson, who paused to ask her hourly temp secretary (me) what she wanted to do with her life. Thank you for believing in me and showing me how it's possible to be a brilliantly busy, kind, compassionate physician author.

I am forever grateful for Dr Mark Mendelson, who introduced me to trauma-informed care (without calling it that) in my residency continuity clinic, modeling how to provide family-centered care and how to consider the whole picture for all our families.

I'm so thankful that Dr Andy Garner encouraged me to turn what I learned from Resilience University (RU) into this book. Thank you, Dr Garner, for connecting me with American Academy of Pediatrics (AAP) Publishing! Thank you to my editor, Chris Wiberg, for helping me make these concepts even clearer as we brought this book into form. Thank you to all the AAP committee, council, section, and department members who reviewed and read draft chapters; I know you are all busy, and I sincerely appreciate your time and insight.

The support of the Maine Chapter of the AAP has been such a wonderful blessing. Thank you to Dee Kerry and my wonderful pediatric colleagues who have embraced the tools and strategies in this book as I developed them.

I would be remiss if I didn't also thank the pediatricians and researchers who led the Maine Youth Overweight Collaborative decades ago, including Michele Polacsek, Lisa Letourneau, and Tori Rogers, who introduced me to the idea of integrating Plan-Do-Study-Act cycles and motivational interviewing into my existing clinical workflow to support families that want something to change.

I am grateful for the support and encouragement from Drs Bob Sege and Dina Burstein, their wonderful team at the HOPE® (Healthy Outcomes from Positive Childhood Experiences) National Resource Center as well as the other participants in the original HOPE Innovation Network.

I am truly thankful for the AAP Addressing Social Health and Early Childhood Wellness (ASHEW) Initiative and specifically for Megan Heavrin, who helped me

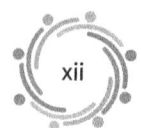

share RU tools and strategies and get valuable feedback. Thank you to Amy King, PhD, and Dr Nerissa Bauer for welcoming me on their podcasts and encouraging me along the path that led to this book.

I want to extend a special thank-you to all the children and families I have worked with. You have shown me how important it is for pediatricians to meaningfully show up for families when things are challenging. Thank you to all the parents who shared with me how they wanted to stop yelling or exit some other frustrating parenting cycle. I didn't tell you this at the time, but I was experiencing so many similar moments in my own journey. You're not alone!

Thank you to all the clinicians who work tirelessly to care for children and support caregivers like me who have experienced trauma and toxic stress. I'm grateful for the young people who are deciding to go into medicine. Thank you for reading this book! The world is a better place with you in it.

And I am forever grateful for my beautiful family for their support and inspiration. Thank you to my children, who put up with me being glued to my computer for hours on end and doing weird things like covering our vacation Airbnbs with giant Post-It notes as I clarified tools and concepts. You showed me how essential it is for all our systems to be trauma informed. Thank you to my loving husband, who never tires of hearing my ideas, is eager to help me sort through provisional thoughts to find the most effective way to share something, and always delights in my often-messy journey. Thank you to my mom for always showing up to help with the kids and feed us, teaching me how to edit my writing, and always celebrating my successes. Thank you to my stepdad, who has always been optimistic about my potential, even when my principal was not. I will be forever grateful for my late sister, who taught me everything. Literally. She always held space for me when things were impossibly hard. Thank you to her wife for coming up with the term *The Anatomy of a Meltdown* as I clarified how parents can shift away from focusing on unwanted behaviors and toward connection. I'm forever grateful to my late father for supporting my dreams, believing in my potential, and teaching me how to be a critical thinker.

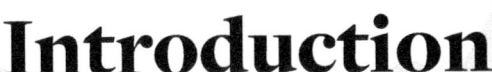

Introduction

Do you remember when you decided you wanted to become a doctor? I remember choosing medicine because I felt joy helping other people feel better when they were suffering. As the first person in my family to go to medical school, I also remember thinking that my career would be sort of like those of my parents, who were professors; only, instead of teaching classes, I would be taking care of patients. I had absolutely no idea what I was getting into.

I had no idea I would need to be on call. I had no idea I would have to spend hours in operating rooms (ORs) and intensive care units. And I had no idea that when I finally got to take care of patients, so much of that care would be dictated by factors I had no control over, like insurance and hospital administrators.

I've now been practicing for more than 20 years and learned to work within the confines of electronic health records (EHRs), administrative demands, insurance restrictions, and variable access to essential services for children and their families. I've learned that it is an immeasurable blessing to be designated someone's primary care provider, so they come to see me when they need help with something. And I've learned that sometimes, the most powerful tool I have is listening—not prescribing medications or ordering imaging studies but validating the journey my patient and their family are experiencing. Of course, prescribing medications, ordering imaging, and setting up referrals are all still an essential part of what I do. But as the years go on, I realize how crucial it is to be more than just the "fancy waitress" who listens to what someone wants or needs and then interprets a complex menu of Western medical options, guiding with recommendations about why and when families might want to choose a specific option.

I also understand how essential it is to take care of myself and how my own stress, especially when it has risen to toxic levels, derails my ability to provide the kind of care I envision when I am imagining my truest, most beautiful practice style—the kind of practice where I can listen fully, connect, and hold space for whatever is going on in the lives of the people I am blessed to interact with, whether they are administrators, staff, parents, or my patients. I remember our dean at the University of Vermont telling us in her "welcome to medical school" speech that we needed to take care of ourselves first or we couldn't take care of anyone else.

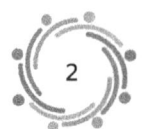
At the time, that sounded to me like I had to make sure I ate lunch or slept well. But after decades of practice, I realize that it also means taking care of the stress associated with practicing medicine that looms as a nearly constant threat and that I strive to mitigate every day.

As you may imagine, although I had taken all the prerequisites and volunteered in clinical settings, I was not prepared for medical school. I'm embarrassed to admit that I thought residency programs and internships were required only if you decided to be a surgeon or a specialist. Throughout medical school, I experienced a massive case of imposter syndrome. I felt like everyone else understood a language I had never been taught. For example, when we were going on rounds in my surgery rotation, I was given the job of taking notes. I was scurrying around after a very tired and short-tempered intern and his senior resident, trying to document everything everyone said and did. The other medical student on the team was trying to help me with my notes. His dad was a surgeon, so this student fit right in. He was leaning over my shoulder, reading what I was writing. On the patient list, under each name, I was writing "eyes and nose" with a set of numbers after them. He laughed and corrected me: "They are saying 'I's and O's,' Gretchen. It's short for 'ins and outs.'" I laughed nervously at my vulnerability, being so obviously seen as someone who didn't understand the language of medicine as I began to realize I was being indoctrinated into a completely foreign culture.

I intentionally chose my surgery elective first, figuring that since I was brand new to clinical settings, everyone had lower expectations, which would be great and could only help me. Up front, I set 3 personal goals:

1. Don't cry on rounds.
2. Don't throw up in public.
3. Don't fall asleep in someone's abdominal cavity.

I did cry on rounds, but I never threw up, even though just thinking about that sound of sawing through bone while in the OR still makes me gag. I continued to frequently not understand the mysterious shorthand or abbreviations peers and preceptors used. I was terrified to hurt someone, which led to a methodical slowness that was not particularly appreciated within the surgical realm. The first time a nurse asked me to prescribe acetaminophen for a patient's postoperative pain, I sat down in front of this exasperated nurse to read the patient's 2-inch–thick paper record from beginning to end before I called the intern to pass along my recommendation. And I was always exhausted. Once, I even missed my alarm, slept through rounds, and materialized sheepishly at a midday conference. I noticed there was no room for me to take care of myself. I thought of what the dean had said and felt like I was probably just getting it wrong again. I was sure everyone else had figured out how to take care of themselves better than I had.

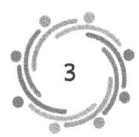

One day when I was on call, we were notified that there was a man with acute appendicitis in the emergency department (ED). We'd been in the OR all day and it was around 4:00 pm. The attending surgeon decided he would stay and operate on this one additional patient before going home. It took some time to prepare an OR, and the patient was having a computed tomographic (CT) scan to confirm the ED doctor's working diagnosis. The CT scan revealed not appendicitis but a bowel obstruction from a soccer ball–sized tumor. All of us were waiting in the surgery lounge when the resident explained this to the attending. The attending thought about it for a few minutes and then announced that the right thing to do was to still operate tonight, since the tumor was blocking the intestines and causing pain.

By the time we went into the OR, it was almost 8:00 pm. In this rotation, medical students took first call every third night. I was not used to staying up all night at all, let alone every third night, and I was beyond exhausted. At first, things were going well and it seemed like I might get to lie down by midnight in the call room. But just when I thought we were almost done, I was told that my next job was to hold the tumor up so the residents and the attending could dissect away the vital organs and vessels from below. I felt like crying but lifted the tumor and held it as steadily as I could.

Around 2:00 am, my arms were literally giving way and I was so tired that I occasionally resorted to a few of those brief, unintentional let's-try-napping-while-we're-standing-up tricks that never work. Each time I did that, I would sway and almost drop the tumor. The residents threw me stern "stop doing that" glares over their masks. Finally, one of them said, "If you keep it up, you're going to contaminate the surgical field! Hold it still or go to bed!"

I don't know what I was thinking. To this day, I remain well aware that these words were not an invitation to be excused. But instead of apologizing and beating up on myself more, I carefully put the tumor down, went to the call room, and fell asleep.

How does it feel when reading my story? Do you cringe? What comes up for you? What are your "holding a tumor at 2:00 am" stories? Did anyone tell you how important self-care is as a doctor? I bet they did. Did anyone support you in actually taking care of yourself? That is not as common. The modern health care system is not designed to allow doctors to honor their own humanness or to care for their own unmet needs. At some point, we're expected to become martyrs to medicine. It's as if an unspoken part of becoming a doctor involves transforming your own humanness into something that can be ignored, suppressed, disposed of... We learn, by imprinting, that our body's needs for food or sleep can be subjugated to the needs of our patients. Yet by ignoring our own fundamental needs, we begin down a slippery slope, which not only increases burnout but also separates us from our patients.

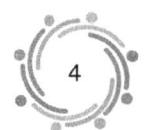

When I developed the clinical approach I describe in this book as "Resilience University" (RU), I was tired of medicine. I was tired of spending my day checking boxes in the EHR to prove I had talked about specific, externally monitored things with the families rather than just talking with them about what they wanted my help with and honoring their strengths and challenges. I was tired of trying to figure out which medication insurance companies approved of instead of being able to offer the one I really thought would help the most and cause the fewest side effects. I was tired of feeling like I was just sticking my finger into the proverbial hole in the dam, watching families go through impossibly hard situations while my role in their time of need was to set up a bunch of referrals and send them off to unfamiliar offices to meet clinicians they didn't know. I was also tired of feeling cornered into prescribing psychoactive medications for children with behavioral problems when families needed so much more.

I was even more tired of seeing these families in follow-up and finding out that none of the referrals had actually resulted in meaningful care or assistance. I was tired of feeling like I'd failed my families when the prescriptions I offered didn't suddenly fix everything as they had hoped. I was tired of feeling like my practice of medicine had been reduced to algorithms other people wrote for systems other people controlled in a world that valued behavior over wellness. I felt like the art of medicine was lost and no longer had a place in the modern medical system. And I was missing time with my own children to do a job I felt was demoralizing. I was well on my way to burnout and found myself frequently dreaming about opening a coffee shop where I could sell really delicious lattes and still have plenty of time to spend sleeping, eating, and hanging out with my own kids.

But instead, as a last-ditch effort before opening Pianka's Prescription Coffee Shop, I decided to see if I could offer something more. I decided that perhaps, before I gave up on a decade of education and 2 decades of practice, I could try to address what I saw happening within my practice by expanding what I could offer instead of forgetting what I'd learned and hiding under an espresso machine. So, I developed a framework and tools so I could work with families, using a quality improvement approach, to help them with the root causes of recurrent suffering. And I was able to create a new way of problem-solving with families that made me love practicing medicine again.

Thank you for giving this idea time and space in your world. I sincerely hope that you find this approach and the tools in this book as energizing and restorative as that delicious latte I might have made for you if I hadn't come up with RU.

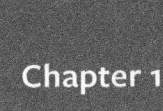

Chapter 1

Offsetting Adversity With Resilience

The approach described in this book relies on well-established models of health and wellness combined with rigorously studied processes for change. Drawing on evidence-informed strategies to lower stress and improve communication, we can help repair relational health ruptures and expand access to positive childhood experiences (PCEs). Using stepwise change strategies, we can address barriers to integrating anticipatory guidance and health promotion recommendations. Focusing on tiny, manageable steps of change, clinicians and families can cocreate individualized paths forward, fostering resilience.

Resilience has been defined in many ways, but the definition I like to use, to paraphrase, is "the ability to adapt to difficult or challenging internal and external life experiences with mental, emotional, and behavioral flexibility,"[1] one messy moment at a time. Complementing ongoing systemic efforts to prevent toxic stress and adversity in childhood, this book teaches a step-by-step meaningful response to mitigate the impact when we identify its presence in existing clinical encounters.

Families often bring behavioral and relational issues to primary care physicians. Yet we may not be accustomed to clarifying whether these issues are symptoms of stress or adversity. When they are related to toxic levels of stress or a history of trauma, traditional guidance may not work and could even make matters worse. With most adults now reporting adversity in their own childhood,[2] trauma-informed parenting advice has become my most common practice. A practice gap exists here since the science is relatively new and this type of advice and guidance remains limited in primary care education. The trauma-informed tools and strategies you will learn from this book are equally useful for families experiencing chronic, potentially toxic levels of stress caused by any number of factors. Approaching family concerns with a resilience lens is equally impactful whether the child, the parent, or both have experienced adversity or if the family is currently experiencing overwhelming levels of stress.

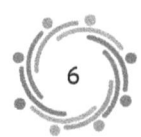

A Cumulative View of Adversity and Resilience

Childhood adversity, including toxic stress, has proven to affect not only bio-logical systems as a child grows but also the developmental processes, including crucial steps in brain development. The adverse childhood experiences (ACEs) studied by Felitti and Anda in their original study[3] have been expanded over the years to include broader sources of adversity such as bullying, community vio-lence, and racism,[4] making it plausible that almost all our patients will, at some point in their lives, experience one or more ACEs.

Positive childhood experiences offset the long-term mental and physical health impacts of childhood adversity,[5,6] giving us evidence to back what we know from our clinical experience: not all adversity has the same impact. Family culture, nurturing relationships, healthy coping skills, adequate resources, community support, and other factors can buffer the impact of adversity and toxic stress. This chapter explores the concept of offsetting adversity with resilience; the chapters that follow will walk you through a step-by-step approach so you can turn this concept into action and meaningfully respond to families experiencing adversity or toxic stress, regardless of the cause.

Many people have attempted to catalog what resilient children and families look like from the outside; I'm not interested in doing that here. If a hurricane swept through a coastal town and the only house left standing was pink with blue shutters on the windows, it wouldn't make any sense to tell everyone that to ensure a hurricane-proof town, we need to just make sure to paint all the houses pink with blue shutters. Focusing on what resilience looks like from the outside doesn't take into account the complex interplay of factors that held that little pink shack with blue shutters together through the hurricane. Many of our families have strengths and protective factors that may be invisible to us; conversely, other families experience invisible adversity. In families, just like in houses, distress tolerance is internal. For humans, it is inextricably linked to access to resources, relational health, emotional agility, and self-care (**Figure 1-1**).

Resilience arises from being able to integrate a core set of protective and stress-mitigating factors that make a child's "house" strong enough to withstand a metaphorical hurricane. Modern research has given us enough data to become "resilience engineers" in helping the families we care for overcome barriers and internalize resilience.

We are finally starting to understand not only what resilience looks like from the inside out but also how to help families find it when things have gone sideways. Understanding what has—and hasn't—happened in a child's life can be the first step in helping them, and their caregivers, heal. We know that parental or guardian ACEs and PCEs can affect relational health, so some practices screen for these.

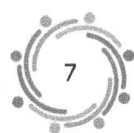

Figure 1-1.

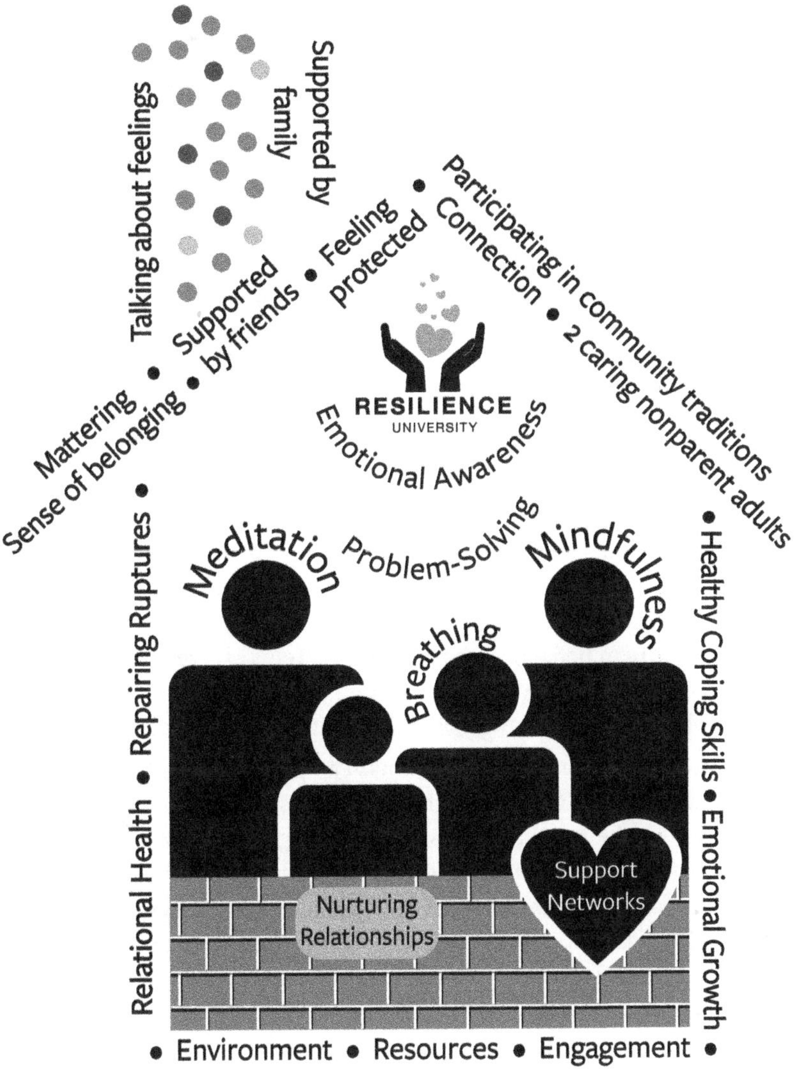

Supported by family

Talking about feelings

Supported by friends

Mattering

Sense of belonging

Feeling protected

Participating in community traditions

Connection

2 caring nonparent adults

Repairing Ruptures

Relational Health

RESILIENCE
UNIVERSITY

Emotional Awareness

Meditation

Problem-Solving

Breathing

Mindfulness

Healthy Coping Skills

Emotional Growth

Nurturing Relationships

Support Networks

• Environment • Resources • Engagement •

ENGINEERING RESILIENCE:
STRENGTH FROM THE INSIDE OUT

Resilience arises from being able to integrate a core set of protective and stress-mitigating factors that make a child's "house" strong enough to withstand a metaphorical hurricane. Modern research has given us enough data to become "resilience engineers" in helping the families we care for overcome barriers and internalize resilience.

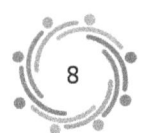

But whether or not we're doing this screening, we can universally support relational and family health. Some families may not feel comfortable sharing their trauma histories, while others may not be able to verbalize how much stress they are actually experiencing. Framing our guidance with stepwise problem-solving strategies grounded in neurobiology helps everyone with a nervous system, regardless of trauma history or acknowledgment of stress level. Supporting parents and caregivers with this guidance shifts the way they interact with their kids even during stressful times or when they find themselves triggered.

For example, consider a mother who brings up at her son's 11-year health supervision visit that she can't get him to clean his room. This family is new to you, and your office does not routinely screen for ACEs or PCEs. Mom is raising him on her own and works hard as a nurse. You ask the mom to explain more about what she is experiencing. She explains that he is supposed to clean his room on the weekends but instead just plays video games all day. It's like he doesn't even hear her when she says he needs to clean his room. He shares that Mom screams at him, and Mom replies, *Well, it's the only way you ever listen.*

Let's deconstruct what is happening here so we can see it within a neurohormonal framework. This mom is stressed and in the "fight" version of a sympathetic nervous system response. Her son is also stressed but experiencing a different form of a nervous system response, the parasympathetic "freeze." We can help both of them befriend their nervous systems and respond differently to each other. Thinking about what is happening through that lens allows everyone to focus on what options are available to mitigate the stress response.

The natural neurohormonal stress response can prevent parents from understanding what is happening in their child's nervous system; in turn, they may inadvertently view their child as the source of danger. **Figure 1-2** is an adaptation of the neurohormonal stress response diagram from Andrew Garner and Robert Saul's book, *Thinking Developmentally: Nurturing Wellness in Childhood to Promote Lifelong Health.*[7] This mom feels like she is being chased by a saber-toothed tiger: the stress of life is compounded when her son appears to be ignoring her requests and his chores. This sympathetic response, mediated by the hypothalamus, results in elevated epinephrine, norepinephrine, and cortisol levels. But it also tells the posterior pituitary to release oxytocin to help Mom remember to bring her son with her as she escapes the imaginary tiger. Her son's

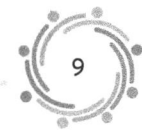
stress response is mediated by the periaqueductal gray matter in his cerebellum, resulting in his inability to move and respond to his mom.

Figure 1-2.

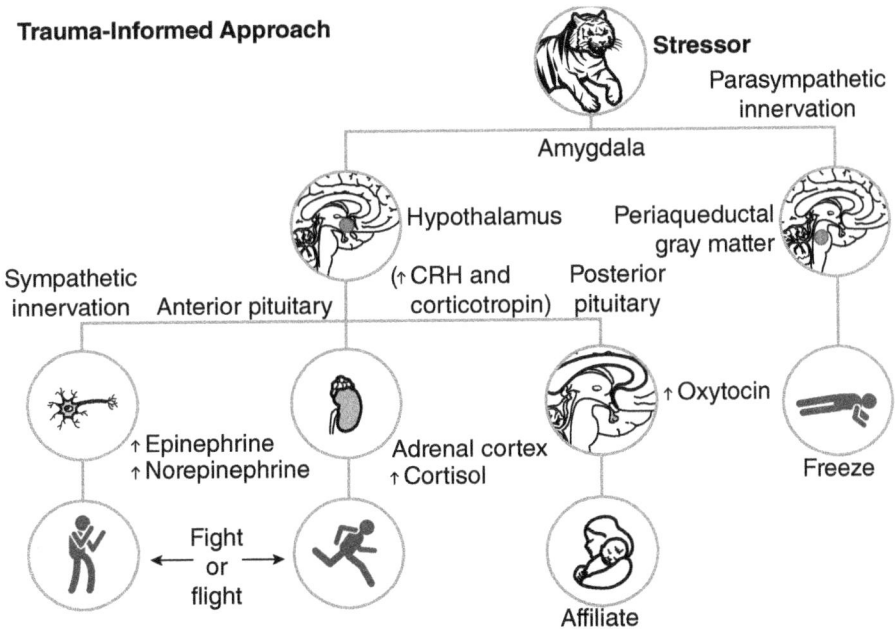

Trauma-informed approach to parenting problems that uses the neurohormonal stress response diagram from Garner and Saul as a framework. ↑ indicates increased level of; CRH, corticotropin-releasing hormone.

Derived from Garner AS, Saul RA. Defining adversity and toxic stress. In: *Thinking Developmentally: Nurturing Wellness in Childhood to Promote Lifelong Health*. American Academy of Pediatrics; 2018:15 and Roelofs K. Freeze for action: neurobiological mechanisms in animal and human freezing. *Philos Trans R Soc Lond B Biol Sci*. 2017;372(1718):20160206.

Preparing families with stepwise problem-solving strategies and tools allows them to respond to each other differently in these settings. We can help repair relational health ruptures and mitigate the impact of the stress on both parent and child. We can encourage the parents to put that affiliate response, or the "tend and befriend" part of the sympathetic nervous system response, to

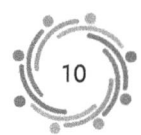

use. Parents can see themselves as "with" their kids rather than pit themselves against their kids in an adversarial stance. We can help the son ground himself back in his body and exit his video game hypnosis so he can respond differently to his mom's requests. We offer support in cocreating a new plan with quality improvement cycles and motivational interviewing (MI) and can support change (**Figure 1-3**).

In our core medical training, we didn't learn about "trauma" or "toxic stress" as organ systems and we didn't do a "resilience" rotation. Symptoms arising from adversity or stress may not be something you feel as confident in assigning to a system as those from the respiratory system or cardiovascular system, because this is a new way of connecting with patients and practicing the art of medicine. That is OK. We are all learning this together.

When humans experience stress, it can affect them in different ways, not all of them negative. Physical stress is necessary for our bodies to gain new levels of fitness. Mental stress can help us learn new material and succeed in new ways. This kind of stress has a beginning and an end and is referred to as *positive stress*. These stressors are experienced within a context of growth and skill attainment. We traditionally have a cultural and social-emotional lattice that prepares us for this stress. It doesn't feel overwhelming unless that lattice is absent and the stress unrelenting. The structure or framework within which we experience stress is what changes the way our bodies physically experience it.

For example, compare studying hard for a test and having a supportive parent who is sitting with you, encouraging you, bringing you nourishment, and checking on you to being told sternly that *If you fail this test, you will be ruined for life!* by a parent who is angry, absent, and unsupportive. The former ends up being experienced as a positive stressor even if a child fails the test; the latter, a negative one even if they pass the test. The test is the same; the task is the same; but the emotional and physical support network, or lattice, is completely different. In the end, it's not actually about the test but about the imprint the stress left on the child.

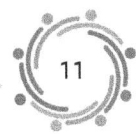
Figure 1-3.

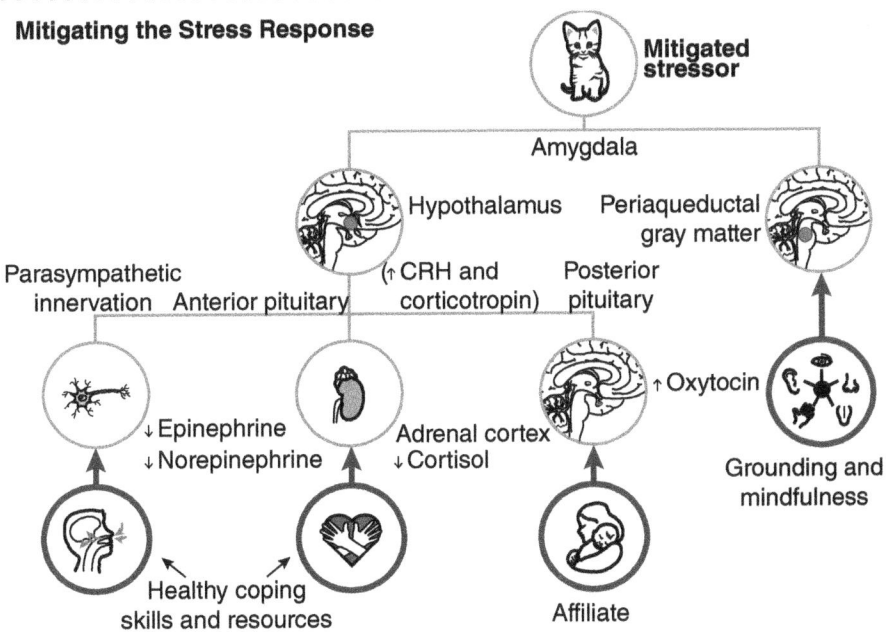

Mitigating the Stress Response

Mitigated stress response, which allows parents to put the affiliate response to use and offset fight, flight, or freeze responses with healthy coping skills and self-care. Both parent and child have access to the affiliate response so they can reframe the experience and no longer see each other as the source of danger. ↑ indicates increased level of; ↓, decreased level of; and CRH, corticotropin-releasing hormone.

Derived from Garner AS, Saul RA. Defining adversity and toxic stress. In: *Thinking Developmentally: Nurturing Wellness in Childhood to Promote Lifelong Health*. American Academy of Pediatrics; 2018:15; Roelofs K. Freeze for action: neurobiological mechanisms in animal and human freezing. *Philos Trans R Soc Lond B Biol Sci*. 2017;372(1718):20160206; and Kearney BE, Lanius RA. The brain-body disconnect: a somatic sensory basis for trauma-related disorders. *Front Neurosci*. 2022;16:1015749.

The experience of the child taking a test without support can be viewed as *tolerable stress*. This kind is neither good nor bad; it simply is. We learn to live with it; perhaps it will help us grow someday in retrospect, but at the time, it is not associated with emotional growth and yet is not experienced in a way that feels unrelenting, even if it temporarily feels overwhelming or negative. For the child taking the test, they may feel unsupported but are able to find their way, and in the end, the experience doesn't result in a lasting intolerable level of stress. Another example of this might be if your parents got divorced and although everyone had everything they needed and there was no violence and no housing or food insecurity, you had to adjust to a new way of living and relating to your parents. With the right supports, this could feel stressful but not be experienced

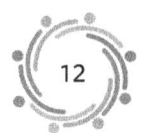

in a way that overwhelms the nervous system. Consider a refugee family[8] that lost their home and all their belongings but they hold on to a certainty that what they are doing and where they are going will bring a better life for everyone. The children in this family will endure hardship and stress, but with the support of their parents as well as essential resources and support, they can endure this stress and adjust to their new life without lasting negative effects. Yet if these protective elements are not present, being a refugee can quickly turn into an intolerable, harmful experience with a lasting mental or physical toll.

When tolerable stress becomes intolerable, it becomes toxic. This type of stress is harmful and is the core of each of the identified ACEs. *Toxic stress* arises when you are experiencing the stress and you have neither adequate coping skills nor necessary resources. The stress is unrelenting and overwhelms your nervous system. Toxic stress activates the fight, flight, or freeze response within our nervous system. This results in an increase in epinephrine and cortisol levels so we can run or fight or an activation of the periaqueductal gray matter so we can hide. The nervous system of a stressed parent reacts as if it is running from a saber-toothed tiger, even if the parent is just trying to get their children to listen to them. When the nervous system is in an overwhelmed state repeatedly or for a prolonged period, it can alter the way genes are expressed (ie, epigenetic regulation), lead to missed crucial experiences during development (as described by developmental neuroscience), and disrupt the immune system's ability to function. These stressors can be so harmful that when they are experienced during sensitive times in development, a child's brain development can be affected.

This sympathetic stress response also includes the affiliate pathway, which is mediated by the posterior pituitary, releasing oxytocin to remind us to pick up our babies and carry them with us as we run away from that saber-toothed tiger. We can help families put this protective pathway to use when we remind them that our children are not the source of danger, even if they are screaming and running away from us when it is time to come inside for dinner. By consistently showing up in a nurturing way, even in the face of stress, parents can promote wellness and a sense of biological safety.

As pediatricians, we are acutely aware of how challenging and dynamic parenting feels even when you're not being chased by a proverbial saber-toothed tiger. What "works" as a parent for a child when they're a baby doesn't "work" when they become a toddler. What a parent uses to manage behaviors when their child is in elementary school doesn't work when they are in high school. And what "works" for the first child may be ineffective with the second. And most parents are trying as hard as they can every single day to provide for their children and keep them from experiencing adversity. Focusing on managing behaviors instead of identifying underlying feelings or unmet needs only increases parental stress levels.

Public health professionals and policymakers have been working for decades to try to shift the political, social, and economic factors that lead to individual- and community-based ACEs. And still, 61% of adults have an ACE score of 1 or higher and 16% have a score of 4 or higher.[9] And when you start to consider "little *t*" trauma as well as "big *T*" trauma, these numbers magnify even more. Adverse childhood experiences and natural disasters are examples of obvious, big *T* traumas, but our families are also experiencing cumulative little *t* traumas. These can go under the radar, unnoticed, and children may not get the same kind of support they would for a big *T* traumatic experience. Caring adults and other family members may not even know that these experiences have been traumatic for the child.

Consider a child who is getting their shoes on to go to school but has only just learned how to tie them. The parent is running behind and worried about getting written up at work for being chronically late. The parent is stressed and says to the child in a pressured voice, *Hurry up and tie your shoes or I'm going to be late again for work!* The child is trying as hard as they can but sees their parent become angrier and angrier with their struggle. The parent, now yelling, expresses how they will lose their job if the child doesn't hurry up and tie their shoes. The child feels overwhelming stress; they are trying as hard as they can, they are unable to accomplish what they need to, and they are being yelled at and told that bad things are about to happen because of them. This relatively mundane experience can be a little *t* trauma that triggers the fight, flight, or freeze response in the same way that being chased by a saber-toothed tiger would. Then imagine that this scene plays out every workday for months and, perhaps, the parent eventually does lose their job. The child's cumulative experience can internally match a big *T* trauma but may remain invisible to the caregivers and family support network, so the child doesn't get the nurturing support they need.

We can help families see how shifting the focus from behaviors to underlying needs and feelings can mitigate this response. Consider how common this type of trauma or toxic stress can be in the lives of our patients. Overwhelming stress can arise in surprisingly mundane situations, like sleep problems or not following directions. Attention problems, hyperactivity, anxiousness, aggression, out-of-control behavior, "losing it," and many other behaviors can be related to these mundane cumulative stressors. The American Academy of Pediatrics (AAP) 2021 policy statement "Preventing Childhood Toxic Stress: Partnering With Families and Communities to Promote Relational Health"[10] highlights the importance of safe, stable, nurturing relationships (SSNRs) in preventing harm from toxic stress. Safe, stable, nurturing relationships are at the core of that protective lattice that has the ability to transform the way children experience stress, from

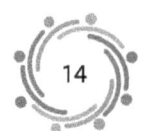
toxic to tolerable or even positive. To provide this relationship, parents must be able to care for their own sympathetic nervous system response and see that their child is actually not the source of danger. At the same time, we must honor how a parent who has experienced trauma themselves may experience a child's behaviors in a way that makes an SSNR harder.

Thankfully, we now have a series of reference books to guide us in how to care for patients and families that have experienced trauma. Garner and Saul's *Thinking Developmentally* provides a solid background in the theory and research underpinning how pediatricians can play a crucial role in fostering resilience in the face of adversity. Heather Forkey, Jessica Griffin, and Moira Szilagyi's *Childhood Trauma and Resilience: A Practical Guide* is a hands-on clinical resource you can keep on your desk as you see patients, to remind you of how to frame what you are seeing when you encounter a family in distress. R.J. Gillespie and Amy King's *The Trauma-Informed Pediatric Practice: A Resilience-Based Roadmap to Foster Early Relational Health* helps you prepare your office to do this most important work and helps clinicians "fill their own buckets" so they have their own inherent resilience to offer patients and parents strength when they are going through hard times.

Garner and Saul explain the theoretical framework underpinning all interventions to foster resilience and offset adversity. One tool they use is the *ecobiodevelopmental (EBD) model* of disease and wellness, which helps us frame all these moving parts so we can wrap our minds around the factors that have potentially affected our patients and families, allowing us to see opportunities to offset adversity with resilience interventions. From the 19th to 20th centuries, Western medicine shifted from a dualistic, mind-versus-body biomedical model of disease to one that took into account the role of psychosocial factors, a biopsychosocial model.[7] Advancements in science after the 1970s led the AAP in its policy statement "Early Childhood Adversity, Toxic Stress, and the Role of the Pediatrician: Translating Developmental Science Into Lifelong Health"[7] to support an even more comprehensive model of both disease and wellness than what the biopsychosocial model could represent. The EBD model accounts for not only the biopsychosocial factors contributing to disease and wellness but also the impact of the environment and ecological milieu on the development of the brain and cognitive function. Using 3 core areas that influence health, the EBD model maps out the relationship between ecology, biology, and development through complex epigenetic, neurodevelopmental, and chemical processes.

Using the EBD model of disease and wellness, we can see how multiple stressors can alter cognitive function, leading to problems with behavior and learning that can have broad and long-lasting implications in a child's life, long after the adversity has ended. Similarly, we can begin to visualize opportunities to mitigate this adversity with resilience-building factors. If adversity can accumulate in tiny moments over time, so can resilience. Protective factors can become more accessible as families develop reliable problem-solving approaches to addressing barriers to adapting to difficult internal and external changes. As clinicians, we can promote "resilience intelligence," or the understanding of what families and children need to do to be able to respond to difficult life experiences in a way that allows them to grow stronger and consistently shift new or recurrent stressors from toxic to tolerable.

We used to debate the extent to which children were affected by "nature" versus "nurture." As with most things, the more we've learned, the more complex the truth has become. If you think about child development and health and wellness within the context of the EBD model, nature is essentially our biology and nurture is our ecology. Pediatricians, of course, knew there was more to the equation and added the element of time, integrating emerging knowledge from developmental neuroscience and epigenetics research. Garner portrays this as an "ongoing, dynamic dance between ecology and biology"[11] over time and encourages clinicians to think both developmentally and ecologically while honoring underlying biological processes.

We now know that what children inherit from their parents is not a static, carved-in-stone entity. Genes can be turned on and off through a fluid process referred to as *epigenetic regulation*.[12] We also know that certain experiences during sensitive periods of development can alter the brain's architecture. Researchers in the field of developmental neuroscience have argued that integrating what we know about cognitive developmental neuroscience into our daily clinical practices has been one of the greatest challenges but holds the potential to greatly benefit youth and society.[13] As Vandenbroucke and colleagues[13] point out, standard research approaches tend to be siloed, with the researchers working separately from community members, organizational leaders, and policymakers. Yet we must translate research findings into language that is widely understandable and useful in daily life. This book will help you convert complex scientific and clinical knowledge into useful daily life skills you can share in existing clinical encounters.

Offsetting adversity with resilience requires that we understand the cumulative neurobiological impact of stress and decipher it for families. Cumulative stress experienced early in life can alter the function of the amygdala[14] and contribute to many disease states later in life.[15] Chronic stress also weakens the immune system in a myriad of ways that can increase the risk for illness by suppressing protective immune responses and by exacerbating pathological immune responses and inflammation.[16] Yet for a parent, this information may feel overwhelming and even come across as judgmental, so we have an obligation to metabolize it, transforming these findings into useful day-to-day strategies.

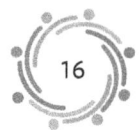

The EBD model (**Figure 1-4**) allows us to think about how each intervention in this book works: these interventions enhance the process of adapting to difficult or challenging internal and external life experiences with mental, emotional, and behavioral flexibility. This end result is what I described earlier in this section of the chapter as resilience intelligence, or the ability to problem-solve around obstacles that arise and seem to keep you from being able to adapt.

Figure 1-4.

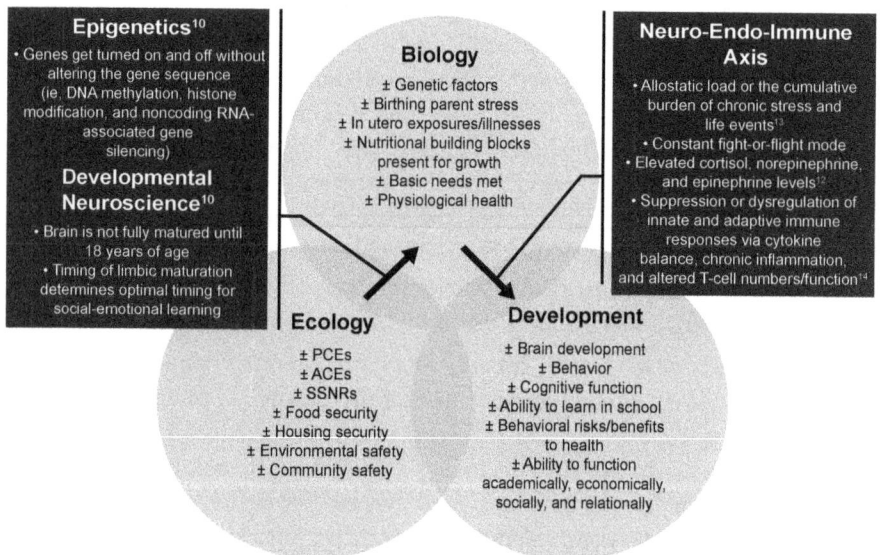

Ecobiodevelopmental model of disease: opportunities to counter adversity and foster resilience. ACE indicates adverse childhood experience; PCE, positive childhood experience; and SSNR, safe, stable, nurturing relationship.

And it's not just parents who can feel overwhelmed by the complexity of this process. To translate the science into actionable strategies in clinical encounters, clinicians need a stepwise approach. Looking at all these factors together when a family presents for care can feel overwhelming for us. In the chapters that follow, you'll learn how to consistently address barriers to integrating protective and stress-mitigating factors and offer strategies for buffering the impact of potentially harmful ecological, biological, and developmental factors by using a stepwise process for change.

How does all of this sound to you? Are you feeling overwhelmed? Are you feeling stressed? Excited? Either way, don't worry. We're going to use an approach that also helps with your own stress level as you begin to integrate these tools. Offsetting the impact of the adversity is not something with immediate results, like a 10-day

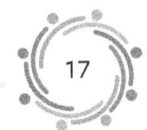
course of medication or a steroid burst. This is going to take time. It took time for stress to have an effect on your patient's family dynamics and neurodevelopment, and it will take time for things to heal. We can address the factors that result in illness and disease with a stepwise process that facilitates the work of consistently supporting relational health and addressing social drivers of health (SDOH) as part of our existing primary care workflow (**Figure 1-5**). This work relies on a multigenerational approach so that both parents and children can learn healthy ways of responding to the ongoing stressors in their lives.

Figure 1-5.

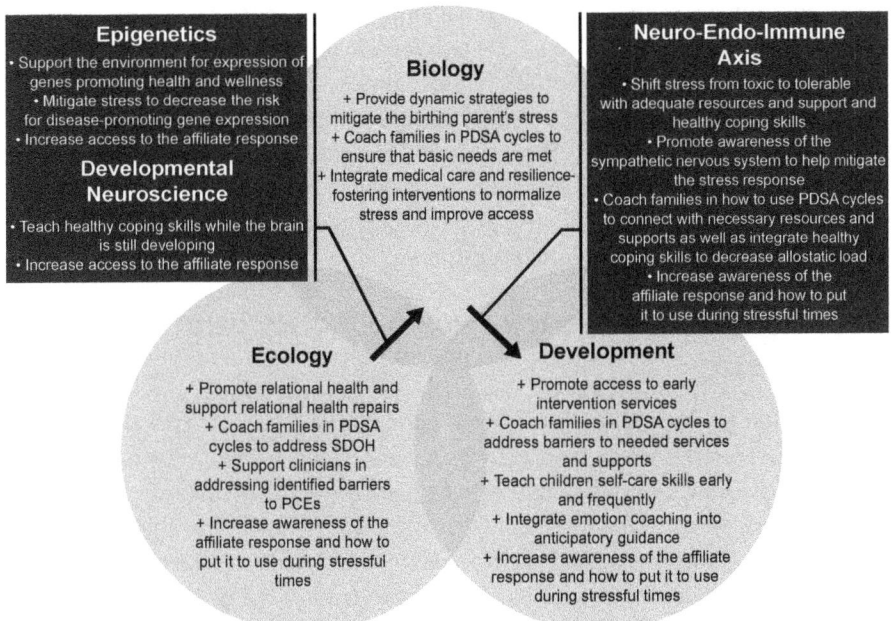

Opportunities for resilience within the ecobiodevelopmental model of disease and wellness. PCE indicates positive childhood experience; PDSA, Plan-Do-Study-Act; and SDOH, social drivers of health.

At first, this may seem overwhelming and perhaps even confusing. Don't worry, we will go through how to leverage each of these opportunities step by step. You may be amazed by how behavior changes and how family dynamics can change in a short interval when the family members are motivated and they have simultaneous access to the resources and tools they need. In my experience, families are quick to develop new responses to their own physiological stress responses, allowing them, over time, to lower stress hormone levels while being more likely to be able to put that precious affiliate response to use. We will be using a

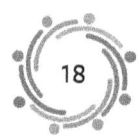

concise version of MI to help leverage our dynamic with the family so they can harness their inherent strengths to bring about our cocreated goals.

Ongoing research is needed to fully understand how biomarkers, epigenetic regulation, cognition, and development change with resilience-fostering interventions after children have experienced adversity and toxic stress. I look forward to seeing the studies on harnessing opportunities in the EBD model (see **Figure 1-5**) to alter gene expression, but we won't have that data for another decade or so. Interdisciplinary clinical experience demonstrates how these interventions can increase resilience,[1] and many argue[13] that we have an ethical obligation to integrate protective findings from neuroscience research into our daily practice while additional research is ongoing. We know that children's development is adversely affected by toxic stress and we can translate the research into interventions. For example, meditation, mindfulness, positive parenting, and other stress-lowering strategies have already independently been studied and proven to offset the impact of stress. It is our moral obligation to offer clinically proven interventions with a first aid approach to patients and their parents while we continue to investigate the precise physiological methods in how they work together as a comprehensive intervention.

See One, Do One, Teach One: A Quality Improvement Perspective

To know how to support resilience in our patients, we have to start with addressing our own toxic stress. When we forget how to live connected to our own emotions and needs, we, too, become more fragile and less resilient. We may try to take care of ourselves in an asynchronous manner, working our butts off for the workweek and then doing lots of yoga and exercise and meditation on the weekends we have off. But this imbalance is unsustainable, and the stress of doing this becomes toxic over time and leads to burnout. To address our own stress, we have to lean in to it and connect with our own unpleasant feelings by applying a series of quality improvement cycles for ourselves. We have to identify and remove our own barriers to healthy coping skills and adequate resources, whatever those may be, before we can do this professionally.

When we try to skip this step, we can't teach it to our children or the families we work with. Remember learning to perform procedures in medical school and residency, specifically how we always used the motto *See one, do one, teach one*? Use

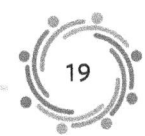

this same approach now. It starts with reading this book; that is how you "see" one. Then you "do" one as you apply this approach first with yourself and your relationships with your own family and loved ones. Then after that, you will be able to "teach" this approach to families so they can use it.

You may be thinking, *But I bought this book to more effectively help my patients. Why do I have to do something for myself first? I'm fine.* Quality improvement is a lifelong process. Even if you feel as though things are "fine" and you are not in the near-burnout space where I was when I started developing these tools and strategies, you will find that you can feel even more fulfilled by the work you are doing when you apply these skills. We have to be careful not to fall into the "ivory tower" trap, which in medicine is sort of a "white coat" trap: thinking that because I am the one with the degree and the position, somehow I am not experiencing the same stressors as my patients.

Our stressors all vary individually, but I encourage you to think about the EBD model and even sketch your own version of **Figure 1-5** with respect to your childhood and, potentially, your own children. Without being judgmental, turn your compassion to yourself. What factors have brought you here, wherever you are right now, and how did they affect you? As Gillespie and King note in their book, *The Trauma-Informed Pediatric Practice*, we must do this work before we can ask our staff or colleagues to do it. And take care of yourself and be gentle with what you find on your journey about how you came to where you are. The culture of a busy, modern medical practice seems to contradict the essence of true self-care. Refer to their roadmap on how being trauma informed as a practice starts within each of us.[17]

To do this work with ourselves and our patients, we need a systematic approach to change, which includes a stepwise approach to addressing barriers. Change is hard for all of us, and when we consider making or recommending a change, we want to make sure it is going to result in an improvement. The formal study of quality improvement goes back to the beginning of the industrial age. One interpretation of one of W. Edward Deming's 1950s lectures led to a Plan-Do-Study-Check cycle that was integral to quality control in Japan. This cycle was designed to allow for continual improvement of products in production in the industrial sector. Deming refined the strategy in 1993 to develop the now widely popular Plan-Do-Study-Act (PDSA) model[18] (**Figure 1-6**).

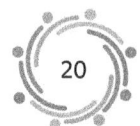
Figure 1-6.

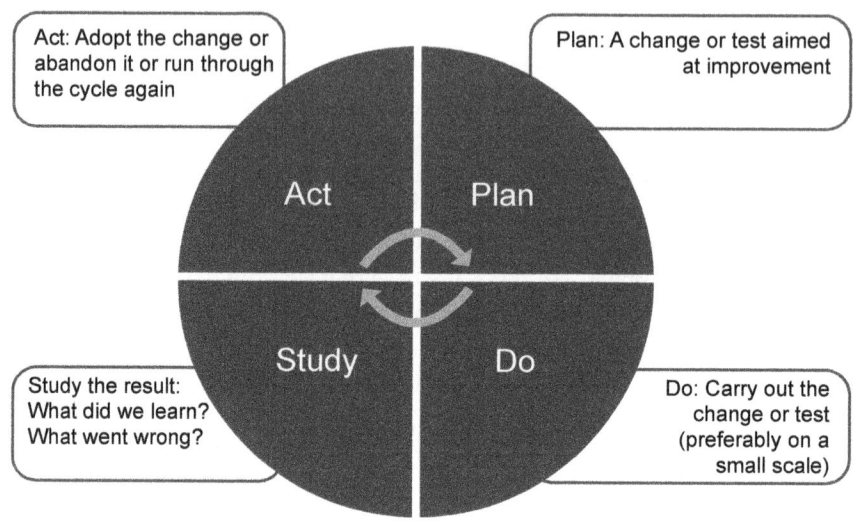

Plan-Do-Study-Act cycle: each cycle, choose something you want to change, try a small test of change, study the results (Did it work?), and then determine if this change was an improvement before you either adopt the change or abandon it and try something else.

This systematic approach to change has been accepted as effective and nimble across different sectors. The health care industry has now widely incorporated continual PDSA cycles as a way to improve quality in settings that involve many different simultaneously crucial factors. Effective interventions in health care are often "complex and multi-faceted and developed iteratively to adapt to the local context and respond to unforeseen obstacles and unintended effects."[19] The Institute for Healthcare Improvement has a toolkit for health care professionals and systems to apply the PDSA approach in quality improvement initiatives. Their Model for Improvement[20] framework begins with 3 questions to guide each PDSA cycle:

1. What are we trying to accomplish?
2. How will we know that a change is an improvement?
3. What change can we make that will result in an improvement?

Keeping these 3 questions in mind when working with families will help you cocreate plans.

Early in my career, I was fortunate to be able to participate in the Maine Youth Overweight Collaborative (MYOC).[21] This initiative, with multiple sites across Maine, applied a chronic care model to youth overweight. The approach was similar to addressing adversity and resilience, in that the barriers were sensitive issues that parents and patients may not have wanted to routinely talk about, so using an MI approach was essential. The MYOC also used PDSA cycles to help change ingrained behaviors, and I have used them as part of my practice style ever since. We will use both these tools in the context of the stepwise process outlined in this book.

Toxic stress is not fixed and unchangeable unless we can't integrate needed coping skills, strategies, and resources.[22] If a family enters into a difficult life event without adequate coping skills or resources, it doesn't mean the family is doomed to experience the adversity as toxic. With a strengths-based, problem-solving approach, we can help identify obstacles preventing our patients and their families from integrating essential skills and protective factors, while using MI to support them in overcoming barriers. Sequential PDSA cycles paired with a concise MI technique represent the core process for change you will learn from this book.

The goal of each PDSA cycle in Resilience University (RU) is to lower stress levels from toxic to tolerable or even positive (**Figure 1-7**). Showing families how they can do this on their own builds their capacity to use the supports and inherent strengths the family has had access to but may not have been able to operationalize because of various intervening factors.

Figure 1-7.

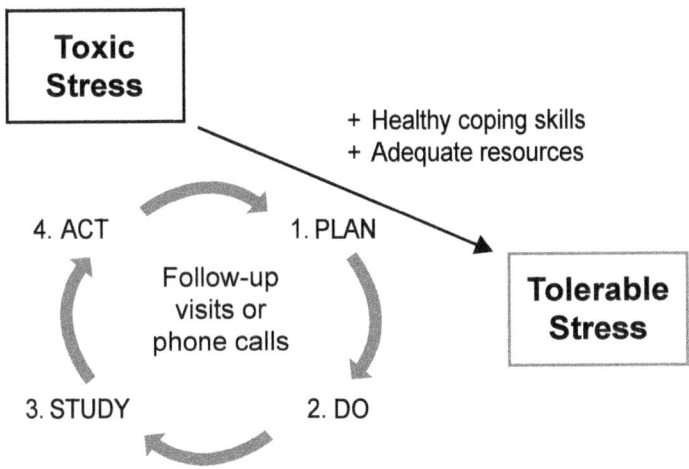

Shifting stress from toxic to tolerable by using a continual quality improvement approach and integrating healthy coping skills, resources, and support.

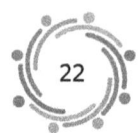

Remember, the goal is to support resilience intelligence, which reflects an ability to respond to a familiar stressor in a new way that facilitates adaptation with mental, emotional, or behavioral flexibility. Toxic stress is the only kind of stress that seems to be linked to illness and biopsychosocial harm. Remember, the actual source of stress is less important than our response to the stress. Using 5 steps consistently with each PDSA cycle helps keep the family's needs at the center (**Figure 1-8**). We have an ethical obligation to translate this for families so they know that even though some adversity or overwhelming stress has happened, it doesn't guarantee that they or their child will experience a negative outcome. Educating families about the power of protective factors helps them understand how to inherently shift stressors from toxic to tolerable, by using a tried-and-true method for change within a complex dynamic system (more on this in Chapter 4, Process for Stepwise Change).

Figure 1-8.

STEPS

1. Identify the family's goals:

_____

_____

2. Cocreate a plan:

_____

_____

3. Try the plan for _____ (amount of time; usually 2 weeks is a good place to start).

4. Evaluate the plan at a return office visit: How did it go?

_____

_____

5. Discuss whether it "worked" or a new strategy is needed:

_____

_____

Five steps in cocreating Plan-Do-Study-Act cycles with the patients and families you care for.

The RU approach described in this book uses a combination of a widely accepted model of disease and wellness (EBD model) and a well-vetted approach to change in the health care setting (MI with PDSA cycles). In addition, each intervention (described throughout this book; Table 6-2 provides exact locations) is grounded in previously established methods for lowering stress and providing healthy coping skills. These include Stephen Porges' polyvagal theory,[23]

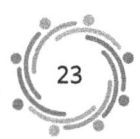

acceptance and commitment therapy,[24] dialectical behavioral therapy[25] and cognitive behavioral therapy,[26] and mindfulness-based stress reduction.[27] In addition, RU applies Charlotte Harper Brown's Strengthening Families approach[28] within the HOPE® (Healthy Outcomes from Positive Experiences) framework developed by Dr Robert Sege and his colleagues at Tufts,[29] which is founded on Bethell and colleagues' breakthrough research showing that 7 key PCEs can offset long-term mental health effects of childhood adversity.[5] These 7 PCEs are as follows:

1. Feeling able to talk with your family about feelings
2. Feeling that your family stood by you during difficult times
3. Enjoying participating in community traditions
4. Feeling a sense of belonging in high school
5. Feeling supported by friends
6. Having at least 2 nonparent adults who took genuine interest in you
7. Feeling safe and protected by an adult in your home

By the end of this book, you will be able to help foster at least 4 of these 7 PCEs (1, 2, 6, and 7), with 6 being you, their clinician, taking a genuine interest in your patients. I've had children say that their favorite part of the sessions (outlined in Chapter 5, A Structured Approach to Resilience Coaching) was knowing I really cared about how they were feeling. By modeling for families how to start conversations about how everyone is feeling (instead of just focusing on how everyone is behaving), you can help shift the dynamic from one of mutual dysregulation and reactivity to one of coregulation and connection. This shift allows parents, even those who have experienced their own trauma, to understand the root cause of their child's behaviors better, which, in turn, allows them to stay connected and helps the child feel safe and protected no matter what is happening around them.

In addition, using the 4 building blocks of HOPE can help simplify things when a family is experiencing overwhelming amounts of stress. The 4 building blocks of HOPE[29] are environment, engagement, relational health, and emotional growth. Think about it like you do a review of systems for SDOH, breaking down the PCEs into categories. This framework can help you identify areas of inherent strength and areas needing a little external support. Each "tower" of blocks will change in size and composition over time in a child's life (**Figure 1-9**). Normalizing the change for families helps validate that variability is an inherent part of life and not pathological.

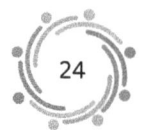
Figure 1-9.

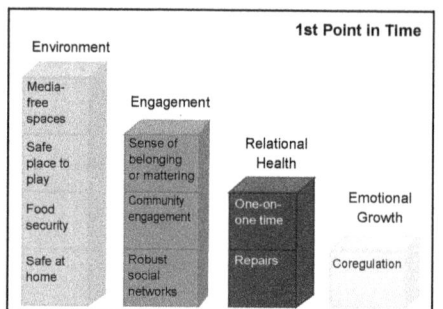
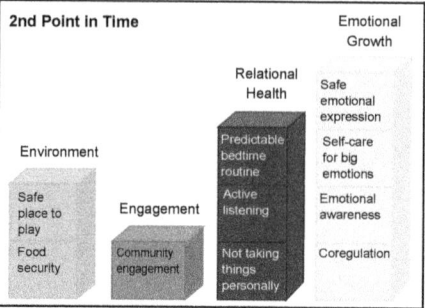

HOPE (Healthy Outcomes from Positive Experiences) building blocks, a dynamic approach to social drivers of health. The left and right panels represent different points in time for the same family.

HOPE (Healthy Outcomes from Positive Experiences) is a registered trademark of Tufts Medical Center.

The systematic approach to integrating stress-lowering strategies into the family culture means that when a family comes back for a follow-up and says, *Doctor, what you told me to do isn't working,* you don't take it personally; you know that this is just part of the change process. You lean in with curiosity, find out where they are in their journey, and help them plan for the next step.

Integrating Nadine Burke Harris' *Roadmap for Resilience* "stress busters"[30] (**Figure 1-10**) into day-to-day clinical care allows you to promote things that we've always known, intuitively, are good for you but we can now say are proven by research. The stress busters include going outside, getting good sleep, eating healthy, having access to mental health care, having supportive relationships, practicing mindfulness, and being physically active. To me, this is a dynamic framework, similar to the HOPE building blocks: on any given day or week, you won't have all of them; they're fluid. But when one isn't working for you, perhaps others are more available. As you learn the tools and strategies presented in this book, you'll feel confident working with families to help them know that at least a few stress-busting strategies are always within reach.

Ready to give "See one, do one, teach one" a try? Start with this approach at home and with your own family or those you spend a lot of time with. Try PDSA cycles to get your husband to put his socks into the dirty clothes basket (sorry for the gendered comment; it is just impossible for my husband, no matter how many PDSA cycles I have tried, so let me know if you figure out how to get him to do it). Start using the stress-buster wheel (more on this in Chapter 4, Process for Stepwise Change) as a new way to respond to your teenager when they're angry. Print the wheel and put it on the fridge, then encourage your teen to try to do something from the wheel when they are having a bad day. Have them write a list of at least 2 healthy coping skills, strategies, or resources they can apply from each section.

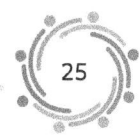
Figure 1-10.

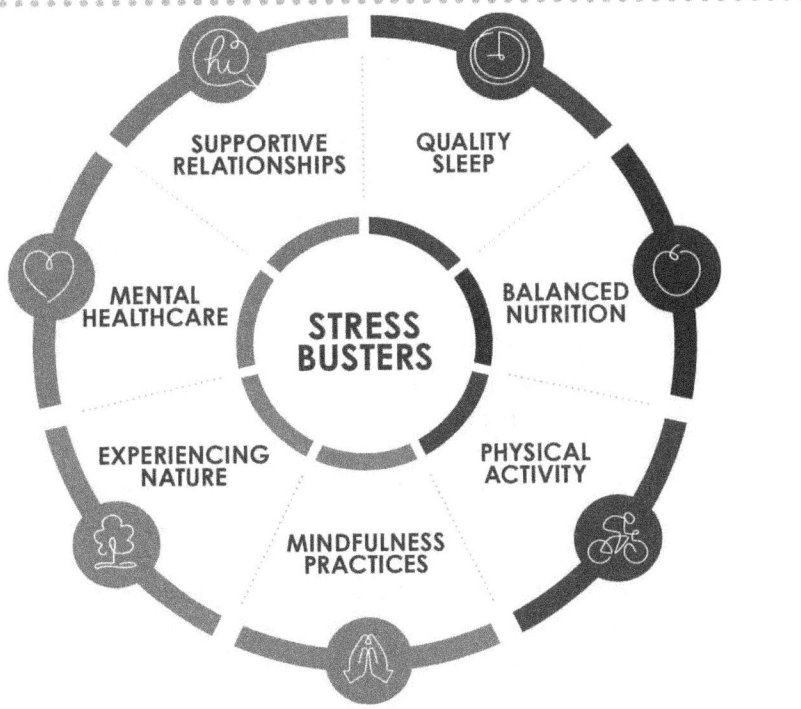

California surgeon general's *Roadmap for Resilience* evidence-based stress-buster wheel.

Reproduced from Office of the California Surgeon General. *The California Surgeon General's Playbook for Stress.* 2022. Accessed October 30, 2024. https://osg.ca.gov/wp-content/uploads/sites/266/2022/05/california-surgeon-general_stress-busting-playbook.pdf.

Is your own family able to talk about feelings? Do you talk about anger? Sadness? If so, with whom? What happens when people get angry in your house? Can you support each other through hard times, or do people get triggered and then the moment gets messy? It's OK. That's how I learned all of this. In my house, all of us got triggered and everything always went sideways. So, I can honestly say this works, and it is OK to start where you are. But you have to practice in your life and at home first. Then you can bring it to your patients. And these tools help at work with grumpy administrators and problematic coworkers just like they help at home with your spouse's dirty socks.

Ready for an example? A mom of 4 children, 4, 6, 8, and 10 years old, is struggling with getting everyone to sit at the table together for dinner. Everyone sits down but then they start fighting before she can even serve the meal. She has tried a reward system, but that worked for only a few days and then became the topic of the fighting. Mom ends up yelling at the kids. She remembers her own mom

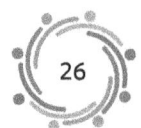

yelling at her around the dinner table and she doesn't want to do the same. She brings her concerns to you; and you just finished reading this book.

Following are the steps you might take to cocreate PDSA cycles with this family, using the **Figure 1-8** template:

1. Identify the family's goals: It might seem at first like this is to eat dinner together at the table, but when you explore it more, it goes deeper than that. You identify that this struggle is a relational health and emotional growth issue, validate Mom's concerns, and talk with the kids about how hard this is. They say they are tired of getting sent to their rooms; then their dinner is cold and gross later. You know Mom just started a new very stressful job because Dad got laid off. You identify their goals: Mom's are to feed her kids and not yell, the kids want to stop getting into trouble, and your goal is to help address the barriers to PCEs (stress, dysregulation, and unrepaired relational health ruptures).

2. Cocreate a plan: You'd next honor the family's strengths and express how stress might be related to what's going on and how, by addressing that, things may get easier. You ask if they want help coming up with a strategy and they say yes. So you suggest that when someone feels angry at the dinner table, they can excuse themselves to take a minute to do toes-to-nose or "box" or "square" breathing or meditate with a glitter jar in the living room (these tools are explained in detail in Chapter 3, Essential Toolkit). Then they can ask Mom for help individually if they need something specific or if they need help with another feeling that led to the anger. If Mom can't address the need in the moment, she can allow the child to eat in the living room or to wait and eat with her while she cleans up after dinner. If Mom feels like she is going to yell, she will see that she is upset, unhook from her traditional response (yelling), and instead take a moment to nurture herself. For this mom, she thinks 3 things that might work would be meditating with the glitter jar, singing to herself, or doing 5 Big Deep Breaths (also explained in Chapter 3).

3. Try the plan for 2 weeks and have a nurse follow up by phone to determine if the family needs to schedule another session with you.

4. Evaluate the plan at a return office visit: How did it go? It worked well; Mom didn't yell and they could eat as a family about twice as often as before.

5. Discuss whether this "worked" or a new strategy is needed: Adopt this plan. Mom will call back if she needs more help, and they will follow up at the 4-year old's health supervision visit in 1 month.

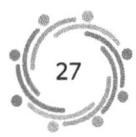

A Strengths-Based Clinical Approach

As primary care clinicians, we are often all too aware of the toxic stress burdens our families are carrying. We may feel frozen in the face of so many problems that we're unable to help with any. This book will help you simultaneously honor the unique strengths of each family and break down the challenges they face into manageable bites so this work doesn't feel overwhelming. Just like we celebrate a child's developmental milestones at the same time we're addressing their diaper rash, RU allows us to celebrate family strengths and resilience while coaching families in continual quality improvement of the areas that are challenging them.

Forkey, Griffin, and Szilagyi introduce a first aid model, known as SPLINT, for working with families experiencing toxic stress.[31] As you develop the skills and strategies presented in this book, you'll feel confident using this model because there are samples for language and tools to use in each step of the response. The acronym SPLINT, when applied within the context of this book, looks like this:

- **Saying that trauma/stress may be the cause:** It seems so simple, but just saying aloud that a child's or family's issue may be related to overwhelming stress or trauma can be validating and comforting when families know something is going sideways and are worried for the well-being of their children. Validating the experience is a powerful way to connect, establish empathy, and call out the elephant in the room. Caregivers may be terrified of acknowledging the potential impact of trauma, so follow up with strengths. Validating and highlighting strengths could sound like *This is hard, isn't it? And I've seen your family do hard things. Remember when Saysha was a baby and you were having trouble getting her to gain weight? You worked so hard and look at how healthy she is now!*
- **Problem-solving:** This step can be challenging since we have only 15 or 20 minutes with the family. They are often there for a health supervision visit or an ear infection or we have something else we have to address as well. That is OK. This book will help you feel confident in efficiently teaching families how to integrate small steps of change, by using the tried-and-true quality improvement technique of continual PDSA cycles. This means that even if the first, second, or third thing they try doesn't "work," you keep on going with evidence-informed interventions until things start to feel less stressful, there is more connection, and they feel the original concern has been addressed. This may sound something like *What I'm hearing you say is that Saysha's behavior is really derailing the day and you'd like some help coming*

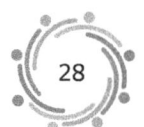

up with a new way to respond. Let's come up with a plan together using these tools I've given you and then you can try it and we'll follow up in 2 weeks and see if it is helping. My experience has been that this is equally effective and mundane. Parents often forget what their original concern was after a visit or two; so, write it down. Then you can remind them and celebrate the change(s) they were able to make. They may come in for a new visit and say nothing is better, but when you remind them of their original concern, they will say, *Oh, yes... Well, I guess that is better, but now this is happening...* Over time, families learn to integrate the strategies themselves and celebrate their ability to make meaningful change, without any coaching from you.

- **Language:** Some of us may have grown up in families that talked openly about feelings, but not all of us did. Certainly, most of us did not do a lot of this talking in formal medical or residency training. So, we need a boot camp in how to talk about trauma, stress, difficult emotions, family dysfunction, dys-regulation, conflict, and other "symptoms" that our families will be experi-encing. It is crucial that we have language that is nonjudgmental, welcoming, and understanding. Resilience University provides you with a wealth of ways to start these conversations in the office as well as give you phrases to model conversations for the family at home when things start to go sideways. One strategy you will learn from later chapters is the VIVA (Validate, Inform, Validate, Ask) approach, which is a validation sandwich. An example of this language may sound like *It is totally normal to feel like Saysha is trying to ruin the day on purpose. Lots of families feel that way about their child's behaviors.* (Validate) *And we know that big unwanted behaviors arise from big unman-ageable emotions or unmet needs.* (Inform) *I understand you feel like you have already tried everything and she won't stop.* (Validate) *Are you interested in trying an evidence-informed approach that many families have found helpful?* (Ask)

- **Investigating further:** With any problem our families and patients bring to us, there is a superficial layer and a deeper layer. For families going through adversity, trauma, and toxic stress, sometimes we may need to go beyond the typical clinical assessment and anticipatory guidance to fully address their needs. We may have been trained (at least a little bit) in asking essential questions about what else we need to know and do. Do we need to call the Department of Health and Human Services? Does the family need help with housing? With food security? What is the urgency of these other contrib-uting factors? What specific needs and situations may make it hard for this family to follow a specific recommendation? Does this guidance or recom-mendation require a "bridging" strategy to make it accessible for the family? (More on this in Chapter 6, Using Relationship-Based and Trauma-Informed Anticipatory Guidance.) We can provide a standard of care in parallel with having these crucial conversations. This book will give you language and tools to help you dig deeper into the emotional/feeling states contributing to whatever problem parents bring to you and help you avoid sending families across a "half-built bridge." This may sound something like *I remember referring Saysha for Child Development Services at our last appointment. Did you ever hear anything?* When the parents say the worker wanted to come to the house and that made the family uncomfortable, you are identifying a half-built bridge, and you can use this opportunity to address it with something like *Of course, that can feel uncomfortable. I can ask them to see her when she is at child care if that will work better for you.*

- **Normalizing:** This seems so easy, yet so often in this type of scenario, we unintentionally say something that is de-normalizing, like *Oh no, it's terrible you have to go through that.* We mean well, but it comes out as sympathy instead of empathy. In those rushed encounters where we have to think and act on our feet, we need to have the language teed up and ready to go so what we really mean to say comes out the way we mean it to. This book will help you internalize how it really is OK to not be OK from adversity or toxic stress, just like it's OK for a child to be sick from an illness. Neither one makes the parent a bad parent or means the family isn't trying hard enough. We can also normalize the protective benefit of PCEs, specifically how these can feel so mundane yet be incredibly powerful. With practice, you'll be able to call out barriers seamlessly, just like you can with nutritional issues or car seat refusal. Finally, this approach helps you with language in the office and for families to use at home that allows everyone to talk about how sometimes, unpleasant moments (eg, yelling, not sleeping, acting out) can be completely normal responses to hard times. When you are using VIVA, this may sound something like *So many parents find themselves yelling at their kids when they are frustrated. Of course you yelled at Saysha.* (Validate) *We know that even the best parents tune in to their child about only 30% of the time, and the rest of the time, they are getting it "wrong" at first and reconnecting later.* (Inform) *I get how stressful parenting can feel.* (Validate) *Would you like to work on a new strategy to help with your own stress and help you respond to Saysha differently in those moments?* (Ask)

- **Therapy, treatment, or guidance:** This is the core of the art of medicine and why RU helps rejuvenate your practice and prevent (or even reverse, as in my case) burnout. When you are talking with stressed families now, it might feel hopeless, draining, and/or exhausting. I used to find myself thinking, *I wish I had something more to offer. All I can do is refer, and who knows if they will ever even get in with these referrals.* I'd see the families a year later, they had never seen anyone, and the problems had just magnified. This book will help your referrals come with a doable action plan and a meaningful message. Just like we're here to help when a child has weird poop or a rash we don't know

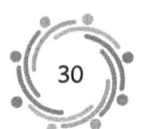

what to make of, we're going to roll up our sleeves and figure this out with our families. We may not have all the answers, but we know where to start. We can tell a family, *This is what you can do until you get in with the therapist/ with the psychiatrist/for neuropsych testing/etc.* In the context of this book, it might sound like *We're in this together. We've got this. You're not alone! I'm here with you as you go through this, just like when Saysha was a baby. Try 5 Big Deep Breaths when you feel like you are going to yell at Saysha, and I'll see you in 2 weeks. I look forward to hearing how things are going. And remember, if it isn't helping, we can always try something else until things feel less stressful, OK?*

Using this approach, you can integrate resilience building into every patient encounter, not only when you embark on a formal 4-session RU with families. Responding to a complex SDOH review of systems and treating symptoms arising from trauma will become as much second nature as caring for the common cold or a blistering case of impetigo. Your comfort with addressing these issues alleviates some of the shame and blame families are carrying and helps them feel like they are not alone in their journey. Just like you were there for the other messy things they didn't know what to do with, you are there for them when adversity, trauma, and stress derail the day.

References

1. American Psychological Association. Psychology topics: resilience. Accessed October 30, 2024. https://www.apa.org/topics/resilience
2. Swedo EA, Aslam MV, Dahlberg LL, et al. Prevalence of adverse childhood experiences among U.S. adults—behavioral risk factor surveillance system, 2011–2020. *MMWR Morb Mortal Wkly Rep.* 2023;72(26):707–715 PMID: 37384554 doi: 10.15585/mmwr.mm7226a2
3. Felitti VJ, Anda RF, Nordenberg D, et al. Relationship of childhood abuse and household dysfunction to many of the leading causes of death in adults. The Adverse Childhood Experiences (ACE) Study. *Am J Prev Med.* 1998;14(4):245–258 PMID: 9635069 doi: 10.1016/S0749-3797(98)00017-8
4. Cronholm PF, Forke CM, Wade R, et al. Adverse childhood experiences: expanding the concept of adversity. *Am J Prev Med.* 2015;49(3):354–361 PMID: 26296440 doi: 10.1016/j.amepre.2015.02.001
5. Bethell C, Jones J, Gombojav N, Linkenbach J, Sege R. Positive childhood experiences and adult mental and relational health in a statewide sample: associations across adverse childhood experiences levels. *JAMA Pediatr.* 2019;173(11):e193007 PMID: 31498386 doi: 10.1001/jamapediatrics.2019.3007
6. Huang CX, Halfon N, Sastry N, Chung PJ, Schickedanz A. Positive childhood experiences and adult health outcomes. *Pediatrics.* 2023;152(1):e2022060951 PMID: 37337829 doi: 10.1542/peds.2022-060951
7. Garner A, Saul R. *Thinking Developmentally: Nurturing Wellness in Childhood to Promote Lifelong Health.* American Academy of Pediatrics; 2018 doi: 10.1542/9781610021531

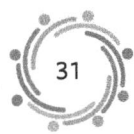

8. Hodes M, Hussain N. The role of family functioning in refugee child and adult mental health. In: De Haene L, Rousseau C, eds. *Working With Refugee Families: Trauma and Exile in Family Relationships.* Cambridge University Press; 2020:17–35 doi: 10.1017/9781108602105.003

9. Centers for Disease Control and Prevention. Adverse childhood experiences (ACEs): preventing early trauma to improve adult health. Vital Signs. November 2019. Updated August 23, 2021. Accessed October 30, 2024. https://www.cdc.gov/vitalsigns/aces/index.html

10. Garner A, Yogman M; American Academy of Pediatrics Committee on Psychosocial Aspects of Child and Family Health, Section on Developmental and Behavioral Pediatrics, and Council on Early Childhood. Preventing childhood toxic stress: partnering with families and communities to promote relational health. *Pediatrics.* 2021;148(2):e2021052582 PMID: 34312296 doi: 10.1542/peds.2021-052582

11. Garner AS. Thinking developmentally: the next evolution in models of health. *J Dev Behav Pediatr.* 2016;37(7):579–584 PMID: 27429356 doi: 10.1097/DBP.0000000000000326

12. Inbar-Feigenberg M, Choufani S, Butcher DT, Roifman M, Weksberg R. Basic concepts of epigenetics. *Fertil Steril.* 2013;99(3):607–615 PMID: 23357459 doi: 10.1016/j.fertnstert.2013.01.117

13. Vandenbroucke ARE, Crone EA, van Erp JBF, et al. Integrating cognitive developmental neuroscience in society: lessons learned from a multidisciplinary research project on education and social safety of youth. *Front Integr Nuerosci.* 2021;15:756640 PMID: 34880735 doi: 10.3389/fnint.2021.756640

14. Hanson JL, Nacewicz BM. Amygdala allostasis and early life adversity: considering excitotoxicity and inescapability in the sequelae of stress. *Front Hum Neurosci.* 2021;15:624705 PMID: 34140882 doi: 10.3389/fnhum.2021.624705

15. Guidi J, Lucente M, Sonino N, Fava GA. Allostatic load and its impact on health: a systematic review. *Psychother Psychosom.* 2021;90(1):11–27 PMID: 32799204 doi: 10.1159/000510696

16. Dhabhar FS. Effects of stress on immune function: the good, the bad, and the beautiful. *Immunol Res.* 2014;58(2–3):193–210 PMID: 24798553 doi: 10.1007/s12026-014-8517-0

17. Gillespie RJ, King A. *The Trauma-Informed Pediatric Practice: A Resilience-Based Roadmap to Foster Early Relational Health.* American Academy of Pediatrics; 2025 doi: 10.1542/9781610027410

18. Moen R, Norman C. The history of the PDCA cycle. Paper presented at: 7th ANQ Congress; September 15–17, 2009; Tokyo, Japan

19. Taylor MJ, McNicholas C, Nicolay C, Darzi A, Bell D, Reed JE. Systematic review of the application of the Plan-Do-Study-Act method to improve quality in healthcare. *BMJ Qual Saf.* 2014;23(4):290–298 PMID: 24025320 doi: 10.1136/bmjqs-2013-001862

20. Institute for Healthcare Improvement. How to improve: Model for Improvement. Accessed October 30, 2024. https://www.ihi.org/resources/how-to-improve

21. Polacsek M, Orr J, Letourneau L, et al. Impact of a primary care intervention on physician practice and patient and family behavior: Keep ME Healthy—the Maine Youth Overweight Collaborative. *Pediatrics.* 2009;123(suppl 5):S258–S266 PMID: 19470601 doi: 10.1542/peds.2008-2780C

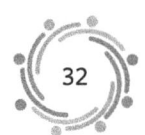

22. Schaeffer B. What you should know about toxic stress. National Alliance on Mental Illness. August 18, 2017. Accessed October 30, 2024. https://www.nami.org/Blogs/NAMI-Blog/August-2017/What-You-Should-Know-About-Toxic-Stress

23. Nationwide Children's. Toxic stress: how the body's response can harm a child's development. *700 Children's* blog. Nationwide Children's. July 13, 2017. Accessed October 30, 2024. https://www.nationwidechildrens.org/family-resources-education/700childrens/2017/07/toxic-stress-how-the-bodys-response-can-harm-a-childs-development

24. Harris R. Embracing your demons: an overview of acceptance and commitment therapy. Psychotherapy.net. Accessed October 30, 2024. https://www.psychotherapy.net/article/Acceptance-and-Commitment-Therapy-ACT

25. Robins CJ. Zen principles and mindfulness practice in dialectical behavior therapy. *Cogn Behav Pract.* 2002;9(1):50–57 doi: 10.1016/S1077-7229(02)80040-2

26. Fenn K, Byrne M. The key principles of cognitive behavioural therapy. *InnovAiT.* 2013;6(9):579–585 doi: 10.1177/1755738012471029

27. Miller JJ, Fletcher K, Kabat-Zinn J. Three-year follow-up and clinical implications of a mindfulness meditation-based stress reduction intervention in the treatment of anxiety disorders. *Gen Hosp Psychiatry.* 1995;17(3):192–200 PMID: 7649463 doi: 10.1016/0163-8343(95)00025-M

28. Harper Browne C. *The Strengthening Families Approach and Protective Factors Framework: Branching Out and Reaching Deeper.* Center for the Study of Social Policy; 2014

29. Burstein D, Yang C, Johnson K, Linkenbach J, Sege R. Transforming practice with HOPE (Healthy Outcomes from Positive Experiences). *Matern Child Health J.* 2021;25(7):1019–1024 PMID: 33954880 doi: 10.1007/s10995-021-03173-9

30. Bhushan D, Burke Harris N, Bethell C, et al. *Roadmap for Resilience: The California Surgeon General's Report on Adverse Childhood Experiences, Toxic Stress, and Health.* Office of the Surgeon General, State of California; 2020. Accessed October 30, 2024. https://www.acesaware.org/wp-content/uploads/2020/12/SG-Report_Draft-Preso_v8_Public_ACEs-Aware_a11y.pdf

31. Forkey H, Griffin J, Szilagyi M. Pediatric management. In: *Childhood Trauma and Resilience: A Practical Guide.* American Academy of Pediatrics; 2021:123–139 doi: 10.1542/9781610025072

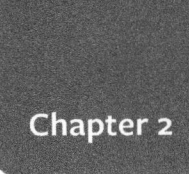

Chapter 2

Overview of Resilience University

The approach to practice I call Resilience University (RU) takes the research on resilience and translates it into a stepwise process you can use in clinical encounters. Ann Masten provides an overview of resilience research in her book *Ordinary Magic*,[1] highlighting so much of what we see in our practices working with families. Her work[2] along with that of others,[3,4] with more research emerging after the COVID-19 pandemic,[5] highlights how resilience is fundamentally accessible to everyone when barriers to essential components are addressed.

Masten identifies several resilience-promoting factors that form the essence of *Ordinary Magic* and are consistently represented in the research for both individual and family resilience. When viewed in conjunction with what we know about the role of "good enough parenting,"[6–8] these include

- "Good enough" parenting or caregiving
- Close nonparent relationships
- Problem-solving and self-regulation skills
- Agency to act and motivation to succeed

In a 2019 keynote address,[9] Masten emphasized how we can support resilience with process-focused methods to "restore, mobilize, and harness the power of *Ordinary Magic*." Resilience University teaches you to support families over time in restoring, mobilizing, and harnessing their own inherent resilience within the context of existing clinical care. The tools and strategies in this book support parents, caregivers, and children in feeling more able to make changes to reach their goals, while promoting nurturing relationships and family health. Individuals and families can integrate new skills and tools for self-care and problem-solving, which support coregulation, self-regulation, self-efficacy, and the repair of relational health ruptures. Of course, RU is just one part of what we need. Mitigating the impact of toxic stress relies on the continued efforts of policymakers and community organizations[10] to ensure that access to necessary resources and supports is available in all communities.

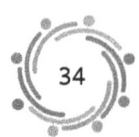

Behavioral Health Guidance

One opportunity for skill building arises when parents are frustrated by a lack of success in how they respond to their child's behaviors. I modeled RU in part after a program we used to have in Portland, ME, known as Potty University, a developmental-behavioral subspecialty clinic where we could refer kids who were struggling with potty training. The kids were referred for the program and worked with the team for as long as they needed. When they had mastered the skill of using the potty, they "graduated." Since toilet refusal is a behavioral issue that is frustrating to parents and contributes to parent stress, it seemed like a good model to start with for other behavioral problems that were frustrating and stressful and often fell through the cracks of different clinicians' comfort zones.

My experience had been that as primary care clinicians, we often need more tools in our behavioral health guidance toolkit. At the University of Virginia, I was trained to counsel parents to use a common counting method and enforce time-outs if the child wasn't behaving by the time the count reached 3. This approach, based on operant conditioning, is intended to discourage unwanted behaviors. I taught this to families and tried it with my own children for years. I kept thinking I must be doing it wrong with my own kids because I didn't feel like it was working; I felt like I was just bartering away our essential connection for improved behavior. I started asking parents about their experiences with time-outs in general. Over and over, parents shared how this method didn't work, that things escalated routinely when trying to enforce time-outs, and that in the end, the child often continued with the behaviors the parents were hoping to extinguish. Sometimes parents reported using harsh discipline (ie, physically restraining or verbally insulting the child) out of sheer frustration from being unsuccessful in enforcing the time-out. After years of these experiences, I began to question: *Why are we sending kids away to their rooms for a time-out just when they need help the most?* I didn't want to teach parents to do something that inadvertently seeded the message that kids were less welcome when they were experiencing big difficult emotions.

This question haunted me for years. A newer version of the time-out, called a *time-in*, encourages parents to stay with the child, lean in with curiosity, and try to find out what is really going on. But both techniques ask parents to try to address big unpleasant feelings in the moment, when the child's prefrontal cortex is "offline," and assume that the parent or caregiver is regulated. Both methods fail when the parent and child are mutually dysregulated. More than half of parents report a trauma history, so I realized we needed a trauma-informed approach. When a frustrated parent's prefrontal cortex goes offline, they resort to whatever parenting skills they have left, which may be harsh discipline: yelling, shaming,

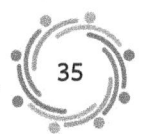

blaming, or physical force. And if caregivers have unhealthy coping responses like substance use, they may gravitate to these behaviors under the stress of being unrealistically told they should be able to control their child's behaviors.

While time-ins acknowledge the need for coregulation and connection and the importance of the child's underlying emotional/physical state, the model needs to also be multigenerationally trauma informed. We can prepare parents and caregivers to use tools and strategies to access coregulation more consistently or hold space for what to do when coregulation is not possible. Ideally, no behavioral problem should feel so insurmountable that parents resort to doing something they will regret later, like insulting their child or modeling an unhealthy coping response. I call this type of situation a "parenting hangover," where you act in exactly the way you promised yourself you would never do and beat yourself up for doing it. Many times, these responses are actually part of our intergenerational trauma, what we inherit from our own parents, just as they inherited it from their parents and so on.

With streamlined motivational interviewing (MI) and serial Plan-Do-Study-Act (PDSA) cycles, we can address barriers to change and support parents to integrate new tools and strategies they may not have experienced themselves. One new behavioral health guidance tool is NICER (Notice, Identify, Connect/coregulate, Explore, Review/repair) parenting and is discussed in detail in Chapter 4, Process for Stepwise Change. In our longitudinal role as primary care clinicians, we can offer key touchpoints for parents as they go through the process of learning how to regulate their own nervous system, even if they rarely experienced coregulation themselves. We can normalize how common it is for parents to feel like they didn't get what they needed as children when they had their own big overwhelming emotions. Parents may not be able to see when they are struggling with frequent dysregulation and may project their feelings onto their child, thinking if the child behaved better, they wouldn't have to yell so much.

A strengths-based approach helps us leverage our trusted relationship to begin to explore barriers to integrating positive childhood experiences (PCEs) and cocreate a path forward with whatever level of support is needed. With a trauma-informed lens, parents can experience their child's behavior differently once they take a minute to care for themselves. This tool is known as SUNBEAM (See, Unhook, Nurture, Breathe, Emotionally Aware, Mindful, Meditation) and is discussed in detail in Chapter 4. With this approach, trauma doesn't have to define parents. Any parent can shift how they respond to their children's unpleasant feelings to being more consistently nurturing and responsive.

Although we're often encouraged to use a multigenerational approach to behavioral health guidance, we lack stepwise strategies to support parents who may be

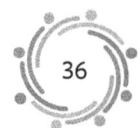

experiencing high levels of stress. A 2017 literature review[11] identified 5 modifiable factors that enhance resilience in pediatric clinical care:

1. Addressing maternal mental health problems
2. Encouraging responsive, nurturing parenting
3. Building positive appraisal styles and executive function skills
4. Teaching children self-care skills and routines
5. Using trauma-focused interventions and educating families about trauma

Of course, the Bright Futures anticipatory guidance reflects all these factors, and, reading the list, we universally agree that these are good things and helpful strategies. Yet a practice gap exists when it comes to translating this research into actionable, trauma-informed steps for families actively experiencing potentially harmful stress levels. Our recommendations may be inaccessible because of previously unidentified barriers, like mutual dysregulation from trauma or stress-related sympathetic nervous system responses. The stepwise process for change outlined in Chapter 4 will prepare you to consistently address these barriers and support families to do so on their own.

One key point is how we respond to situations where mutual dysregulation disrupts relational health. When everyone's nervous system is detecting a threat, we can help parents and children put the sympathetic nervous system's affiliate response to use, which is discussed in more detail in Chapter 1, Offsetting Adversity With Resilience. Inequitable access to nurturing relationships arises without a trauma-informed approach when families are stuck in fight-or-flight mode without an exit path. *Emotional regulation* refers to the process by which individuals modify their emotions, their response to emotions, or the situations that elicit emotions to allow them to respond to other demands.[12] It typically develops as children experience consistent coregulation,[13] where an adult maintains a space for calm external soothing and understanding. Yet many adults did not experience coregulation when they were little and experience varied responses to their own emotions. And parents who are experiencing toxic levels of stress may consistently find themselves in fight-or-flight mode during a typical day of parenting. Bringing our awareness to these stress responses is the first step in addressing them as barriers to maintaining the nurturing relationships children need for healthy development.

We generally have 3 primary strategies we use to regulate emotions: being mindful, applying cognitive reappraisal, and suppressing emotion expression.[14] Suppressing emotional expression in general is thought to be detrimental over time. Studies focus on teaching reappraisal, or using the mind to reframe the experience that led to the unpleasant emotion so as to make it more tolerable.[15] Yet this strategy is inaccessible to young children or to anyone who is in sympathetic overdrive with fight, flight, or freeze mode. For these reasons, the strategies you will learn from this book rely primarily on a mindfulness approach to emotions, which focuses on being emotionally aware and accepting the emotion with curiosity and openness.[16] When parents and children can befriend their nervous systems and learn how to work with them, they can feel encouraged to change stuck patterns in how they relate to each other.

The multigenerational trauma-informed approach you will learn here takes those 5 factors that promote resilience, listed earlier in this section of the chapter, and makes them more accessible even to families where parents and children may be repeatedly triggered and mutually dysregulated. We can help promote equitable access to these modifiable factors for all families, even if they are facing multiple social drivers of health (SDOH), have a history of trauma, and/or are enduring toxic levels of stress.

Consider integrating these resilience factors in the context of neuroception. In 2009, Dr Stephen Porges coined the term *neuroception* and developed the polyvagal theory,[17] which essentially explains how our nervous system is constantly surveying the landscape and asking the question "Am I safe?" The answer that the body gets back when we are overwhelmed by stress is "No." Our vagus nerve is bringing information to the brain from the body (often referred to as *vagal tone*) and modulating our responses to our environment all the time. Teaching parents and children to tap into this resource and use the vagus nerve instead to bring in information that says "Yes, you are safe" can foster nurturing relationships and PCEs. This resource tapping takes time and practice and is a completely new concept for many families. This is where you come in, helping them clarify a specific scenario they want help working on (streamlined MI practice I call VIVA [Validate, Inform, Validate, Ask]; more on this in Chapter 4) and then developing a small test of change (PDSA cycle, also in Chapter 4) before you call or see them back for follow-up.

Our nervous systems are constantly in flux, and this is true for all of us, not only for people who have experienced lots of adversity. Notice the next time you feel anxious in a foreign setting; that is your body's neuroception in action. Once you notice the worried or anxious feeling, what happens? If you've had difficult or traumatic experiences in a similar environment, it is somewhat common to be triggered and end up in fight, flight, or freeze mode. Translating this response into something that parents and children can understand normalizes the human stress system, bringing mitigating factors within reach. Next time you are in an uncomfortable situation, acknowledge your vagus nerve trying to help you. Reassure it with 5 Big Deep Breaths (this tool is explained in detail in Chapter 3, Essential Toolkit) and see how you feel. Once you feel comfortable with this strategy on your own, practice it with parents. This might sound something like *Bring to mind the last time you parented in sympathetic stress mode, known as "fight"*

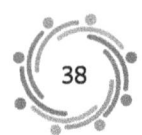

or "flight." Do you think you would have parented differently using this strategy? When we are in parasympathetic stress mode, or "freeze," calm parenting may come easier; but it's still possible to connect with and nurture your child more in sympathetic than parasympathetic mode—since you can put the affiliate response, or "tend and befriend," to use.

Leveraging the Physician-Caregiver Relationship

For many parents, pediatricians are a trusted source of advice when it comes to parenting.[18,19] Most modern parents with young children also use social media for parenting advice,[20] and given the overwhelming amounts of information available on these sites, it can be daunting at best for parents to decipher which discipline strategy is best or how they should respond to worrisome behaviors. Polished approaches to child behavioral problems often look good on someone else's TikTok video but don't work when the parent tries them at home. My experience has been that parents often want our advice about other people's advice before they try it with their child.

Many parents are more aware now than prior generations of how important it is to stay connected with their children even when things are hard and to try to respond to them in a calm manner. They're searching for ways to stay connected with their child, especially when disciplining them, to make sure their child doesn't feel alone. Sometimes this search leads to parents adopting a more permissive parenting style if they are afraid that any conflict might come between them and their child. These parents can struggle with the balance of connection, boundaries, and rules and may bring these questions to you. Simply suggesting time-outs or other "cry it out" methods may mean our guidance is one of those "half-built bridges" that don't actually bring any benefit to the family. Parents will often say they've already tried everything to solve a specific problematic behavior, and they're so frustrated, they feel like there is nothing left to do. And then that frustrated feeling triggers their sympathetic nervous system and they unintentionally end up in fight, flight, or freeze mode, perhaps even with one of those dreaded parenting hangovers.

Supporting nurturing connections requires that we be prepared with evidence-informed guidance for obstacles families might experience. A compassionate approach to stress and trauma-related parenting predicaments helps build any necessary bridges with active listening, clarifying questions, and problem-solving strategies (the combination of PDSA cycles with the strategies and tools we will discuss in Chapters 3, Essential Toolkit, and 4, Process for Stepwise Change). This shifts our practice from solely mitigating risks and managing diseases to also promoting wellness and protective factors.

Parents are often asking for help with challenging parenting situations related to stress or trauma even if they cannot articulate it. Unrepaired relational health ruptures and disconnection are often an underlying component of the primary reason for the family's visit (eg, defiance, aggression, school refusal). Parenting problems are often integral to the family feeling like they cannot address behaviors effectively on their own. When parents bring their kids to us in these scenarios, it is often not to ask for our parenting advice but rather for us to put their child on a medication or to clarify a perceived diagnosis (eg, bipolar disorder or attention-deficit/hyperactivity disorder [ADHD]).

I've been well trained in prescribing medications and determining the best way to clarify mental health diagnoses. But no one taught me how to recognize relational health ruptures or help families feel supported as they go through hard times. I was not trained in how to support families in talking about their feelings. I had incredible mentors who taught me so many things, but these skills were not included, perhaps because until recently these factors had not been fully studied and found to be protective.

Strategies for fostering resilience and PCEs haven't been integrated into traditional pediatric training, partly because the research in this area is so new. The chapters that follow will provide what you need to meaningfully respond when parents bring you behavioral and emotional health concerns that currently feel daunting. The families we care for that are experiencing poverty and multiple SDOH often feel stuck and as though no matter what they do, things won't change.[21] As you learn the tools and strategies presented in this book, you will be able to support families in self-actuation and promote autonomy.

In a 2016 Zero to Three survey,[22] parents said our help with parenting problems was widely turned to (89% of the time) but useful only 62% of the time. In this same survey, parents expressed that 2 of the major struggles they wanted help with were having enough patience with their child and controlling their own emotions. They are asking for help with their own emotional regulation, which is foundational to nurturing relationships and PCEs.

We know that pediatricians are perfectly poised to provide concrete support for parents in challenging times. We already do this. The chapters that follow will help you feel confident in including positive parenting and stress-busting strategies in your toolkit of advice and confident in the power of these simple techniques. Many pediatric clinicians have a limited menu of strategies to offer families experiencing multiple SDOH and adversity. Some may feel like they have nothing more to offer than a list of community resources or a referral out of the practice. Perhaps you've given up on trying to help and you're tired of hearing parents say that your advice isn't working. Just like we don't give up on getting a baby to sleep

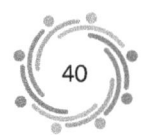

on their back, once we understand barriers to healthy coping skills and relational health repairs, we can work with the family to address them.

Parental emotional regulation is crucial and relies on healthy coping skills,[23] but we're not yet learning these as part of our medical education. This emotional support is a thing we can learn, just like biochemistry or neuroanatomy. We're just not taught how to help parents be more patient or what it means to "control" their own emotions. A history of trauma and ongoing toxic levels of stress can further limit any parent's patience or emotional regulation. The chapters that follow will teach you how to offer a multigenerational system for integrating healthy coping skills and address barriers to access in resources and support. Over time, this new framework will become as natural as discussing bottle weaning, toilet training, or school readiness. You'll develop a depth and breadth of guidance and recommendations as well as tools and strategies to overcome obstacles and setbacks around relational health and emotional growth.

Bridging the Practice Gap

Historically, pediatricians face a chasm between what we know about the impact of adversity on the children we care for and what we feel prepared to do in the clinical setting to offset this impact. While the American Academy of Pediatrics (AAP) doesn't endorse routine screening for adverse childhood experiences, many health systems have integrated this as a quality measure along with screening for SDOH. Many clinicians find themselves uncomfortable with the conversations that follow these screenings. Without a context and framework, we're reluctant to start conversations about adversity,[24,25] understandably concerned that talking about certain issues might make families feel worse, not better. Yet families are already coming to us to talk about things they wouldn't talk about with anyone else: the weird rash, the green poops, the odd smell to the baby's pee. Whatever it is, we are there, welcoming their miracles and their messes, all with open arms and an open mind.

The AAP has been calling for "thorough anticipatory guidance, active screening for at-risk children, knowledge of local resources, identification and implementation of interventions to decrease sources of toxic stress, and development of comprehensive treatment plans for mitigation of toxic stress effects."[26] The strategies and tools in this book will help you bring these calls for action to life in your day-to-day practice. Prepared to approach relational health and behavioral problems with a trauma-informed lens, we can normalize and validate these experiences while using our precious longitudinal relationship with families to problem-solve and help them feel less alone. When we combine this approach with a stepwise process for change that is integrated within a habit-stacking framework, we have a powerful toolkit for resilience.

With this toolkit, supporting families in using systematic approaches to decision-making and change becomes part of clinical care. We know that people living in poverty can struggle with a lower sense of agency or the ability to actively determine how their life unfolds as well as feel unable to advocate for their children, adopt new skills, or bring about change in their lives.[21] Perhaps you're comfortable using PDSA cycles in your offices to improve metrics but you're not used to using this change strategy at home or in direct clinical care. The chapters that follow will illuminate how to integrate a host of trauma- and evidence-informed tools and strategies into your practice as well as provide you with an approach to share these tools and strategies with the patients and families you work with.

Resilience University's core 4-session structure allows us to dive deeper into specific behavioral issues and parent concerns. This is particularly helpful if a family is reluctant or unable to accept referrals out of the practice and wants to work with just you. The chapters that follow will guide you through a process to work intensely with a family over time on a specific issue if they are declining other services. I notice I rarely have a visit where I don't reach for at least one of the tools or strategies outlined in the next few chapters.

I understand if this approach feels confusing or overwhelming at first. But don't worry. The process allows you to integrate this into your practice at your own pace. All of us find ourselves in situations where we aren't sure if we have it in us to help with one more thing. We feel pushed from all sides to screen for more things and document more topics and to "do it all" in the same amount of time. The approach you learn here will help you get out of the proverbial weeds and get right to the heart of the issue, streamlining your conversations around behavior and relational health issues and strengthening your ability to concisely and meaningfully address whatever arises in the room.

Remember, this book is not trying to make you into a counselor or motivational interviewer. Rather, think of this as a boost so you can take a small step toward restoring the art of medicine within today's world. If you want to use counseling with your teens and young adults, there are programs to train doctors to use cognitive behavioral therapy in the office with their patients. But that is not the intent of this book. These chapters introduce an array of easy-to-share coping skills and stress-lowering interventions from a broad range of evidence-informed, trauma-informed strategies, including some elements from accepted therapeutic interventions.

Resilience University in Action

Wondering what RU looks like in practice? Just like any new process, it may take time to integrate this approach into your daily routine, but you can start using individual tools and strategies immediately. Using habit stacking, you can begin

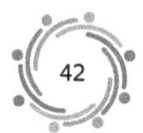

to offer one coping skill with each prescription or one trauma-informed parent-ing strategy with each referral. Becoming comfortable with addressing barriers to healthy coping skills, resources, and necessary support encourages you to lean into SDOH even when you previously felt there was little you could do about these factors you knew were affecting your patient's health.[27]

At times, it may be clear that a family needs all 4 sessions of RU (eg, if a child is repeatedly getting kicked out of preschools, the parents are at their wits' end, and you've already tried all the available community resources). Other times, it may just seem like there is a single strategy that might help, such as teaching the family a mindfulness practice to help with sleep problems or encouraging a parent to start using SUNBEAM when they habitually yell at their child for being slow in the mornings. For other visits, perhaps you offer 1 or 2 strategies or tools, cocreate a PDSA cycle, and then plan a follow-up within a few weeks. Remember, never do these cycles or interventions *instead of* referrals, prescrip-tions, or other services you would traditionally offer. Rather, they're something you can do in parallel with the family while all of you are waiting for other appointments and in addition to any appropriate screenings and prescriptions.

They're also something you can use when a parent feels strongly that their child should be put on medications for their out-of-control behaviors when it is not clear if the child has a diagnosis that warrants medication. When you elicit the history, you note a lot of stress and mutual dysregulation and wonder if that is part (Or all?) of the reason the child is not following the parent's directions. You'll still refer for counseling and, perhaps, neuropsychological testing; but in my region, these referrals take months to a year to happen. Offering to work directly with the family on the problematic behaviors in the context of RU while waiting for the referrals and/or clarifying the underlying diagnosis is often well received. You will also become comfortable with teaching children coping skills they can use even when they cannot get the nurturing response they need from a stressed parent as the parent is working on integrating their own self-care skills.

It's possible caregivers may become comfortable enough with managing things in a new way that they no longer feel like the child requires the referral or prescription, just from being offered healthy coping skills, trauma-informed parenting strategies, and a problem-solving approach. Once caregivers feel confident that they know how to respond and the child has a set of coping skills they can use, behaviors are less disruptive and can actually be used as a launchpad for family resilience.

I'll walk you through a sample case so you can visualize what this process looks like in practice. (All the cases in this book are composite examples and do not reflect individual patients. Names and identifying information have been changed to protect the privacy of patients and their families. Any similarity to specific individuals is spurious and unintentional.)

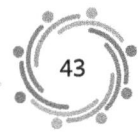

Case Scenario

A colleague referred a 5-year-old boy specifically for RU after he started hitting and displaying other behavioral problems. He didn't have any mental health diagnoses and had previously always been healthy. His older sister had autism and had just gotten to the point where her behaviors were more manageable when the son started acting out. Mom felt like he was imitating what he had seen his sister do, but when she tried time-outs, his emotions just escalated and his behaviors worsened.

Resilience University Session 1

At the first session, I used active listening to hear what had been going on and clarify what the hardest thing had been. I asked open-ended questions to find out what tools this family had found useful so far and celebrated those (strengths based). Mom commented that she didn't see how this process was going to help. She said in helping her daughter, she was sure she had "been everywhere and done everything" and they were really only here because his doctor had referred him. I used VIVA, my form of MI (see Chapter 4, Process for Stepwise Change), to ask for permission to explore and see if there were any other useful tools or strategies we could find. Mom was agreeable to try since things were so hard and I emphasized that if at any point, this exploration didn't seem to help, they could share that with me and we could stop.

I drew a time-versus-emotion curve on the exam table paper (**Figure 2-1**; more on this in Chapter 3, Essential Toolkit) and illuminated for Mom how her son's big unmanageable emotions were likely driving his big unwanted behaviors; it wasn't like he was trying to ruin the day.

Figure 2-1.

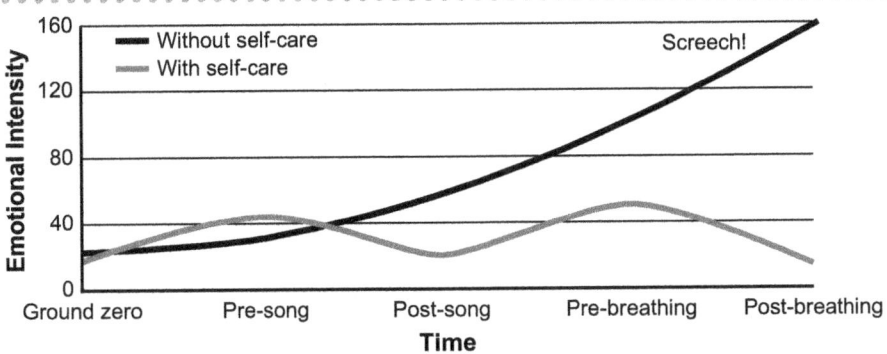

Time-versus-emotion curve. Left unregulated and uncared for, a child's emotions can quickly careen out of control. If parents or caregivers help them apply self-care strategies when the emotions are smaller, the day looks more like the sine wave on the bottom of the diagram and less like the "zero to screech" trajectory over and over.

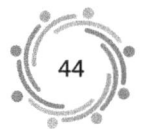
Mom looked skeptically at me and replied adamantly: "Oh no. You don't know him. He is totally trying to ruin the day. Trust me." I asked for his favorite color and we made a glitter jar together. We talked about how he was feeling when he acted out as I taught him how to meditate and how to do toes-to-nose (a child's version of the body scan; these tools are explained in detail in Chapter 3). I told him these were his "superpowers" and he could use them anytime he had big unpleasant emotions. I then explained NICER parenting to Mom. This is covered in Chapter 4 and is a trauma-informed parenting approach that breaks down a parent's response to unwanted behaviors into a stepwise process: first, what they do in the moment (Notice that there is more to this behavior than the behavior itself; Identify what that is, whether an unmet need or unmanageable emotion; and Connect with the child around self-care and coping skills) and later, what they do when everyone is regulated (Explore what else they could have done when that big experience happened, and Review if there are any other necessary apologies to make or consequences to give). I encouraged her to connect with her son's feelings rather than keep trying to discipline him while the unwanted behavior is happening. I provided handouts to reinforce what we had discussed ("Glitter Jar Meditation: Your Body Will Thank You," from Appendix E; "NICER Parenting," from Appendix W; and "SUNBEAM: A Parent's Antidote to Meltdowns," from Appendix X).

Figure 2-2.

Family Feelings Chart		
Angry Mad Frustrated Annoyed Irritated		
Sad Lonely Left out		
Hungry Famished Starving		
Confused Worried Scared Overwhelmed		
Cold Freezing		
Tired Sleepy Exhausted		
Happy Joyful Loved		
Overwhelmed Stressed Freaking out		

Add a sticker, a check mark, or a comment when you notice you are feeling a certain way. Have each person in the family use a different sticker or color. See if you can start talking with each other about your feelings.

A family feelings chart can help families begin to talk about feelings when no one is used to doing so. It can also expand talking about different feelings that have previously been off-limits.

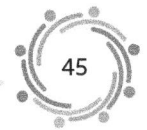

They were excited to try a family feelings chart (**Figure 2-2**; more on this in Chapter 4) and scheduled a 2-week follow-up.

Resilience University Session 2

At the second RU session, Mom had started to see how her son might be feeling lonely, bored, or frustrated and that those feelings might need some self-care strategies. She said it was impossible, however, to get him to do anything to take care of himself when he was having these feelings. I drew the time-versus-emotion curve again and we discussed the "back the bus up" approach (covered more in Chapter 4), realizing he may already be too dysregulated by the time she asks him to try a coping skill. We problem-solved about how they could integrate nervous system–soothing activities throughout the day as well. Using VIVA, we cocreated a plan for Mom to model simple self-care strategies, like singing or pausing for a few big deep breaths, on a regular basis and reinforced the trauma-informed parenting self-care strategy SUNBEAM (also covered more in Chapter 4). We made a self-care superpowers sticker chart (**Figure 2-3**; more on this in Chapter 5, A Structured Approach to Resilience Coaching) to celebrate whenever he could do these things or even remember, after the fact, that he could do these things. I provided Mom with handouts to reinforce what we discussed ("Back the Bus Up: A Parenting Problem-Solving Approach," from Appendix R, and the sticker chart) and they scheduled a follow-up for 2 weeks.

Figure 2-3.

How I feel...	What I can do...	I did it!	RESILIENCE UNIVERSITY
Angry Mad Frustrated Annoyed Irritated	• Squishy ball • Run outside • Take a break • 5 big breaths		
Sad Lonely Left out	• Cuddle pets/stuffies • Hug Mom/Dad • Glitter jar • Listen to music		
Confused Worried Scared Overwhelmed	• Glitter jar • 5 big breaths • Sing • Blow bubbles		
Tired Sleepy Exhausted	• Take a break • Toes-to-nose • Rest • Sleep		

Self-care superpowers sticker chart.

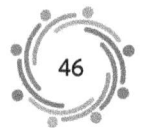

Resilience University Session 3

At the following session, Mom said she had started to see things change. She had begun to integrate SUNBEAM and NICER parenting into her day. She would suggest that her son sing a favorite song (the ABCs) or take a few deep breaths when she noticed he was starting to get frustrated with his sister. This usually happened when his sister didn't want to play with him or asked him to leave her room. Mom reiterated that he still occasionally hit his sister and sometimes got so angry that Mom couldn't get him to calm down. We worked on strengthening tools around NICER parenting, by using language focused on emotion coaching and self-care (*I wonder if you're feeling frustrated? What can you do to take care of that feeling?*) instead of the traditional demand-focused language she had been using (*Stop it! Calm down! Don't do that!*). We made him a *My Little Book of Big Feelings* (**Figure 2-4**), pairing different emotions with helpful coping skills. I told them that their "homework" was to work on adding emotions and skills to the book and to use it as a guide when things were hard. I gave Mom the handout on emotion coaching ("Resilience University Emotion Coaching," from Appendix Y), they took home a blank list of "10 Things I Can Do When I Feel Yucky" (**Figure 2-5**; more on this in Appendix Y) to finish at home, and they scheduled a follow-up within 2 weeks.

Figure 2-4.

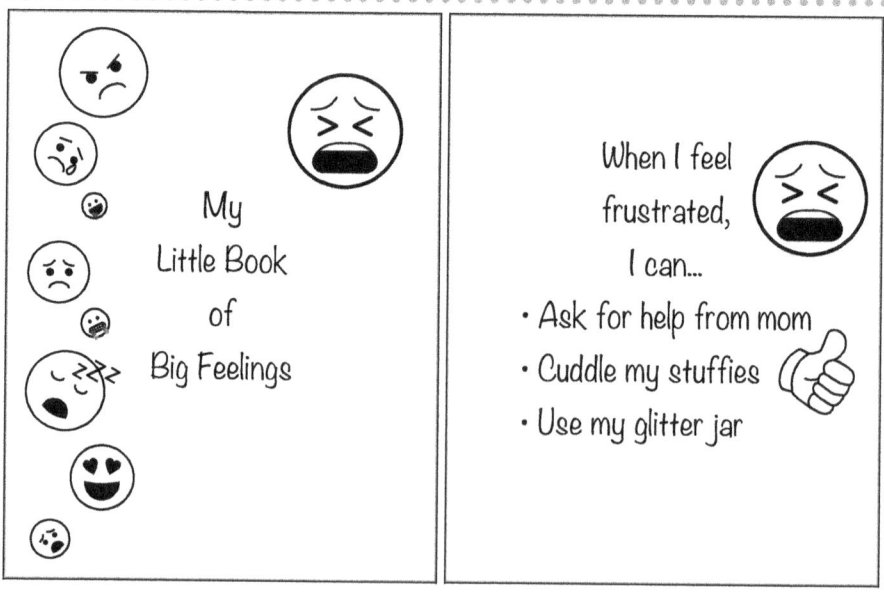

Example of *My Little Book of Big Feelings*; you can make your own with printer paper and stickers from the dollar store.

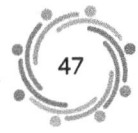

Figure 2-5.

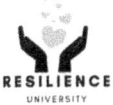

RESILIENCE
UNIVERSITY

10 THINGS I CAN DO
WHEN I FEEL YUCKY!

1. _____

2. _____

3. _____

4. _____

5. _____

6. _____

7. _____

8. _____

9. _____

10. _____

A "10 Things I Can Do When I Feel Yucky" list can help prompt younger kids to use healthy coping skills.

Resilience University Session 4

At the fourth session, Mom reported things were good. The family had COVID-19, so there had been a longer stretch between the third and fourth appointments until everyone could leave the house. When I asked if the boy was still hitting his sister, Mom looked confused: "Oh no, he hasn't done that in ages." When he couldn't practice self-care, Mom modeled it with singing and he would imitate her. We went over the 4 building blocks of HOPE (Healthy Outcomes from Positive Experiences) worksheets from Chapter 3, Essential Toolkit, and using VIVA, we came up with strategies for when Mom needed a break and identified more environmental factors they could control to help him regulate his emotions. Mom identified a grandmother and a neighbor who could help when she felt frustrated herself so she could have time to practice her own self-care (using SUNBEAM). I asked if she left like they needed any other referrals or services. Mom said no, things felt much more manageable and she would let me know if anything new arose.

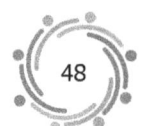

Honoring Family Structure

Obviously, not all children are living with their parents. I have attempted to alternate the terms *parent(s)* and *caregiver(s)* throughout this book. Similarly, many families have much more complex living arrangements and social structures, where it may not be just one set of adults raising the child. Discipline and emotional support may involve aunties, uncles, and other extended family networks. You may become aware of these relationships as you're filling out the building blocks worksheets, but it is also important to ask if anyone else in the family may want to come to a session or have their own set of handouts.

Family needs and family structure affect how the RU sessions are done and how the tools are implemented at home. For many families, teaching the skills to just one parent is not nearly as powerful as sharing them with both parents and/or grandparents, if possible, and other babysitters and caregivers. Stay curious, ask who else might appreciate trying these strategies with the kids, and remember, you don't have to get it all figured out at the first session. Depending on how well you know the family, you may need time to understand whom the adults are in the child's life.

We can support families and mitigate the transmission of trauma through generations. Often this transmission happens through subconscious wording or habits of the people who are caring for the kids. Supporting caregivers necessarily involves an awareness of how intergenerational trauma influences the extended family dynamic. Percentages vary between surveys and with questions asked, but it is common for parents across different international surveys to regret having children, and that percentage increases with financial difficulties.[28] For some caregivers, the role is unexpected and this may add to the stress. Family systems are complex and dynamic, and the perceptions of others in the family may limit the support a caregiver can connect to at any moment.

Cultivating a Self-Care Nook

Have you ever thought about what life would be like if we didn't have a kitchen? Everyone would be "hangry" all the time. We have a dedicated space where we keep the pots and pans and food and cooking appliances so we are prepared for one of our potentially unpleasant feelings: hunger. That way, we can care for ourselves (we hope) before the hungry feeling morphs into anger and frustration.

Encourage families to make what I call a "self-care nook" to plan for other kinds of unpleasant feelings that arise during the day. This can be a corner of the living room or the back of a closet or even outside or in the basement. They can use an old shower curtain and some holiday lights to demarcate it from the rest of the house. This is where the glitter jar, squishy balls, weighted blanket, favorite stuffies, play dough, drawing or journaling supplies, and other self-care resources

live, so children know where they are and can take care of themselves when they don't feel good. Parents can model using this space, which can teach even pre-verbal children to use it as a resource. The kitchen analogy described previously can help them understand why this is helpful.

Following are the steps for a family to create a self-care nook (see Appendix CC for a handout):

- Choose your location: Inside or outside; you can set this nook up in a bedroom, the basement, the backyard, or even a closet. Hang up an old shower curtain or regular curtain and some holiday lights or fairy lights.
- Glitter jar: Be creative; your family's glitter jar lives here, on the floor or a little footstool, small table, box, or windowsill. It should be easy to see it when sitting.
- Comfy seat: Cushions and more cushions; add a few squishy pillows and a favorite soft blanket. Your child can also bring a few favorite stuffed animals for cuddling.
- Favorite photo: Any photo that helps the family member using the nook feel loved; try a photo of you or your child as a baby or toddler. If you don't have something to put it on, you can simply stick it to the wall with tape.
- Journal or pad of paper: For drawing or writing or just doodling; include a pad of paper, a journal, or scraps of paper to write or draw on. For the family member using the nook, draw how you are feeling or write about your feelings and thoughts.

Summary

The overall outcome of RU honestly can feel pretty mundane, an example of Ann Masten's "ordinary magic." There are no fireworks and no spontaneous transformations before your eyes. But sometimes months later, when the child is in the office for a cough or a rash, the caregiver will stop you and comment how "that resilience stuff really works," or the kid will tell you about how they used their glitter jar during a scary thunderstorm when their home lost power. Sometimes they will still end up needing medication for ADHD or anxiety, but the family won't be relying on the medication to fix everything. The family will go into the process of responding to any stressor, behavioral problem, or mental health concern with a full toolkit of healthy coping and communication skills.

References

1. Masten AS. *Ordinary Magic: Resilience in Development.* Guilford Press; 2015
2. Masten AS, Barnes AJ. Resilience in children: developmental perspectives. *Children (Basel)*. 2018;5(7):98 PMID: 30018217 doi: 10.3390/children5070098

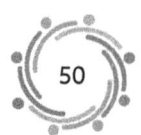

3. Center on the Developing Child. *InBrief: The Science of Resilience.* Harvard University; 2015. Accessed October 31, 2024. https://developingchild.harvard.edu/resources/ inbrief-the-science-of-resilience

4. Guo T, Jiang D, Kuang J, et al. Mindfulness group intervention improved self-compassion and resilience of children from single-parent families in Tibetan areas. *Complement Ther Clin Pract.* 2023;51:101743 PMID: 36913906 doi: 10.1016/j. ctcp.2023.101743

5. Davidson B, Schmidt E, Mallar C, et al. Risk and resilience of well-being in caregivers of young children in response to the COVID-19 pandemic. *Transl Behav Med.* 2021;11(2):305–313 PMID: 33236766 doi: 10.1093/tbm/ibaa124

6. Winnicott DW. Transitional objects and transitional phenomena; a study of the first not-me possession. *Int J Psychoanal.* 1953;34(2):89–97 PMID: 13061115

7. Smith M. Good parenting: making a difference. *Early Hum Dev.* 2010;86(11):689–693 PMID: 20846799 doi: 10.1016/j.earlhumdev.2010.08.011

8. Ratnapalan S, Batty H. To be good enough. *Can Fam Physician.* 2009;55(3):239–242 PMID: 19282524

9. Masten A. Ordinary magic: advances in developmental resilience science. Presented at: Miami International Child & Adolescent Mental Health Conference; February 22, 2019. Accessed October 31, 2024. https://youtu.be/YcfWZU2cfp8

10. Masten AS, Motti-Stefanidi F. Multisystem resilience for children and youth in disaster: reflections in the context of COVID-19. *Advers Resil Sci.* 2020;1(2):95–106 PMID: 32838305 doi: 10.1007/s42844-020-00010-w

11. Traub F, Boynton-Jarrett R. Modifiable resilience factors to childhood adversity for clinical pediatric practice. *Pediatrics.* 2017;139(5):e20162569 PMID: 28557726 doi: 10.1542/peds.2016-2569

12. Gross JJ. Antecedent- and response-focused emotion regulation: divergent consequences for experience, expression, and physiology. *J Pers Soc Psychol.* 1998;74(1):224–237 PMID: 9457784 doi: 10.1037/0022-3514.74.1.224

13. Paley B, Hajal NJ. Conceptualizing emotion regulation and coregulation as family-level phenomena. *Clin Child Fam Psychol Rev.* 2022;25(1):19–43 PMID: 35098427 doi: 10.1007/ s10567-022-00378-4

14. Brockman R, Ciarrochi J, Parker P, Kashdan T. Emotion regulation strategies in daily life: mindfulness, cognitive reappraisal and emotion suppression. *Cogn Behav Ther.* 2017;46(2):91–113 PMID: 27684649 doi: 10.1080/16506073.2016.1218926

15. Gross JJ, John OP. Individual differences in two emotion regulation processes: implications for affect, relationships, and well-being. *J Pers Soc Psychol.* 2003;85(2):348–362 PMID: 12916575 doi: 10.1037/0022-3514.85.2.348

16. Chambers R, Gullone E, Allen NB. Mindful emotion regulation: an integrative review. *Clin Psychol Rev.* 2009;29(6):560–572 PMID: 19632752 doi: 10.1016/j.cpr.2009.06.005

17. Porges SW. The polyvagal theory: new insights into adaptive reactions of the autonomic nervous system. *Cleve Clin J Med.* 2009;76(4)(suppl 2):S86–S90 PMID: 19376991 doi: 10.3949/ccjm.76.s2.17

18. Standford Center on Early Childhood. In their own words: parents speak on how their children are doing, their family's supports, and their goals. Fact sheet. Rapid.

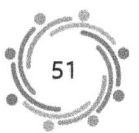

January 27, 2023. Accessed October 31, 2024. https://rapidsurveyproject.com/our-research/parents-on-how-their-children-are-doing-supports-goals

19. Taylor CA, McKasson S, Hoy G, DeJong W. Parents' primary professional sources of parenting advice moderate predictors of parental attitudes toward corporal punishment. *J Child Fam Stud*. 2017;26(2):652–663 PMID: 28529440 doi: 10.1007/s10826-016-0586-3

20. Report MP. Sharing on parenting: getting advice through social media. *Mott Poll Rep*. 2023;44(3). Accessed October 31, 2024. https://mottpoll.org/reports/sharing-parenting-getting-advice-through-social-media

21. Sheehy-Skeffington J, Rea J. *How Poverty Affects People's Decision-Making Processes*. Joseph Rowntree Foundation; 2017

22. *Tuning In: Parents of Young Children Tell Us What They Think, Know and Need*. Zero to Three, Bezos Family Foundation; 2016. Accessed October 31, 2024. https://www.zerotothree.org/resource/national-parent-survey-report

23. Bethell C, Gombojav N, Solloway M, Wissow L. Adverse childhood experiences, resilience and mindfulness-based approaches: common denominator issues for children with emotional, mental, or behavioral problems. *Child Adolesc Psychiatr Clin N Am*. 2016;25(2):139–156 PMID: 26980120 doi: 10.1016/j.chc.2015.12.001

24. Pearce J, Murray C, Larkin W. Childhood adversity and trauma: experiences of professionals trained to routinely enquire about childhood adversity. *Heliyon*. 2019;5(7):e01900 PMID: 31372522 doi: 10.1016/j.heliyon.2019.e01900

25. Screening for adverse childhood experiences (ACEs) in pediatric practices. Center for Community Health and Evaluation. December 2019. Accessed October 31, 2024. https://www.kpwashingtonresearch.org/application/files/7415/7618/7560/CCHE_ACEs_screening_lessons_12-2-19.pdf

26. Franke HA. Toxic stress: effects, prevention and treatment. *Children (Basel)*. 2014;1(3):390–402 PMID: 27417486 doi: 10.3390/children1030390

27. Maani N, Galea S. The role of physicians in addressing social determinants of health. *JAMA*. 2020;323(16):1551–1552 PMID: 32242894 doi: 10.1001/jama.2020.1637

28. Piotrowski K. How many parents regret having children and how it is linked to their personality and health: two studies with national samples in Poland. *PLoS One*. 2021;16(7):e0254163 PMID: 34288933 doi: 10.1371/journal.pone.0254163

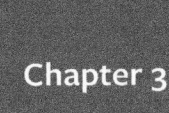

Chapter 3

Essential Toolkit

The Resilience University (RU) approach described in Chapter 2, Overview of Resilience University, relies on a set of core tools that you can apply in any setting once you become comfortable with using them. If you start by working through 4 formal RU sessions with families, over time, you'll notice how the same tools and strategies come in handy in many other clinical encounters. One of the first steps is identifying how you are going to establish a level of trust and connection with the parents or caregivers as you clarify if they want to do this work with you. Many families are struggling with family discord escalating to yelling and unwanted behavioral issues, but not all these families may be prepared to talk about it with you. Pathologizing yelling, without being curious about what might be leading to it, is a form of judgment that can limit our capacity to offer meaningful support. Yelling is like the canary in the coal mine, signaling something else is going on.

As we learn more about the harmful long-term impacts of parental yelling,[1] we know we need to support parents in finding alternative ways to respond to their child in the moment. Financial stressors have been correlated with maternal yelling at children younger than 5 years,[2] so we can offer Plan-Do-Study-Act (PDSA) cycles (see Chapter 4, Process for Stepwise Change) to help improve access to essential resources. Since you are already the one they come to about their child's health when things fall out of alignment, you're perfectly poised to coach them through other change processes when they need support. Throughout this book, I use the terms *parent(s)* or *caregiver(s)* for simplicity to refer to the person caring for the child when this person may actually be a foster parent or, through a kinship care arrangement, another relative.

Overwhelming, intolerable toxic stress is pervasive and insidious. Many families experience it silently, feeling shame for the stressors they are experiencing, and this creates an invisible, impermeable barrier to asking for help. Many parents know they shouldn't be yelling but also don't have access to any strategies that can alter their responses to difficult situations. The goal of this book is to support you in meaningfully connecting around yelling or any other stressor, offering language and strategies to remain curious and avoid inadvertently invalidating the family's experience or heightening their shame.

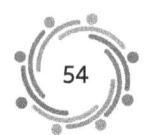

When you inevitably put your foot in your mouth and say something you didn't mean to, you can also normalize the repair process with the family and model how to do it. As we know from Tronick and colleagues' research, good parenting involves these types of mismatched interactions and relies on repairs.[3] The brain-aligned tools discussed in this chapter help lower stress in a nonjudgmental way that doesn't pathologize typical responses to trauma and stress, like yelling, but instead helps clarify where these responses come from. This prepares you to help parents and caregivers work with their own nervous systems and change how they respond to their children. As you feel more prepared to help families integrate healthy coping skills and connect to essential resources, responding to overwhelming stress naturally becomes a rewarding part of your practice. Lowering the felt stress of parenting is an unspoken ask from so many families that struggle with having enough patience with their children.[4] You may worry that this approach sounds like it will take forever. Instead of extending appointment times, getting right to the heart of what a family actually needs help with means you connect more efficiently, helping the family feel heard and making the encounter even more meaningful for everyone.

For RU to be effective, families have to be coming to you ready to make changes. I use a concise motivational interviewing approach combined with PDSA cycles to cocreate a plan with families after we determine that they would like to try something different. Our goal as clinicians may be different from that of the parents and the children. Parents may be hoping behaviors will change, and children may be hoping to get in less trouble. We are hoping to support more resilience-building strategies in their family culture. Regardless, all of us can cocreate a developmentally appropriate plan to support a sense of agency in achieving these goals.

Remember, the goal is not for the family to eradicate worried feelings or all problematic behaviors or for the parents to never yell again. Those goals would be unrealistic—and unhealthy! I tell parents that everyone is still going to be a normal human and, as such, will have a myriad of normal emotions and experiences, some of which may be unpleasant and loud. Resilience University creates space so these experiences can feel more tolerable and less toxic, no longer generating the overwhelming sense of stress that the family had previously been used to. With awareness of how emotions come and go and how we can always do something to take care of ourselves and help lessen the impact of an unpleasant experience, families can learn to bend and not break with heavy stress loads. Your role is supporting the family as they work toward their goals while simultaneously increasing access to positive childhood experiences (PCEs) and protective, buffering factors.

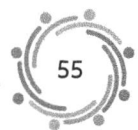
Motivational Interviewing

We are used to encouraging our families to adopt behaviors and strategies that help promote the health and well-being of their children. If a caregiver says a child hates their car seat, we don't just abandon the plot and say, *Never mind, they can just sit in the car without it.* We work with the parent, kind of taking the role of a car salesperson, asking, *What can I do to help your kid tolerate a car seat today?* Of course, we are not trying to become experts in motivational interviewing (MI) (or car salespeople, for that matter). We are instead using the basic tenets of this approach to help clarify what families want help with and assist in removing barriers, with anything from using car seats to talking about feelings.

Resilience University incorporates a simplified form of MI. Motivational interviewing has been studied and proven to help change challenging behaviors that resist other interventions and traditional advice giving.[5] Motivational interviewing is an interpersonal style that helps focus on the priorities of the patient and family and mobilizes their intrinsic values to motivate change. In the RU framework, parents are motivated by the long-term goals and hopes they have for their child. Although each family and child is unique, a recent survey[6] elicited the following overarching themes:

- Parents care deeply about children's safety, health, and well-being.
- Parents want their children to find success, stability, and fulfillment in their academic, professional, and personal relationships and endeavors.
- Parents also hope their children will work to address inequities, which requires emotional intelligence and empathy.

Reframing behavioral problems for parents can illuminate how these behaviors are arising from unmanageable emotions or unmet needs. Then parents can connect how caring for the unmet needs or emotions (instead of just stopping the behaviors) is essential to achieving their long-term goals for their children. Many parents already see this, and that is why they ask for our help with behaviors, because they know what they are doing (ie, yelling) isn't helping. We can share the science behind how responding to these emotions and needs within the context of PCEs promotes protective factors. Addressing behavioral problems this way supports the child's mental and physical health as they become an adult. We can feel confident that the evidence-informed tools and strategies we're sharing will support the child's overall wellness and goals while enhancing their ability to act with empathy when they encounter inequities.

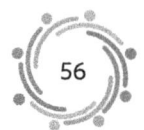

With MI, we assume a coach-like role instead of the traditional "doctor knows best" attitude. This aligns with patient- and family-centered care models (**Figure 3-1**), and we can support the family's decision-making process as we cocreate a path forward. The family are the only ones who can discern what works and might be sustainable in their household. There are many options they can choose from; our role is to understand what their needs, goals, and challenges are and then help them problem-solve while considering different options that could promote family health and child wellness. We are taking the role of a guide during MI, not deciding for the family. The parents and the child have more detailed data about what may or may not be a fit with their needs in their current environment.

Figure 3-1.

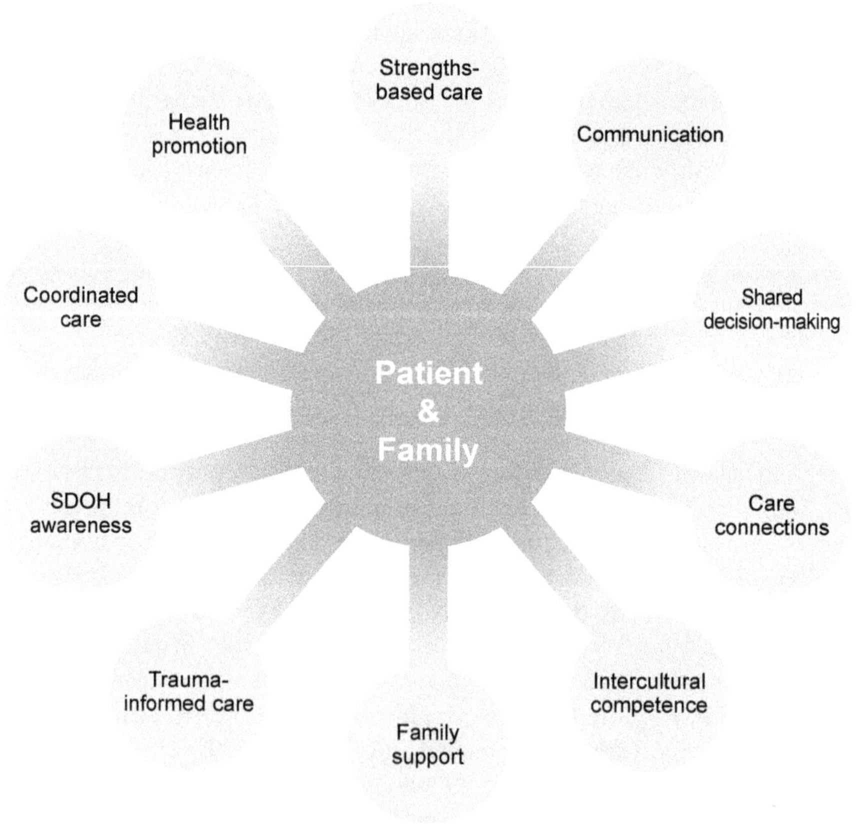

Resilience University Patient- and Family-Centered Care model. We can use motivational interviewing to respond to patient and family concerns, keeping their needs at the center. SDOH indicates social drivers of health.

To work with the essence of MI, it helps to know how the pros use it as you become comfortable with adapting it to each clinical encounter. Formal MI requires 4 broad categories of connection: engaging (creating a *welcoming* space), creating focus (identifying the *what*), evoking purpose or intention (clarifying the *why*), and planning for change (*cocreating a path*).[7] If this feels overwhelming at first, just stay with me. You'll be amazed at how much of this you are already doing in the context of anticipatory guidance.

The first step, engaging, involves creating a welcoming, accepting, nonjudgmental, normalizing space for whatever is happening within the family. As the child's pediatrician, you likely have already done this if you have an established, longitudinal relationship with the family. You've helped with all sorts of things without making them feel judged or like they're doing something wrong. You may find that you need to extend this welcoming, normalizing approach to social-emotional stressors, which is part of the first RU session.

Creating focus, or identifying the *what*, involves everyone—you, parents and caregivers, and children. Focusing on *what* the caregiver and/or child would like to see change in this setting often involves acknowledging unwanted behaviors or unrepaired relational health ruptures. Children are often tired of "getting into trouble" all the time and would like to be yelled at less and get their "privileges" back. Parents may have unreasonable expectations for their child, not taking into account developmental stages, and may need validation that things are hard as well as education around what is developmentally appropriate. From that shared understanding, you can cocreate a new goal. Problematic patterns can evolve over time within the context of any family's culture. *Family culture*, for the purposes of this book, refers to the values and traditions that shape the behaviors and practices in a family and are transmitted from one generation to the next. You support families when they want to integrate new ways of responding to unpleasant circumstances into the family culture, using a toolkit of strategies. On one level, this is no different from talking about strep throat. In that scenario, the plan includes taking antibiotics, using a new toothbrush, staying home for 24 hours, and not sharing dishes. In one where you're talking about behavior problems, it includes a family feelings chart, a new parenting strategy, and a glitter jar, the first of which we will review in Chapter 4, Process for Stepwise Change, and the second and third of which we will review in the Healthy Strategies and the Science Behind Them section later in this chapter. Families can begin to use these new strategies to increase PCEs, lower stress, and integrate healthy coping skills into their day. The family will choose what works for them; your role is to coach them in addressing obstacles that arise during the process of cocreating a plan with developmentally appropriate goals.

During this process, it is natural for the next step to happen seamlessly. An underlying larger purpose or goal often comes through from the parent or caregiver; this is the *why*. Within the context of MI, this is referred to as *evoking*, or using open-ended

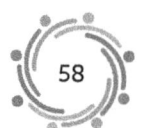

questions to help find the true motivation for the change. You're helping parents clarify *why* the *what* is important. Parents will often express something like wanting to stop the behaviors so they can keep their child in school. Other parents may say they want to see the child stop lying about homework because they don't want them to repeat their own difficulties from not finishing high school. Or perhaps they want to stop yelling because they want to be more connected to their child.

Cocreating a path forward is where applying the PDSA cycles and integrating coping skills and resources come in. The key here is to reflect back what the parents and the child say during each session and then plan small steps forward toward their goals. Your role is to consistently illuminate how stress and unmet physical and/or emotional needs are an integral part of each challenge or unwanted behavior. The family members express what they think might work for them and you cocreate a plan, collaboratively setting goals for integrating new responses to frustrating, problematic situations.

The essential elements of interpersonal style in MI may at first feel a little different from how you usually elicit a traditional medical history. You're expected not to come away from reading this book an MI expert but just to have a seamless way of using this type of strategy when it is necessary. Asking a bunch of yes/no questions (as we may be used to doing when we are taking a traditional medical history) doesn't result in collaborative decision-making. Actively listening with an MI approach allows us to lean in with curiosity (modeling what we are asking parents to start doing), asking open-ended questions about what is going on and how things are going. These elements of dynamic interpersonal style are often known as OARS for short[8]:

- Ask **OPEN-ended questions:** "How are things going?" "Tell me what is hard." "What is hardest?" "What are you proud of?"
- Offer **AFFIRMATIONS:** Celebrate "superpowers" (ie, a child's or parent's ability to integrate healthy coping skills), validate experiences and celebrate with the child or parent, or point out changes and any attempts or successes at integrating positive parenting and trauma-informed parenting skills.
- Practice **REFLECTIVE listening:** "It sounds like it's hard when he won't get into the car." "I hear you saying you really don't want to yell like your parents did."
- **SUMMARIZE** the visit: "Do you think helping Johnny with his hunger and frustration after school might help keep him from throwing his schoolbooks when he gets home?" and then later "OK, so we came up with a plan to try letting Johnny take a break from homework when he gets frustrated—to go outside and kick the soccer ball for 15 minutes—and see if that helps keep him from yelling and giving up. At our next visit, I look forward to hearing how things go."

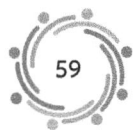

In the context of RU, this 2-way approach becomes the foundation of communication. You'll find that it allows the family to share what is important to them more fluidly, and you can get right to the heart of what they would like help with sooner. You may notice that you start using these strategies in other patient encounters and that it enhances your ability to connect and empathize with families. My concise version of MI is called VIVA (Validate, Inform, Validate, Ask; see Chapter 4). You may even realize that this way of communicating helps the strep throat visit feel more meaningful.

Healthy Strategies and the Science Behind Them

The following toolkit comprises the fundamental essence of RU. Once you've mastered what it looks like to share these concepts and strategies and address barriers that arise to integrating them, you will have a stepwise approach to supporting the integration of protective factors into a family's culture. This approach parallels and complements all the other things you have offered historically (eg, referrals, prescriptions, evaluations). The strategies and tools provided here become a form of first aid, the immediate bridge to help families address things keeping them from arriving where they intended to go on their growth journey.

The strategies and tools all work together but are introduced at different sessions, as you will see in Chapter 5, A Structured Approach to Resilience Coaching. Starting with the foundation and building from there, families can begin to lessen their overall burden of stress and respond to each other's needs rather than react to behaviors. Each tool takes only a few minutes to explain, depending on how in depth you want to go, and demonstrating them in the office is simple. (In the Appendix, you'll find patient- and family-facing handouts for many of the tools discussed in this chapter, as well as a link to downloadable versions.)

Each one of the modularized interventions in RU is evidence informed, meaning that it comes directly from an evidence-based strategy (**Table 3-1**). Resilience University translates resilience science into something families can understand and use, by packaging the interventions up into an accessible toolkit with a systematic approach to facilitate change. As you coach families for resilience, you want to know that what you are suggesting is actually based in science. Some families may even ask, *What is the science behind this?*; you will be ready to respond. The goal is not to become a therapist or meditation instructor but to simply apply immediate first aid when you identify trauma-related symptoms as well as help foster a healthy response to stressors.

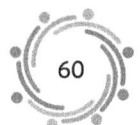

Table 3-1. Strategies and Tools Used in Resilience University

Tool/Strategy	Rationale for Inclusion	Evidence-Based Foundations/References
Breathing exercises[9]	Breath control, using the vagus nerve to return to "rest and digest"	Polyvagal theory, 4-7-8 breathing[10]
Meditation	Breath control, watching the mind, taking a break	Multiple studies, polyvagal theory
Mindfulness	Grounding oneself in the body or using the senses to bring calming information into the brain	Multiple studies, MBSR, trauma informed
NICER parenting	Allows time for the prefrontal cortex to come back "online," focuses on connection and emotional awareness	Trauma informed, positive parenting, MABT,[a] cognitive reappraisal[b]
SUNBEAM	Acknowledges that parents are triggered; lowering parental stress; helps integrate self-care, thus modeling it for kids	Cognitive defusion,[c] cognitive reappraisal, trauma informed, positive parenting, polyvagal theory, box breathing,[11] 4-7-8 breathing, MBSR, MABT
"TikTok/YouTube brain"	Places distance between oneself and one's thoughts	Cognitive defusion and reappraisal, ACT[d]
Validate, Validate, Validate	Emphasizes the importance of emotion and connection, lowers stress, helps foster regulation/coregulation space	DBT,[e] CBT[f]
Time-versus-emotion curve	Catching an emotion when it is small/early; can help lower intensity with self-care	Social-emotional learning,[g] emotional awareness, physiology of emotion, polyvagal theory
"10 Things I Can Do When I Feel Yucky" list	Supporting children to integrate healthy coping skills	Medical disease research that models looking at preparing children with self-care strategies, polyvagal theory
Family feelings chart	Encourages families to begin talking about feelings	PCEs, social-emotional learning, CBT
Strengths-based (HOPE) building blocks	Encourages discussion around what strengths and opportunities the family has to foster more PCEs	PCE research, protective factors research

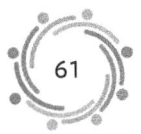

Table 3-1 (*continued*)

Tool/Strategy	Rationale for Inclusion	Evidence-Based Foundations/References
Stress-buster wheel/ stress reduction plan	Proactively maps 1st/2nd/3rd option in each area so families are more likely to be able to apply something	Self-care strategy research, California surgeon general's *Roadmap for Resilience* (multiple studies included in this report)
Emotion coaching	Facilitates a meaningful response from parents for their child's emotions (decreases dismissive and disapproving responses)	Social-emotional learning, Gottman emotion coaching research, Zahl-Olsen and colleagues' emotionally oriented parenting review article,[12] CBT

Abbreviations: ACT, acceptance and commitment therapy; CBT, cognitive behavioral therapy; DBT, dialectical behavioral therapy; HOPE, Healthy Outcomes from Positive Experiences; MABT, mindful awareness in body-oriented therapy; MBSR, mindfulness-based stress reduction; NICER, Notice, Identify, Connect/coregulate, Explore, Review/repair; PCE, positive childhood experience; SUNBEAM, See, Unhook, Nurture, Breathe, Emotionally Aware, Mindful, Meditation.

[a] MABT "develops the distinct interoceptive awareness capacities of identifying, accessing, and appraising internal bodily signals that are identified in physiological models as the critical components of interoception for emotion regulation" (Price CJ, Hooven C. Interoceptive awareness skills for emotion regulation: theory and approach of mindful awareness in body-oriented therapy [MABT]. *Front Psychol*. 2018;9:798).

[b] Refers to "altering the personal meaning of an emotional event to enhance attention to emotional responses" (Wang YX, Yin B. A new understanding of the cognitive reappraisal technique: an extension based on the schema theory. *Front Behav Neurosci*. 2023;17:1174585).

[c] The process of looking at your thoughts instead of focusing on their content.

[d] The definition of ACT according to Psychology Today is "...an action-oriented approach to psychotherapy that stems from traditional behavior therapy and cognitive behavioral therapy. Clients learn to stop avoiding, denying, and struggling with their inner emotions and, instead, accept that these deeper feelings are appropriate responses to certain situations that should not prevent them from moving forward in their lives. With this understanding, clients begin to accept their hardships and commit to making necessary changes in their behavior, regardless of what is going on in their lives and how they feel about it" (www.psychologytoday.com/us/therapy-types/acceptance-and-commitment-therapy).

[e] The definition of DBT according to Psychology Today is "...a structured program of psychotherapy with a strong educational component designed to provide skills for managing intense emotions and negotiating social relationships. Originally developed to curb the self-destructive impulses of chronic suicidal patients, it is also the treatment of choice for borderline personality disorder, emotion dysregulation, and a growing array of psychiatric conditions" (www.psychologytoday.com/us/therapy-types/dialectical-behavior-therapy).

[f] The definition of CBT according to Psychology Today is "...a form of psychotherapy that focuses on modifying dysfunctional emotions, behaviors, and thoughts by interrogating and uprooting negative or irrational beliefs. Considered a 'solutions-oriented' form of talk therapy, CBT rests on the idea that thoughts and perceptions influence behavior" (www.psychologytoday.com/us/basics/cognitive-behavioral-therapy).

[g] According to the Child Mind Institute, *social-emotional learning* refers to "...the way children acquire social and emotional skills. It includes things like managing difficult emotions, making responsible decisions, handling stress, setting goals, and building healthy relationships" (https://childmind.org/article/what-is-social-and-emotional-learning).

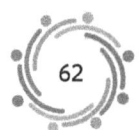

A Note About Referrals and Emergencies

Continue to use your existing plan for referrals for counseling, neuropsychological evaluations, psychiatry referrals, and other interventions. If a child is in crisis, continue to call and refer to the crisis system in your area. If you need to send a patient to the emergency department and you anticipate a long wait for the evaluation and/or placement, providing a set of healthy coping skills and strategies to use while the parents/caregivers and child are waiting can help normalize the stress associated with this difficult experience and help allow families to stay connected and support each other through this specific hard time. The strategies and tools you're learning from this book are in addition to any necessary referrals and consultations, never instead of them.

For many families, a simple shift in how they are approaching behaviors and responding to mental health needs may go a long way toward restoring family health, and you can follow up with additional support and help cocreate different PDSA cycles over time as concerns arise at subsequent follow-ups, health supervision checkups, or acute care touchpoints. When you place counseling, formal neuropsychological evaluation, or psychiatry referrals in parallel with this work, make sure you follow up with the family and ensure that the referral was successful, being mindful to address any barriers to obtaining the desired care. Barriers may be related to social drivers of health (SDOH) such as transportation insecurity or not having a device that accepts incoming phone calls to schedule appointments. Barriers for families may also include limited mental health awareness, perceptions of health seeking, social stigma, and embarrassment; concerns about confidentiality and the ability to trust someone they don't know; and financial barriers and professional availability.[13]

Breathing Exercises

We may conceptually understand the power of using our breath for relaxation, yet as clinicians and parents ourselves, we may not really believe it will help; or if we do want to use it, we may forget in the moment. Deep breathing and breath control have been studied, and we know that these techniques calm our nervous systems.[14] Three core breathing exercises are part of RU. Families may find one or multiple breathing exercises helpful. Sometimes parents gravitate to different ones than their children. If teaching breathing exercises to families is not something you are familiar with, this section will help you feel more confident in teaching this practice to patients and parents.

5 Big Deep Breaths

Using the "See one, do one, teach one" approach, I invite you to try this breathing exercise. First, notice your stress level and how your body is feeling right now. Then, after you read these instructions, close your eyes (if that is accessible to you) and take a big deep breath. Breathe in through your nose all the way to your belly as if you are smelling something delicious, then blow out slowly through your mouth with pursed lips like you're blowing out a birthday candle. Do this 5 times and then notice again how you feel. Did how you feel change after the exercise? I tell kids that big deep breaths are one of their most amazing superpowers; they just have to get in the habit of using them when they first notice any unpleasant feeling (eg, frustrated, annoyed, overwhelmed). Remind kids that if they can do this, they can often change the way the entire day goes and end up in a lot less trouble and keep those privileges they work so hard to have. The goal is not to suppress or change the unpleasant feeling but rather to simply focus on self-care while the feeling is there. See Appendix A for a handout on this exercise.

I teach families that breathing is one of the ways they can use their bodies to tell their brains that everything is OK when they're feeling stressed. If you need a script to help convey this in the office, the language I use sounds like this: *It's like using the body to check the surroundings and report back to the brain: "Hey, I checked. And actually, there are no monsters under the bed, the sky is not falling, and we are not surrounded by saber-toothed tigers."* Remind them that if we were surrounded by saber-toothed tigers, chances are we would be running, our legs would be moving as fast as they could, and we would be breathing fast from the effort. By bringing our mind's attention to the fact that our breath is slow and steady, our vagus nerve tells our brain that everything is OK. The vagus nerve is the longest nerve in the body and brings information from the body back to the brain, telling it that we have literally checked and verified safety. This is an example of polyvagal theory at work: the vagus nerve is constantly scanning for danger, but if it finds conditions suitable for "rest and digest" instead of "fight" or "flight," we can use it to help lower stress.

Box Breathing

"Box" or "square" breathing has been shown to calm and regulate the nervous system, help the body cope with stress, ease panic and worry, and bring more oxygen to the body.[15] Families may be interested to know that box breathing is what Navy SEALs use when they are under stress.[16] Have the family practice it in the office, tracing the square on the diagram (**Figure 3-2**; also available as a handout in Appendix B) or just on the exam table or the wall while you walk them through the breathing pattern.

Starting at the bottom right corner, where the star is: *Breathe in to the count of 4.* Then, turning the corner and heading up the left side: *Hold your breath to the count of 4.* Going across the top: *Breathe out to the count of 4.* Finally, going down the right side: *And now, wait to the count of 4. I recommend doing it at least 4 times, but you can keep going as long as you need to.*

The specific shape used to visualize the technique isn't that important; you can also encourage families to use a circle if that works better for them. The idea is

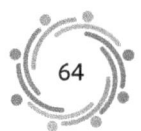

to use something palpable and proprioceptive to help regulate breathing so the body tells the brain that the person is safe.

This technique is particularly helpful for kids who feel like they can't tolerate distress in a confined physical situation (eg, when they are feeling irritated or frustrated in the car or on the school bus). They can trace the square on the window or the seat in front of them while doing the exercise. Tell them, *You can do this until the person next to you stops bothering you or you get to your bus stop.*

Figure 3-2.

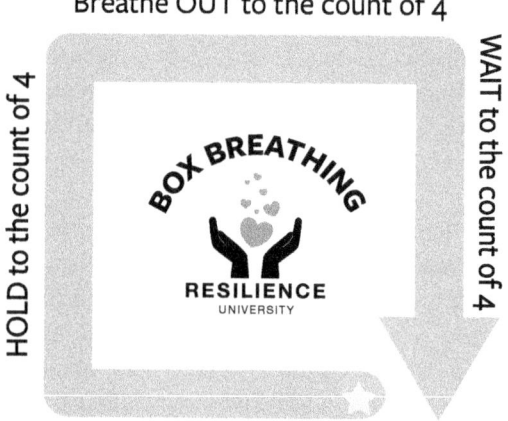

Diagram for "box" or "square" breathing.

Relaxation Breathing

Relaxation breathing is modeled after Andrew Weil's 4-7-8 breathing,[17] a counting-based technique that facilitates a calm state. Researchers have identified a potential genetic explanation for why this works.[18] For years, I tried to teach kids 4-7-8 breathing and they would come back to see me triumphantly proclaiming they were using my "7-5-9 breathing!" While I am sure any breath control is helpful, I have found that using a mantra instead of just counting helps children and parents remember the numeric rhythm as well as drown out the subconscious mind's often unhelpful suggestions.

This is a good one for older kids, teens, and parents. I explain relaxation breathing this way: *A simple mantra that uses the cadence of 4-7-8 breathing with reassuring words to reprogram our subconscious when things are feeling overwhelming or you're stressed out. When we do this, we use our brain to remind us that we are loved, that this feeling will come and go (it won't last forever), and that even though things feel*

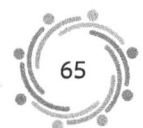
unpleasant, we are not alone and we can do hard things. All the breathing exercises are similar in how they calm our neurohormonal stress response. I say to the kids, when they're doing a breathing exercise, *It's like your body is telling your brain this: "I checked under the bed and there are no monsters!"*

To practice relaxation breathing, have the parent or older child breathe in while saying to themselves, *I am OK.* Then, they hold their breath, saying to themselves, *This feeling will come and go.* Finally, they exhale while saying to themselves, *I am loved and I can do this.* Many adults have a very negative inner voice, and when things start to go sideways, they start to beat themselves up about it. This is often a carryover from their own childhood that they may inadvertently pass on to their kids. By reprogramming this inner voice that arises in times of stress from something that is negative to something that is supportive and loving, parents can apply the calming power of their breath while quieting their negative inner voice. See Appendix C for a handout on this exercise.

Other Ways to Use the Breath

Using the breath is a thing we already do in many common activities with our own kids as well as our patients.

Singing is an example of an activity that requires big deep breaths, which makes it as soothing to the singing parent (or clinician) as it is to the distressed child. Research about the impact of singing on the singer themselves has been largely done in the context of choirs; in this setting, singing has been shown to lower cortisol levels.[19,20] The stress-lowering benefits of singing extend to listeners, including children as young as infants. Studies show that infant-directed singing helps support social learning and development[21] and foster emotional regulation.[22] Singing also causes the release of oxytocin and endorphins, which lowers stress.[23] Furthermore, singing has been shown to help people attain a state of mindfulness,[20] a key element in the tools and strategies that follow.

For a child, songs can also serve as a measure of time, and a predetermined set of songs (playlist) can be more helpful for a parent than just asking the child to "wait" when the parent needs time for completing another task or for managing their own stress level. For older children and adults, listening to music is a powerful emotional regulation strategy[24] that can be used to enhance existing strategies.[25] Educators have used this for some time, and a recent review confirmed that the benefits of music on a child's development include greater emotional intelligence, academic performance, and prosocial skills.[26]

Another way we can use our breath to calm our nervous system is by blowing bubbles. This simple technique is something nurses[27] and pediatricians[28] have used to help children with pain and fear for decades. It has also been studied as an anxiety- and stress-lowering strategy.[29] The type of breathing required to blow bubbles involves the

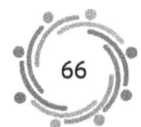

same kind of deep, slowly exhaled breaths that have been studied and shown to lower cortisol levels.[30] See Appendix D for a caregiver-facing handout on using the breath.

Encourage parents to think of these simple techniques as interventions they can use during the day to intentionally help lower stress in situations where either child or parent (or both!) consistently has a hard time. They can make their own bubbles with the following recipe from occupational therapist Anne Zachary[31]:

Mix the following ingredients together in a container:

- ¼ c baby shampoo
- ¾ c water
- 3 tbsp corn syrup

If they don't have a bubble blowing wand, they can make one with pipe cleaners or just have their child dip one or more drinking straw(s) into the bubble mixture and blow through the other end.

Meditation

> **mindfulness meditation:** [A] type of meditation in which a person focuses attention on his or her breathing and [then his or her] thoughts, feelings, and sensations are experienced freely as they arise. Mindfulness meditation is intended to enable individuals to become highly attentive to sensory information and to focus on each moment as it occurs.[32]

While many families are aware that meditation is helpful, not as many have figured out a way to incorporate meditation into their day-to-day activities or their parenting. For example, using a glitter jar, you can easily and efficiently teach families how to meditate, while providing them with a visual reminder of how to incorporate this into their family culture. Very young children, even 2-year-olds, can meditate this way if older siblings or caregivers are modeling it.

Breath awareness meditation has been shown to lower blood pressure and alter sodium excretion in African American youth.[33,34] Research has also shown that people who meditate have better capacity to moderate intense emotions.[35] Many studies have confirmed the benefits of meditation and mindfulness techniques over the past 30 years, including as an approach to treat symptomatic anxiety, depression, and pain in youth.[36] Meditation can serve as a trauma-informed technique to help parents calm their own nervous systems so they can coregulate. In a study of women trauma survivors, meditation facilitated emotional regulation.[37] In times of stress, meditating may be more accessible than cognitive reappraisal since the latter relies on the prefrontal cortex being both "online" and developed enough to reframe an experience.[38]

Meditation here can be defined as a form of mindfulness or a mind-body practice where a person lightly focuses their attention on an object, a word, a phrase,
or breath to mitigate the impact of stressful thoughts or feelings.[39] Teaching
meditation with a plastic glitter jar in the context of a clinical encounter allows
children and adults to focus on the glitter and their breath. When teaching this
to families, make sure you emphasize that for younger children, the parent may
need to do the meditation exercise with the child.

How to Teach Meditation With a Glitter Jar

The first step is to make a glitter jar with the following supplies:

- 1 plastic Voss still water bottle
- 1 or 2 small packets of nontoxic glitter
- 2 small tubes of nontoxic glitter glue

Open the bottle of water, then you or the child adds the packets of glitter and
squeezes in each tube of glitter glue. Close the top of the bottle and have the
child shake it as hard as they can, advising them to be careful not to hit themselves in the forehead with it.

Next, place the glitter jar onto a flat surface in front of the child. Have the child
(with or without you) sit in a comfortable position with their feet on the ground
and hands on their knees facing the glitter jar. Encourage them to rest their
gaze on the falling glitter in the jar. As they watch the glitter settle, have them
breathe in through their nose and then out through their mouth. The "out"
breath should be through pursed lips and last longer than the "in" breath. I use
the same language as with 5 Big Deep Breaths: *Breathe in through your nose like
you are smelling something delicious and blow out through your mouth like you are
blowing out a birthday candle.*

As the glitter settles, encourage the child and/or parents to just keep repeating
the breathing. Once all the glitter has settled, if they still are struggling with a big
emotion or feel unsettled, they can shake the bottle again and repeat the cycle.
Tell the parents they can do this when they feel anxious/worried or frustrated/
annoyed. When parents model this for their children, the kids will learn that this
is a healthy coping skill for unpleasant feelings. I encourage parents with language
like this: *Just like you teach them to get food when they are hungry or a blanket when
they are cold, you can teach them to meditate this way when they feel anxious, worried,
frustrated, or annoyed or when any other unpleasant feeling arises.* I emphasize to
parents that the glitter jar is meant to be used not as a time-out timer but rather
as a physical reminder to access this healthy coping skill. Appendix E features a
handout with instructions for making a glitter jar and doing this meditation.

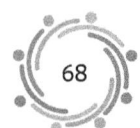

Emotional Awareness

When we are in the middle of a big unpleasant emotion, it feels like it is going to last forever and never leave. One major factor that can push stress beyond what is tolerable and into the toxic range is if the stress is not perceived to be time limited.[40] This interpretation of the feeling as permanent leads to increased stress and compounds whatever situation has arisen. Encouraging families to recognize the feeling as temporary and shift their focus to how they can take care of themselves while that big feeling is there can help shift the experience from toxic back to more tolerable. Emotional awareness has been studied in the context of metacognition, or the process of using thoughts to alter a child's experience of unpleasant emotions.[41] The goal of this brief intervention is to help children and parents understand emotions, including their physical impact on the body,[42] and learn to work with emotions rather than just reject or ignore them.

A key element in understanding our feelings is what I refer to as the *time-versus-emotion curve* (**Figure 3-3**). I will sometimes draw this on the exam table paper as we are talking. Each feeling arises, and according to neuroscientist Jill Bolte Taylor, if our minds don't grab on to the feeling, it will last for about 90 seconds.[43] One example Taylor suggests is to watch the second hand on the clock and just observe the emotion rather than engage with it.[44] This can be hard to implement when the feeling seems overwhelming. Our thoughts can amplify the emotion and perpetuate it, but an alternative approach is to practice some form of self-care and allow each feeling to come and go with its own rhythm. For children and adults alike, being aware of this 90-second rule and practicing catching themselves in the early stage of an unpleasant emotion, so they can engage in a healthy form of self-care, can alter the trajectory not only of that specific emotion but of the family's entire day.

Figure 3-3.

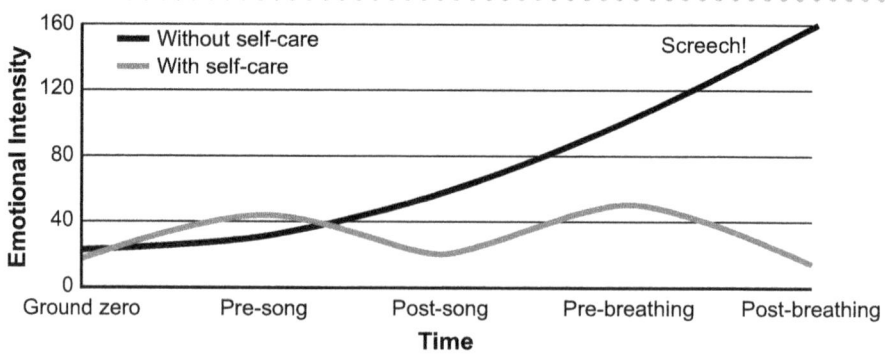

Time-versus-emotion curve.

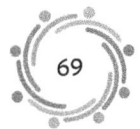

If it helps to have language around responding to our own triggers, this is one way to talk about it. I explain to families that our scary or traumatic experiences are essentially stored in our senses. Emotions associated with those experiences can resurface unexpectedly with sensory stimuli. Knowing this is helpful when caregivers are fixated on the fact that the child is "getting upset for no reason"; it allows the caregiver to remain curious and coregulate instead of becoming frustrated and risking dysregulation. Explaining this in the context of Porges' polyvagal theory is often helpful and sounds something like this: *When that thunderstorm happened and the branch hit the roof over your room, you felt scared, and your body stores that scared feeling in the sound you heard. So, when you heard the loud noise on vacation and all of a sudden felt terrified and then your parents were like, "What on earth are you crying about?" you didn't really know, but something was truly going on in your body. Your nervous system is constantly scanning the environment for potential dangers, and that sound signaled danger. That scared feeling popped up because it was linked to something that happened a long time ago. You can use your vagus nerve to help tell your brain that it's actually OK and the sky is not falling, by doing breathing exercises, meditation, or a mindfulness practice.*

I am amazed at how often children are aware that their unpleasant emotions are leading them to behave in a way that gets them into trouble. Self-care strategies help children with unpleasant emotions long before they are developmentally ready to regulate their emotions. The importance of emotional regulation is a core concept in social-emotional learning curricula in schools.[45] These later, more complex regulation skills are supported by the seemingly simple coping skills in this book. For children and adults, learning about emotional regulation is different from actually being able to work with big unpleasant emotions in the moment. The language I use when discussing how to begin to regulate during unpleasant emotions can sound something like *Do you have big yucky feelings that sometimes take over and then you act in a way that gets you into trouble? Are you tired of getting into trouble?* They appreciate having a proactive plan for what to do the next time they feel "yucky" so they can break the cycle of getting into trouble. Caregivers also appreciate having something to do if they are stuck in a cycle of yelling when their child is engaging in an unwanted behavior or is getting emotional for "no reason." Helping address barriers to healthy coping skills can enhance accessibility to PCEs by making mutual dysregulation less likely.

I explain to children and families that each emotion is like an ocean wave and encourage them to remember that emotions will come and go with their own rhythms. I emphasize that when a big yucky feeling is there, it is their job to try to figure out how they can take care of themselves so they don't hurt themselves or anyone or anything else. Younger children may need their parents' coregulation space to help them do this, and parents may need help calming their own

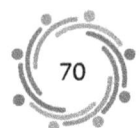

nervous systems. Sample language here may sound something like *Some feelings are bigger than others. Some feelings last longer than others. But we know for a fact that none of the feelings will last forever, and it's our job to take care of ourselves while those big feelings are there so we don't hurt anyone else, anything else, or ourselves.* See Appendix F for a helpful handout on this concept.

This shifts the focus away from caregivers trying to constantly figure out what is "the cause" of the feeling or whether it is valid. Parents often express that they worry the most when their child has outbursts "for no reason." So, we spend time talking about how all our feelings are valid, even when they do not seem to make sense to those around us. By building caregivers' capacity to validate feelings and connect around self-care, the stress of the moment decreases because the child knows what their role is in that unpleasant moment and doesn't feel alone. This is an example of removing barriers so more families can put the affiliate response to use.

Now, just because everyone knows they have a job to do doesn't mean that everything will go smoothly. We will discuss this ebb and flow more in detail later, in the Emotion Coaching section of Chapter 4, Process for Stepwise Change, but the idea is to further support caregivers with an "emotion coaching" approach. Remind parents that *If your child wants to learn to play a sport, you don't expect them to immediately be able to make it to the Olympics. First, you play with them in the backyard, and if the ball goes through the neighbor's window, you may rethink things and move to a different playing field. But when it's important to you, you will problem-solve and keep going until they get it.*

When caregivers or older kids/teens are caught in a big wave of emotion, it can help to have a more focused practice that allows them to care for themselves while the big emotion is there. In these scenarios, I routinely share loving-kindness meditation and walking meditation with them. Loving-kindness meditation is an ancient Buddhist practice; Sharon Salzberg updated the terminology to help make it more accessible. The way I teach it is to start with oneself at the center and move out in concentric circles to those one loves (Appendix G models this meditation for caregivers; Appendix H, for older kids and teens). This is a wonderful practice for those who are feeling worried or anxious, especially when parents are feeling worried about their children or when teens are feeling worried about their peers. My script to introduce this practice goes like this:

• • • • • • • •

You can sit with your eyes closed or simply recite this affirmation as you go about your regular day. You say quietly to yourself, *May I be safe, May I be healthy, May I be happy, May I live with ease.* Then you move out in concentric circles: *May my children be safe, May my children be healthy, May my children be happy, May my children live with ease.* You can include relatives, friends, neighbors,

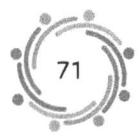

your community, etc. There are no rules; just think of yourself at the center, as though you are radiating love out to those you mention. This practice can feel very soothing, and you can just repeat the same 3 concentric circles if that feels comfortable.

For teens, the first circle may sound more like *May I be safe, May I be healthy, May I be happy, May I live with ease.* Then the next circle may sound like *May my family be safe, May my family be healthy, May my family be happy, May my family live with ease.* And the next circle may be friends or relatives and sound like *May my friends be safe, May my friends be healthy, May my friends be happy, May my friends live with ease.*

• • • • • • • •

Walking meditation is a good option for parents when they are feeling worried or angry. I introduce it as follows:

• • • • • • • •

Imagine hearing your children fighting upstairs and then charging up the stairs, worried and angry, ready to yell, versus using the following meditation practice to arrive more calmly: As you walk, breathe in to the cadence of your steps (*in 2, 3, 4*) and then out to the cadence of your steps (*out 2, 3, 4*). Keep repeating this technique until you arrive at the chaos.

• • • • • • • •

See Appendix I for a handout on this technique. This is also great for us clinicians to use when we're walking between exam rooms and feeling stressed or behind schedule or, as another example, if we're heading to a meeting with our hospital administrators or our child's principal.

Mindfulness Practices

mindfulness: [A]wareness of one's internal states and surroundings. Mindfulness can help people avoid destructive or automatic habits and responses by learning to observe their thoughts, emotions, and other present-moment experiences without judging or reacting to them.

Mindfulness is used in several therapeutic interventions, including mindfulness-based cognitive behavior therapy, mindfulness-based stress reduction, and mindfulness meditation.[46]

Mindfulness uses the body to bring specific information to the brain that helps lower stress and calm the nervous system. In addition to mindfulness meditation, other mindfulness exercises can be particularly helpful when someone is panicking or otherwise unable to regulate or control their breathing. The language I use around this often sounds something like this: *The power*

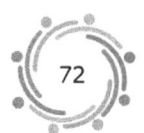

of mindfulness techniques comes from the fact that we are using our senses to bring calming new information into the brain, which lowers our stress level. Our bodies are wired to know that when we are running away from molten lava, we are not stopping to smell the roses or admire the blueness of the sky. By co-opting this nervous system function, we can use a multigenerational approach to mitigate the neurohormonal stress response, surreptitiously bringing calming information to our nervous system and addressing common barriers to nurturing relationships.

Research suggests that mindfulness techniques also improve cognitive and social-emotional skills.[47] For many parents, it's a shift in mindset to think that the most important thing they can teach children is to take care of themselves when big emotions arise. Caregivers are often instead focusing on the cause of the feeling so they can "fix" that or just get rid of the unpleasant feeling as soon as possible. A mindfulness approach to unpleasant feelings has been well studied with pain and fear in the acute care setting,[48–50] and we can help bring it to all the feelings a child and parent may experience and apply it in any setting. One of my favorite approaches to introducing the idea of self-care for kids and their caregivers is to start by asking how they take care of themselves when they feel hungry, tired, or cold. These responses are very predictable. Children will say that when they're hungry, they ask for a snack or get some food. When they are tired, they may rest or go to sleep. When they are cold, they get a blanket or a sweater. But then I ask, *How do you take care of yourself when you are sad or worried?* They often respond with something like watching a video or going on TikTok, and they will say clearly that this is to distract themselves from the sad or worried feelings. The idea of kids being able to do something in the moment to take care of themselves when they feel yucky is at the core of RU. This is help-ful, since we know from research that parents often respond asynchronously to their children even in the context of healthy safe, stable, nurturing relationships (SSNRs).[3] Angry feelings are similar to sadness and worry but are so strong that they're even more likely to overwhelm the nervous system. In my work with parents and children, I've noticed that families often come in with no inherent understanding of what they can do with angry feelings other than to take them out on the person or thing that made them feel angry.

Introducing the fact that for all unpleasant feelings, including anger, our bodies need us to take care of ourselves while the feeling is there is a game changer for many families. Just like we take care of ourselves by eating when we are hungry or sleeping when we are tired, we can recognize when other yucky feelings arise to tell us something. Just distracting ourselves from the feeling only makes it pop back up again later and, probably, bigger. Instead of focusing on something "out there" causing the anger, encourage parents and kids to welcome the feeling as a natural part of being a human. Some feelings are a lot more pleas-ant to experience than others, but they are all a normal part of life. Once we no

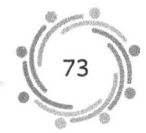

longer dread and reject more than half our emotional experience as humans, we can start to learn how to remain mindful and practice self-care no matter what arises. Emotional awareness helps maintain nurturing, warm connections between parents and children that support family health and adaptability when the family is faced with new stressors or changing internal or external demands.

Sensory Grounding

Just for a moment, try to imagine you're a mom running away from a saber-toothed tiger. Think about your instantaneous neurohormonal stress response. In that moment, you are fearing for your life and running as fast as you can. Your nervous system is in full-tilt fight-or-flight mode, but the affiliate response helps you remember to bring your babies with you as you run. All sensory input coming into your body at that point is stored related to "tiger" to try to protect you from this experience the next time it happens (ie, if you are lucky enough to survive and unlucky enough to get chased by *another* saber-toothed tiger).

After that experience, when you are out picking berries on a calm, sunny day, if you smell something that reminds you of how the tiger smelled, you may immediately go into fight-or-flight mode, even if the smell is something else and you are not in real danger. Explaining this possibility to children helps them understand that sometimes, their brains offer them information that is old and attached to a different experience and may not be terribly helpful in that moment. If you are searching for language here, I like to remind them of the following 2 wise sayings:

- *Don't believe everything you think.*
- *Just because your brain thought it, does not make it true.*

A relatable way to explain this to kids and parents is to refer to this as our "TikTok/YouTube brain." I say something like *Our brains are just constantly bringing up thoughts based on what we usually think, just like TikTok and YouTube offer us videos based on what we usually watch. When we can see our thoughts like this, we distance ourselves ever so slightly from what we are thinking. This distancing can help lessen the chance that our thoughts will fuel our emotional state, and we can give our brains a job, like using the senses to ground ourselves.*

Parents who are having trouble reassuring their children during times of overwhelming stress can use this technique as one of The Three Rs promoted by the American Academy of Pediatrics: Reassure, Return to Routine, Regulate.[51] Using the senses in a methodical way is one way to mitigate the neurohormonal stress response, lessening the impact by bringing in calming sensory information to challenge what the amygdala says is happening.

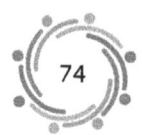
5-4-3-2-1

One quick way kids can use their senses to ground themselves is to simply find 5 things they can see that are blue or 4 things they can touch. 5-4-3-2-1 uses all 5 senses and is a good way to teach caregivers and children how to incorporate this concept into their daily routine. Remember, healthy coping skills can include distraction, but not all distractions are healthy. In scenarios where parents and/or children cannot apply all 5 senses, the practice can be tailored on an individual level.

When you teach this, have kids practice in the exam room; the handout in Appendix J may be helpful too. I prompt them to find

- *5 things you can see (you, Mom, the exam table, the stethoscope, the door)*
- *4 things you can touch (the exam table paper, the rolling stool, Mom's hair, the stuffy you brought)*
- *3 things you can hear (me talking, the noise machine, the helicopter outside)*
- *2 things you can smell (my mask, the cleaning wipes)*
- *1 thing you can taste*

For the taste prompt, I have them imagine something, since in the COVID-19 era families do not usually bring food or drink into the exam room. I suggest here that they imagine how their favorite food tastes, but at home, they could try actually tasting something. Similarly, with smells I often have them use their imagination to bring to mind the smell of the ocean, an apple, a fresh Christmas tree, a campfire, or something else they really like.

Alternatively, you can focus solely on one sense. For example, one strategy I use is to have a child use their sight to focus on a linear task such as finding all the letters of the alphabet on the signage in the room or all the numbers. Another way to share this technique is to have the child name everything they can see that is green or to share all the things they can hear in this moment.

Body Scan for Kids: Toes-to-Nose

Bringing awareness to the body as a way to ground oneself is another helpful stress-mitigating tool for kids and parents. Toes-to-nose is my child-friendly version of the body scan, adapted from John Kabat-Zin's mindfulness-based stress reduction[52] for more accessible use by kids. Like these other strategies, toes-to-nose also uses sensations from the body to notify the brain that, in fact, we are not being chased by saber-toothed tigers and we are safe. It's a helpful tool when children are feeling tired but don't want to sleep, if they are bored and stuck in a car, or if they have to wait for their caregivers to be ready to do something.

Encourage the child to sit or lie down in a comfortable way. It may help for them to start with 5 Big Deep Breaths to settle into the practice and fully arrive in their body. Remind them that mindfulness means using your body to ground

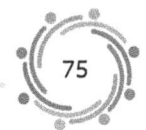

you, and they can use this tool whenever they feel yucky or nervous or are having trouble sleeping or when other strategies aren't working. Once they are comfortable, guide them through the following 6 steps (illustrated in Appendix K):

Step 1: How are your toes? Bring your attention to your toes. Notice your left toes and then your right. Lightly bring your attention to each toe, one at a time. How are they? Does anything hurt? Then go up to your feet. How are they feeling? Your ankles? If anything hurts or feels tight, thank it for all its hard work and keep moving on up your body. If you are trying to fall asleep, say good night to each body part as you notice it.

Step 2: How are your legs? How are your calves feeling? Are they fidgety? Tingly? Numb? Notice if they ache and thank them. Keep moving up to your knees. How are your knees? If your knees hurt, thank them for all their hard work carrying you around and move on. Move up. How are your thighs? Your hips? Does anything hurt? If so, notice it lightly and move on. Check in with your stomach. How does it feel? Is it tight? Or achy? Are you hungry?

Step 3: Check in with your heart. Move up to your chest. How is your heart? Place your hand on your heart and feel it beating. Do you notice any tightness or heaviness? Thank your heart for all its hard work.

Step 4: Check in with your lungs and then your hands and arms. How are your lungs? Are you breathing easily? Breathe deeply. Notice your breath moving in and out. Thank your lungs for all the work they do. Notice how they know just what to do with the air you breathe. Move on to your fingers and hands, clenching and relaxing your fists, and then up your arms. Bend and straighten your elbows. How are your arms? Your shoulders?

Step 5: Check in with your shoulders and neck. How are your shoulders? Are they all the way up to your ears? Try to relax them and drop your shoulders or roll them forward and then backward a few times. Check in with your neck. Is it tight? Does it hurt? Thank it for holding your head on so well.

Step 6: Check in with your head. How is your jaw? Are you clenching it? Are your teeth sore? How is your nose? Can you breathe through it easily? How are your eyes? Are they tired? Heavy? What about your forehead? Does your head hurt? How are your ears? Just notice, lightly, if anything is bothering you, and then, take a big deep breath as you thank your body for all its hard work.

Toes-to-nose can be modified at bedtime to help a child put their "body to bed": *Good night, toes; good night, feet; good night, ankles,* and so on. It is also a good tool for parents to use when their child has experienced a minor injury and needs validation but is not seriously hurt. For a child in pain, it sounds something like this: *Are my toes OK?* Yes. *Are my feet OK?* Yes. *Are my ankles OK?* My left ankle hurts a little. My right ankle is OK. *Are my legs OK?*

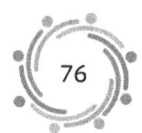

As you guide them up their body, they will notice that although some parts hurt, other parts are OK. Taking the focus away from the pain and redirecting it to healthy, non-painful spots can lessen the intensity of the moment and helps caregivers stay compassionate and connected even if they feel the child is overreacting.

Applied Mindfulness: Mitigating a Multigenerational Neurohormonal Stress Response

Mindfulness is one way to reset things when you have "flipped" your proverbial "lid" as Dan Siegel explains in his classic 2010 book *Mindsight*.[53] Many teachers share this simple model of brain function with their students, and quite a few families are already familiar with it.

I prefer to use an even more simplified version, what I call the "fire-truck brain" analogy (illustrated in Appendix L), as this is even more broadly accessible to families and children. Simplifying the complex fight, flight, or freeze state helps everyone understand the impact that overwhelming stress has on our brains and the reason why it's so hard to try to use our words, explain what is going on, or ask for help in that moment. Parents who feel tired of kids not being able to use their words are reassured that this is a normal stress response. Kids who feel tired of getting into trouble for not being able to ask for what they need also understand that this is a normal stress response. And both children and parents can more consistently identify these moments when you explain the response this way.

Using the analogy of a fire truck, I explain how the part of the brain that's usually tucked away in a "garage" (the amygdala) acts like a first responder. Just like a fire truck showing up with lights flashing, horns blaring, and hoses ready, this part of the brain takes over, ready to respond to danger. This takeover is helpful if your house is actually on fire, but if you just burned the toast, it's not so helpful. Normalizing that our fire-truck brain is quite responsive but sometimes shows up when it is not necessarily needed helps parents and kids alike to understand that this is simply a nervous system adaptation related to when we were hunter-gatherers and we had to protect our babies from getting crushed by stampeding woolly mammoths.

I point out to families that the part of our brain that we use to analyze and talk about our feelings, in order to explore why we feel this way and what this feeling is trying to tell us, is not online when we are in the middle of overwhelming stress (eg, a big unmanageable emotion). As parents begin to consistently notice when their child is in this fire-truck brain state, they can focus on their own healthy coping strategies and not make things worse by trying to get a dysregulated child to explain themselves. A parent asking their child to "use your words" when the child is unable to apply language in their distressed state risks

the parent becoming dysregulated too. With parents learning to model self-care strategies in the context of this approach as well, the chance of having a bidirectionally dysfunctional, mutually dysregulated interaction is much lower. This leads to 2 trauma-informed parenting strategies, NICER (Notice, Identify, Connect/coregulate, Explore, Review/repair) parenting and SUNBEAM (See, Unhook, Nurture, Breathe, Emotionally Aware, Mindful, Meditation), which we will cover more in Chapter 4.

A New Review of Systems Approach

I think of resilience as a human system, and just like we review the organ systems in the body, it is helpful in medicine for us to be able to have a tailored resilience review of systems (ROS) approach. We're used to screening for community engagement as well as emotional and relational health in pediatrics. Over the past decade, we've also begun screening for environmental stressors (ie, housing insecurity, food insecurity, in addition to safety or violence in the home). We commonly refer out or connect families with services when we, with the family, mutually identify a concern in these areas. Part of what you will learn from this book is how to offer a meaningful bridge strategy for families while they are awaiting necessary referrals and resources. But first we need a systematic approach to review the dynamic system of resilience.

The HOPE (Healthy Outcomes from Positive Experiences) framework helps unify our screenings as parts of a dynamic whole so we can cocreate paths forward when families are asking for our help. This framework encompasses 4 building blocks core to the 7 studied PCEs: emotional growth, relational health, engagement, and environment.[54] The building blocks break down resilience factors into categories, so we can use an ROS approach like we are accustomed to elsewhere in medicine. Bringing HOPE to life in primary care means regarding the 7 PCEs more like a symphony and less like a grocery list in our work with families (more on this in the 9-5-2-1-0 section later in this chapter).

We simultaneously celebrate strengths and respond to barriers to protective factors in the same way we might assess a child's respiratory system, noting that the oxygen saturation is 97% and there are diffuse bilateral expiratory wheezes. Addressing barriers is the same as prescribing a nebulizer treatment for this child's wheezing, only our role is to help the family clarify what a child needs in order to shift stress from potentially toxic to tolerable. For example, strong emotional and relational health can maintain resilience amid housing and food insecurities. Asking about sports, activities, and family connections is often already part of our routine, and these kinds of questions explore the building block of engagement. Exploring the building blocks of relational health and emotional growth goes

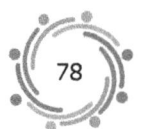

beyond screening for adolescent and postpartum depression. Behavioral problems are often an indicator that something has shifted within the individual and/or family resilience system, and we can support families in identifying this core element rather than focus entirely on how the child is behaving.

In Chapter 4, we'll review how to cocreate serial family-centered PDSA cycles to meaningfully support families through their experiences with resilience and variable SDOH. The strategies in this chapter more specifically focus on exploring emotional growth and relational health, which are 2 of the 4 HOPE building blocks. These foundational skills support the SSNRs we know are crucial to healthy child development[17] and a parent's ability to apply The Three Rs at any moment.

I use worksheets (**Figures 3-4 and 3-5**; also included in Appendixes M and N) to lean in with curiosity about all 4 building blocks. These strengths-based tools allow for a deeper and broader, more meaningful conversation than a yes/no questionnaire. One worksheet prompts the family to think of sources of resilience and strength in their current situation, by using the HOPE building blocks. A second option challenges the child and their caregivers to build "towers" out of these blocks. I give the worksheets either directly to children if they are old enough to write or to the parents if the kids are not yet in elementary school. For teens, I provide them with a stress reduction plan (**Figure 3-6**; also included in Appendix O) and challenge them to try to add at least 2 healthy coping skills, strategies, or resources in each stress-buster area[55] (Friends/Family, Sleep, Nutrition, Mental Health, Mindfulness, Nature, and Movement). This can include one that is perhaps preferred or easiest and then a backup if the preferred one is not accessible at the time. Both of these prompt parents and children to think about how they can take care of themselves under stress and how they are connected and to identify strengths and supports.

Sometimes families have trouble coming up with anything for one or more of the building blocks; but with a little coaching, you may be able to help them identify assets they hadn't considered. If they feel they truly don't have anything in a given area, you can cocreate a path forward. For example, with relational health, maybe they don't feel like they have someone to help when things are hard and they're feeling isolated. In this scenario, you can ask if they might be able to reconnect with Grandma via video chat or have an auntie start regularly picking the kids up from school. Another area where you can support families in reaching their goals is emotional growth. The tools in this chapter paired with the strategies in the next chapter will help you consistently coach families in a stepwise approach for addressing barriers to talking about feelings.

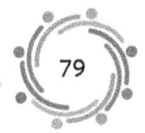

Remember, not everyone needs to have mile-high block towers in each quadrant to offset long-term toxic stress. In fact, for many families, if one building block tower is solid, it sustains them when all the others may be "wobbly." Following are questions we can ask to explore resilience factors in each building block:

- Engagement
    - What is one thing you like to do as a family outside the home?
    - Where do you feel most connected to others?
    - Describe a favorite outing.
    - What is your favorite sport or activity?
- Environment
    - Describe places you love to go.
    - Where do you like to play?
    - Describe your safe space(s).
    - What is your favorite place in your home? Outside your home?
- Emotional growth
    - What feelings do you talk about at home?
    - With whom can you talk about feelings?
    - How can you take care of yourself when you don't feel good?
    - What always helps you feel better when you feel yucky?
- Relational health
    - What do you like to do at home with your family?
    - Who outside your family would always help you if you needed something?
    - Which family story are you proud of?
    - What is your favorite book or movie?

We are honoring each family's unique journey, even with the messy moments. We can remind them that at times, some things may feel more pleasant or unpleasant than others, but unpleasant experiences are nothing to be ashamed of. Instead of rejecting them or trying to avoid acknowledging them, we can support families in radical acceptance, making space for what is happening without judging it while addressing any barriers to resilience and supporting the family's goals. As we become more comfortable with doing so, we can validate unpleasant experiences while supporting healthy coping skills and addressing barriers to resources so a family's health doesn't get derailed by the experience of adversity.

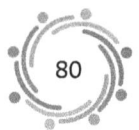
Figure 3-4.

Building Blocks for Health	These 4 building blocks are important factors in growing up healthy. Share what's working and your provider will brainstorm with you for solutions to anything that's not working.

Engagement

What is one thing you like to do as a family outside the home?
Where do you feel most connected to others?

Environment

Describe a place you love to go or play. Where is your safe space?

Relational Health

What do you like to do at home with your family?
Who is someone outside your family that really cares about you?

Emotional Growth

What feelings do you talk about at home? With whom do you talk about feelings? How can you take care of yourself when you have big feelings?

Build a "tower" with your blocks!

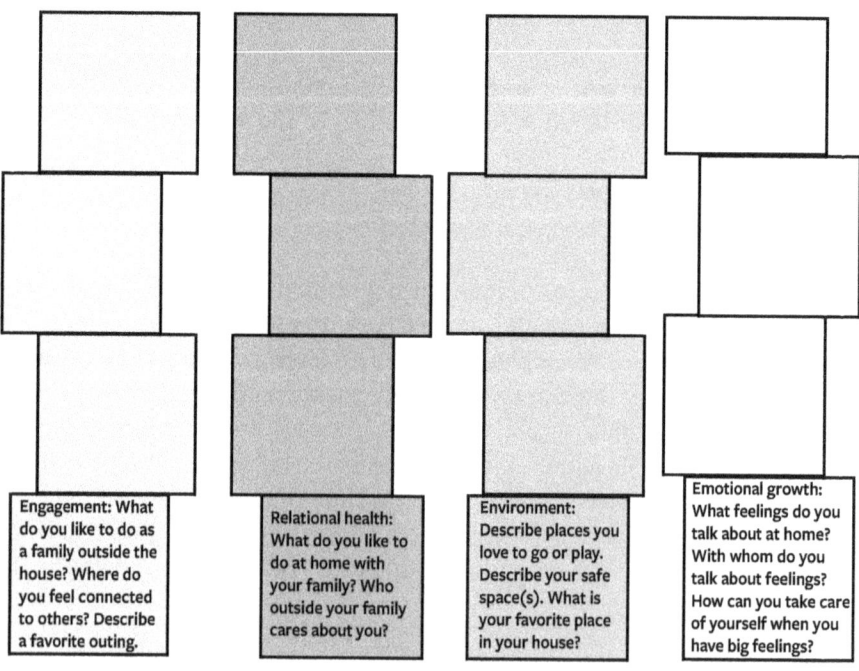

Engagement: What do you like to do as a family outside the house? Where do you feel connected to others? Describe a favorite outing.

Relational health: What do you like to do at home with your family? Who outside your family cares about you?

Environment: Describe places you love to go or play. Describe your safe space(s). What is your favorite place in your house?

Emotional growth: What feelings do you talk about at home? With whom do you talk about feelings? How can you take care of yourself when you have big feelings?

Building block worksheets using the HOPE (Healthy Outcomes from Positive Experiences) framework.
HOPE (Healthy Outcomes from Positive Experiences) is a registered trademark of Tufts Medical Center.

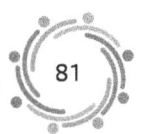

Following are some strategies to address areas that might be feeling a bit wobbly (**Figure 3-5**); in Chapter 4, you will learn how to cocreate small tests of change with families when they want to strengthen a tower:

- Engagement
  - Suggest after-school programs.
  - Explore summer camps and community programs.
  - Identify a local YMCA: Can the family connect to this resource? Are there scholarships? Are there transportation barriers to address?
  - Offer parenting resources (eg, positive parenting resources, community groups).
  - Identify youth programs, outreach, and school and community groups.
  - Offer a list of local places of worship or spiritual centers and resources.
  - Identify parent support groups, online or in person.
- Environment
  - Provide a list of local housing resources.
  - Provide a list of food banks.
  - Provide a list of transportation options.
  - Review gun safety.
  - Review medication safety.
  - Brainstorm about safe play areas.
  - Brainstorm about options for trips and outings.
  - Offer a list of community resources for outdoor activities.
  - Offer trail/park maps and resources (eg, state park passes).
- Relational health
  - How are things at home? What is hard for the parents?
  - Are the parents able to play with their kids? Read with them?
  - What is the parent proud of?
  - How high is the stress level at home?
  - Are there specific things or times of day that are hardest?
  - Name the nonparent adults who can help; identify barriers to asking them for help.
  - Identify community resources that can reduce barriers and decrease isolation.
  - Provide a list of community groups and supports.
  - Provide books and library resources.

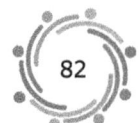
- Emotional growth
  - Ask the parents if they feel like they know how to help their child when their child is angry, frustrated, worried, or scared.
  - Ask the parents how they take care of themselves when they are stressed, sad, angry, or frustrated.
  - Make a family feelings chart and encourage them to ask, *How do I know I am feeling this way?* and *How can I take care of myself while this feeling is here?* (See Chapter 4.)
  - Teach at least one breathing exercise (glitter jar, box breathing, or 5 Big Deep Breaths).
  - Teach one strategy for anger (eg, playing "angry" ball with a Nerf ball, going outside to run around).
  - Teach one mindfulness strategy, such as toes-to-nose or 5-4-3-2-1 (ie, using all 5 senses).

When we have these discussions, we have to be mindful that we may also need to address barriers to participating in or connecting to resources or support, such as language barriers, transportation insecurity, phone service instability, lack of internet access, and others. Making a list of community resources that your office may be able to use for a warm handoff to address these barriers can support resilience. For example, if you refer a family for help with parenting but they have a device that works only with a specific messaging app, they may not be able to receive a call and therefore can't implement your recommendation. If your office has a community health worker, you can ask them to follow up with PDSA cycles with the family until all essential needs are met.

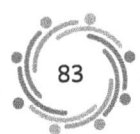

Figure 3-5.

Strengths-Based Building Block Conversations

Engagement

- Suggest after-school programs.
- Explore summer camps and community programs.
- Identify a local YMCA: Can the family connect to this resource? Are there scholarships? Are there transportation barriers to address?
- Offer parenting resources (eg, positive parenting resources, community groups).
- Identify youth programs, outreach, and school and community groups.
- Offer a list of local places of worship or spiritual centers and resources.
- Identify parent support groups, online or in person.

Environment

- Provide a list of local housing resources.
- Provide a list of food banks.
- Provide a list of transportation options.
- Review gun safety.
- Review medication safety.
- Brainstorm about safe play areas.
- Brainstorm about options for trips and outings.
- Offer a list of community resources for outdoor activities.
- Offer trail/park maps and resources (eg, state park passes).

Relational Health

- How are things at home? What is hard for the parents?
- Are the parents able to play with their kids? Read with them?
- What is the parent proud of?
- How high is the stress level at home?
- Are there specific things or times of day that are hardest?
- Name the nonparent adults who can help; identify barriers to asking them for help.
- Identify community resources that can reduce barriers and decrease isolation.
- Provide a list of community groups and supports.
- Provide books and library resources.

Emotional Growth

- Ask the parents if they feel like they know how to help their child when their child is angry, frustrated, worried, or scared.
- Ask the parents how they take care of themselves when they are stressed, sad, angry, or frustrated.
- Make a family feelings chart and encourage them to ask, "How do I know I am feeling this way?" and "How can I take care of myself while this feeling is here?" (See Chapter 4.)
- Teach at least one breathing exercise (glitter jar, box breathing, or 5 Big Deep Breaths).
- Teach one strategy for anger (eg, playing "angry" ball with a Nerf ball, going outside to run around).
- Teach one mindfulness strategy, such as toes-to-nose or 5-4-3-2-1 (ie, using all 5 senses).

Conversation topics to support the HOPE (Healthy Outcomes from Positive Experiences) building blocks.

HOPE (Healthy Outcomes from Positive Experiences) is a registered trademark of Tufts Medical Center.

Figure 3-6.

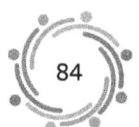

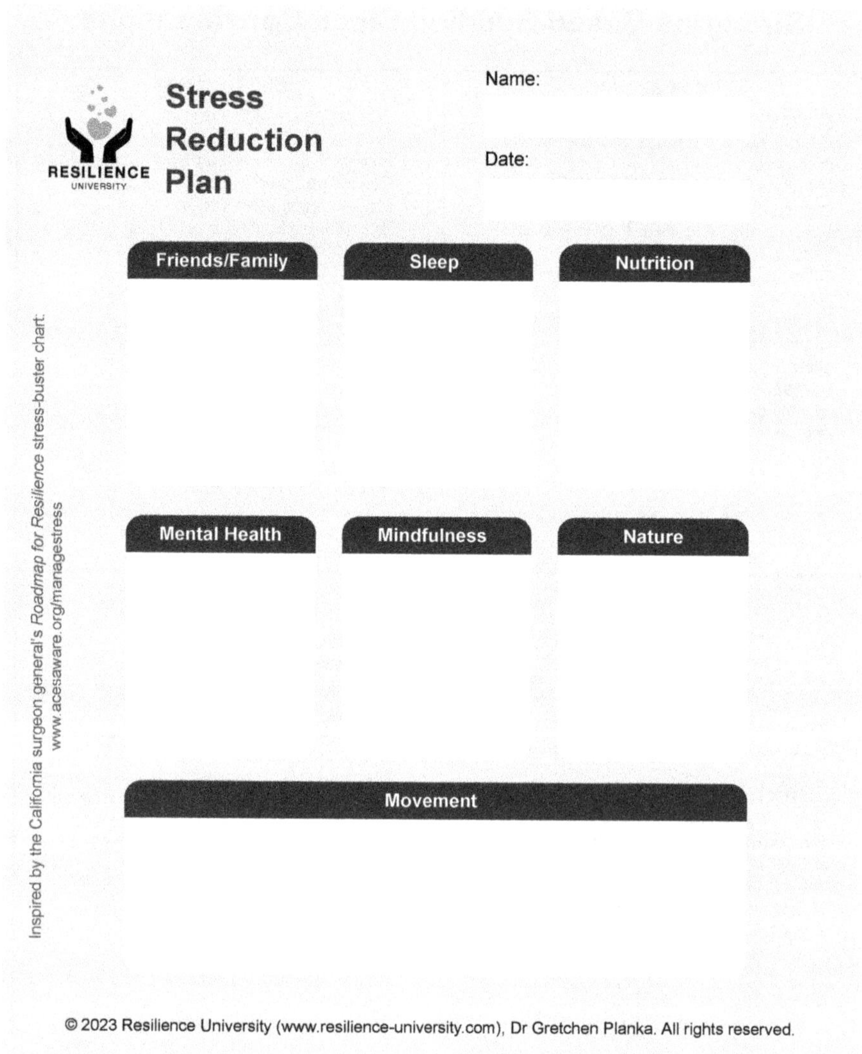

Stress Reduction Plan

RESILIENCE UNIVERSITY

Name:

Date:

Friends/Family

Sleep

Nutrition

Mental Health

Mindfulness

Nature

Movement

Inspired by the California surgeon general's *Roadmap for Resilience* stress-buster chart: www.acesaware.org/managestress

Stress reduction plan for teens.

9-5-2-1-0

The stress-buster strategies from **Figure 3-6** can be distilled into a sticker chart (**Figure 3-7**) for younger kids and their families to make taking care of themselves and lowering stress more tangible. Researchers have developed the 9-5-2-1-0 framework to support youth wellness,[56,57] giving families simple guidelines for elementary/middle school/high school sleep, screen time, nutrition, and

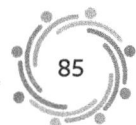

exercise. The guidelines call for 7 to 9 hours of sleep a night, 5 or more servings of fruits or veggies each day, 2 hours or less of recreational screen time, 1 hour or more of physical activity or active play, and no sugary sweetened drinks.

Figure 3-7.

9-5-2-1-0		Monday	Tuesday	Wednesday	Thursday	Friday	Saturday	Sunday	RESILIENCE
	7–9 hours of sleep								✓ = I totally did it.
	5 or more servings of fruits or veggies								☆ = I tried to do it.
	2 hours or less of screen time (doesn't include homework!)								✗ = I didn't try this one.
	1 hour or more of physical exercise or active play								
	No sugary sweetened drinks								

9-5-2-1-0 checklist.

When we are working with families on addressing factors that commonly worsen behaviors, this format encourages them to integrate healthy strategies while honoring barriers. Studies have shown that not all families have equal access to the assets that will allow them to follow this recommendation.[58] If families bring the chart back to share with you and they are having trouble with one or more factors, you can support them with PDSA cycles (more on this in Chapter 4) to address barriers.

Although screen time is ideally limited to less than 2 hours a day, we can use some of the popular video resources to coach families for resilience and integrate these into the family's media use plan. For example, *Daniel Tiger* is a Public Broadcasting Service (PBS) series. When Daniel gets angry, there is a song (available at www.pbs.org/video/daniel-tigers-neighborhood-when-you-feel-so-mad-song) that helps him remember to take deep breaths so he can calm down. He "takes a deep breath and counts to 4" in the song, and in a coloring page (available at cms-tc.pbskids.org/daniel-tiger-website/printables/DTN_Calming-Down. pdf), he models giving a squeezy hug to help oneself calm down. Curiously discussing how the family is currently using screen time can help you cocreate a realistic plan to use videos like this one to integrate healthy coping skills.

Another resource for families with young children is a video on YouTube from PBS where *Sesame Street*'s Elmo uses a strategy similar to toes-to-nose to put himself to bed (https://youtu.be/yhRWpowOLyo). We can help families integrate this into their media use plan if they feel it might be helpful with their child's sleep.

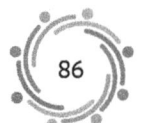

For older children and teens as well as parents, I often recommend the Headspace or Calm app. These apps have options for guided meditation and breathing exercises and can expand the options for families that are either not resonating with the specific tools in this chapter or are looking for other resources and ideas in addition to these strategies. YouTube also has guided meditations and mindfulness practices that many teens and parents find helpful and accessible when trying to make changes to shift stress from toxic to tolerable.

Discussions around screen use as a form of self-care are an opportunity to celebrate family strengths and build a bridge to your recommendations. Be careful not to immediately judge the use of screens. As we will discuss more in Chapter 6, Using Relationship-Based and Trauma-Informed Anticipatory Guidance, and Chapter 8, Universal Integration in Practice, screen time may already represent a strategy used by families to mitigate the impact of stress. For many teens, devices may represent one of their healthier methods of coping.

When we introduce these tools and strategies to parents along with the evidence that informs them, be cognizant that families often do a mental checklist of their own experience and criticize themselves when they aren't able to immediately check off all the boxes for their own children. When I talk about this with parents and caregivers, I use the analogy of a music equalizer app or an equalizer on an old-fashioned stereo system. I make sure to say that fostering resilience is more like composing a symphony than a grocery list and the building blocks are like the sound components. You don't want music to always have the same amount of bass and treble, percussion and strings, or alto and soprano. The best music has variation.

References

1. Dube SR, Li ET, Fiorini G, et al. Childhood verbal abuse as a child maltreatment subtype: a systematic review of the current evidence. *Child Abuse Negl.* 2023;144:106394 PMID: 37586139 doi: 10.1016/j.chiabu.2023.106394
2. Arai T, Goto A, Komatsu M, Yasumura S. Incidence of and improvement in inappropriate parental behaviors of mothers with young children: a retrospective cohort study conducted in collaboration with a local government. *Arch Public Health.* 2021;79(1):37 PMID: 33731221 doi: 10.1186/s13690-021-00558-8
3. Tronick E, Als H, Adamson L, Wise S, Brazelton TB. The infant's response to entrapment between contradictory messages in face-to-face interaction. *J Am Acad Child Psychiatry.* 1978;17(1):1–13 PMID: 632477 doi: 10.1016/S0002-7138(09)62273-1
4. *Tuning In: Parents of Young Children Tell Us What They Think, Know and Need.* Zero to Three, Bezos Family Foundation; 2016. Accessed November 11, 2024. https://www.zerotothree.org/resource/national-parent-survey-report

5. Rubak S, Sandbaek A, Lauritzen T, Christensen B. Motivational interviewing: a systematic review and meta-analysis. *Br J Gen Pract.* 2005;55(513):305–312 PMID: 15826439

6. Stanford Center on Early Childhood. In their own words: parents speak on how their children are doing, their family's supports, and their goals. Fact sheet. Rapid. January 27, 2023. Accessed November 11, 2024. https://rapidsurveyproject.com/our-research/parents-on-how-their-children-are-doing-supports-goals

7. Levounis P, Arnaout B, Marienfeld C. *Motivational Interviewing for Clinical Practice.* American Psychiatric Association Publishing; 2017 doi: 10.1176/appi.books.9781615371860

8. Stewart EE, Fox CH. Encouraging patients to change unhealthy behaviors with motivational interviewing. *Fam Pract Manag.* 2011;18(3):21–25 PMID: 21842805

9. Bentley TGK, D'Andrea-Penna G, Rakic M, et al. Breathing practices for stress and anxiety reduction: conceptual framework of implementation guidelines based on a systematic review of the published literature. *Brain Sci.* 2023;13(12):1612 PMID: 38137060 doi: 10.3390/brainsci13121612

10. Aktaş GK, İlgin VE. The effect of deep breathing exercise and 4-7-8 breathing techniques applied to patients after bariatric surgery on anxiety and quality of life. *Obes Surg.* 2023;33(3):920–929 PMID: 36480101 doi: 10.1007/s11695-022-06405-1

11. Balban MY, Neri E, Kogon MM, et al. Brief structured respiration practices enhance mood and reduce physiological arousal. *Cell Rep Med.* 2023;4(1):100895 PMID: 36630953 doi: 10.1016/j.xcrm.2022.100895

12. Zahl-Olsen R, Severinsen L, Stiegler JR, et al. Effects of emotionally oriented parental interventions: a systematic review and meta-analysis. *Front Psychol.* 2023;14:1159892 PMID: 37519350 doi: 10.3389/fpsyg.2023.1159892

13. Radez J, Reardon T, Creswell C, Lawrence PJ, Evdoka-Burton G, Waite P. Why do children and adolescents (not) seek and access professional help for their mental health problems? a systematic review of quantitative and qualitative studies. *Eur Child Adolesc Psychiatry.* 2021;30(2):183–211 PMID: 31965309 doi: 10.1007/s00787-019-01469-4

14. Gerritsen RJS, Band GPH. Breath of life: the respiratory vagal stimulation model of contemplative activity. *Front Hum Neurosci.* 2018;12:397 PMID: 30356789 doi: 10.3389/fnhum.2018.00397

15. Jha RK, Acharya A, Nepal O. Autonomic influence on heart rate for deep breathing and Valsalva maneuver in healthy subjects. *JNMA J Nepal Med Assoc.* 2018;56(211):670–673 PMID: 30381762 doi: 10.31729/jnma.3618

16. Kumar K. Why do Navy SEALs use box breathing? MedicineNet. Accessed November 11, 2024. https://www.medicinenet.com/why_do_navy_seals_use_box_breathing/article.htm

17. Weil A. 4-7-8 breathing: health benefits & demonstration. Weil Lifestyle. Accessed November 11, 2024. https://www.drweil.com/videos-features/videos/the-4-7-8-breath-health-benefits-demonstration

18. Yackle K, Schwarz LA, Kam K, et al. Breathing control center neurons that promote arousal in mice. *Science.* 2017;355(6332):1411–1415 PMID: 28360327 doi: 10.1126/science.aai7984

19. Kreutz G, Bongard S, Rohrmann S, Hodapp V, Grebe D. Effects of choir singing or listening on secretory immunoglobulin A, cortisol, and emotional state. *J Behav Med.* 2004;27(6):623–635 PMID: 15669447 doi: 10.1007/s10865-004-0006-9

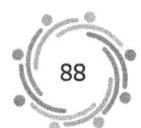

20. Lynch J, Wilson CE. Exploring the impact of choral singing on mindfulness. *Psychol Music*. 2018;46(6):848–861 doi: 10.1177/0305735617729452

21. Lense MD, Shultz S, Astésano C, Jones W. Music of infant-directed singing entrains infants' social visual behavior. *Proc Natl Acad Sci USA*. 2022;119(45):e2116967119 PMID: 36322755 doi: 10.1073/pnas.2116967119

22. de l'Etoile SK. Self-regulation and infant-directed singing in infants with Down syndrome. *J Music Ther*. 2015;52(2):195–220 PMID: 25957338 doi: 10.1093/jmt/thv003

23. Sanal AM, Gorsev S. Psychological and physiological effects of singing in a choir. *Psychol Music*. 2014;42(3):420–429 doi: 10.1177/0305735613477181

24. Cook T, Roy ARK, Welker KM. Music as an emotion regulation strategy: an examination of genres of music and their roles in emotion regulation. *Psychol Music*. 2019;47(1):144–154 doi: 10.1177/0305735617734627

25. Nwokenna EN, Sewagegn AA, Falade TA. Effect of educational music intervention on emotion regulation skills of first-year university music education students. *Medicine (Baltimore)*. 2022;101(47):e32041 PMID: 36451437 doi: 10.1097/MD.0000000000032041

26. Blasco-Magraner JS, Bernabe-Valero G, Marín-Liébana P, Moret-Tatay C. Effects of the educational use of music on 3- to 12-year-old children's emotional development: a systematic review. *Int J Environ Res Public Health*. 2021;18(7):3668 PMID: 33915896 doi: 10.3390/ijerph18073668

27. Küçük Alemdar D, Yaman Aktaş Y. The use of the Buzzy, Jet lidokaine, bubble-blowing and aromatherapy for reducing pediatric pain, stress and fear associated with phlebotomy. *J Pediatr Nurs*. 2019;45:e64–e72 PMID: 30711327 doi: 10.1016/j.pedn.2019.01.010

28. Lavin A. Blowing bubbles, calming patients. *Pediatrics*. 1998;102(3):661 PMID: 9738197 doi: 10.1542/peds.102.3.661b

29. Bahrololoomi Z, Sadeghiyeh T, Rezaei M, Maghsoudi N. The effect of breathing exercise using bubble blower on anxiety and pain during inferior alveolar nerve block in children aged 7 to 10 years: a crossover randomized clinical trial. *Pain Res Manag*. 2022;2022:7817267 PMID: 35082960 doi: 10.1155/2022/7817267

30. Ma X, Yue ZQ, Gong ZQ, et al. The effect of diaphragmatic breathing on attention, negative affect and stress in healthy adults. *Front Psychol*. 2017;8:874 PMID: 28626434 doi: 10.3389/fpsyg.2017.00874

31. Zachary A. OT Corner: why bubbles are a wonderful therapy tool! *PediaStaff* blog. April 29, 2014. Accessed November 11, 2024. https://www.pediastaff.com/blog/slp/ot-corner-why-bubbles-are-a-wonderful-therapy-tool-20860

32. American Psychological Association. Mindfulness meditation. Updated November 15, 2023. Accessed November 11, 2024. https://dictionary.apa.org/mindfulness-meditation

33. Gregoski MJ, Barnes VA, Tingen MS, Harshfield GA, Treiber FA. Breathing awareness meditation and LifeSkills Training programs influence upon ambulatory blood pressure and sodium excretion among African American adolescents. *J Adolesc Health*. 2011;48(1):59–64 PMID: 21185525 doi: 10.1016/j.jadohealth.2010.05.019

34. Barnes VA, Pendergrast RA, Harshfield GA, Treiber FA. Impact of breathing awareness meditation on ambulatory blood pressure and sodium handling in prehypertensive African American adolescents. *Ethn Dis*. 2008;18(1):1–5 PMID: 18447091

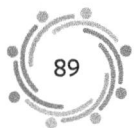
35. Aftanas L, Golosheykin S. Impact of regular meditation practice on EEG activity at rest and during evoked negative emotions. *Int J Neurosci.* 2005;115(6):893–909 PMID: 16019582 doi: 10.1080/00207450590897969

36. Simkin DR, Black NB. Meditation and mindfulness in clinical practice. *Child Adolesc Psychiatr Clin N Am.* 2014;23(3):487–534 PMID: 24975623 doi: 10.1016/j.chc.2014.03.002

37. Lee MY, Eads R, Hoffman J. "I felt it and I let it go": perspectives on meditation and emotional regulation among female survivors of interpersonal trauma with co-occurring disorders. *J Fam Violence.* 2022;37(4):629–641 doi: 10.1007/s10896-021-00329-7

38. Hehr A, Iadipaolo AS, Morales A, et al. Meditation reduces brain activity in the default mode network in children with active cancer and survivors. *Pediatr Blood Cancer.* 2022;69(10):e29917 PMID: 35927934 doi: 10.1002/pbc.29917

39. National Cancer Institute. Meditation. NCI Dictionary of Cancer Terms. Accessed November 11, 2024. https://www.cancer.gov/publications/dictionaries/cancer-terms/def/meditation

40. Bucci M, Marques SS, Oh D, Harris NB. Toxic stress in children and adolescents. *Adv Pediatr.* 2016;63(1):403–428 PMID: 27426909 doi: 10.1016/j.yapd.2016.04.002

41. Davis EL, Levine LJ, Lench HC, Quas JA. Metacognitive emotion regulation: children's awareness that changing thoughts and goals can alleviate negative emotions. *Emotion.* 2010;10(4):498–510 PMID: 20677867 doi: 10.1037/a0018428

42. Dennis TA, Buss KA, Hastings PD, et al. Physiological measures of emotion from a developmental perspective: state of the science. *Monogr Soc Res Child Dev.* 2012;77(2):i–204. Accessed November 11, 2024. https://www.jstor.org/stable/23256638

43. Taylor JB. *My Stroke of Insight: A Brain Scientist's Personal Journey.* New American Library; 2009

44. Robinson BE. The 90-second rule that builds self-control: the key to greater happiness and peace of mind. Psychology Today. April 26, 2020. Accessed November 11, 2024. https://www.psychologytoday.com/ca/blog/the-right-mindset/202004/the-90-second-rule-builds-self-control

45. Housman DK. The importance of emotional competence and self-regulation from birth: a case for the evidence-based emotional cognitive social early learning approach. *Int J Child Care Educ Policy.* 2017;11(1):13 doi: 10.1186/s40723-017-0038-6

46. American Psychological Association. Mindfulness. Accessed November 11, 2024. https://www.apa.org/topics/mindfulness

47. Filipe MG, Magalhães S, Veloso AS, et al. Exploring the effects of meditation techniques used by mindfulness-based programs on the cognitive, social-emotional, and academic skills of children: a systematic review. *Front Psychol.* 2021;12:660650 PMID: 34867573 doi: 10.3389/fpsyg.2021.660650

48. Sinha IP, Brown L, Fulton O, et al. Empowering children and young people who have asthma. *Arch Dis Child.* 2021;106(2):125–129 PMID: 32709687 doi: 10.1136/archdischild-2020-318788

49. Sharpe D, Rajabi M, Harden A, Moodambail AR, Hakeem V. Supporting disengaged children and young people living with diabetes to self-care: a qualitative study in a socially disadvantaged and ethnically diverse urban area. *BMJ Open.* 2021;11(10):e046989 PMID: 34645656 doi: 10.1136/bmjopen-2020-046989

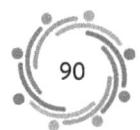
50. Wallwork SB, Noel M, Moseley GL. Communicating with children about "everyday" pain and injury: a Delphi study. *Eur J Pain*. 2022;26(9):1863–1872 PMID: 35829711 doi: 10.1002/ejp.2008

51. *The Three Rs: Ways to Support Your Child's Resilience*. Parent handout. American Academy of Pediatrics. Accessed November 11, 2024. https://www.aap.org/en/patient-care/trauma-informed-care/resources-for-families

52. Kabat-Zinn J. Mindfulness-based stress reduction (MBSR). *Constructiv Hum Sci*. 2003;8(2):73–83

53. Siegel DJ. *Mindsight: The New Science of Personal Transformation*. Bantam; 2010

54. Burstein D, Yang C, Johnson K, Linkenbach J, Sege R. Transforming practice with HOPE (Healthy Outcomes from Positive Experiences). *Matern Child Health J*. 2021;25(7):1019–1024 PMID: 33954880 doi: 10.1007/s10995-021-03173-9

55. Bhushan D, Burke Harris N, Bethell C, et al. *Roadmap for Resilience: The California Surgeon General's Report of Adverse Childhood Experiences, Toxic Stress, and Health*. Office of the Surgeon General, State of California; 2020. Accessed November 11, 2024. https://www.acesaware.org/wp-content/uploads/2020/12/SG-Report_Draft-Preso_v8_Public_ACEs-Aware_a11y.pdf

56. Rogers VW, Hart PH, Motyka E, Rines EN, Vine J, Deatrick DA. Impact of Let's Go! 5-2-1-0: a community-based, multisetting childhood obesity prevention program. *J Pediatr Psychol*. 2013;38(9):1010–1020 PMID: 23933841 doi: 10.1093/jpepsy/jst057

57. Paruthi S, Brooks LJ, D'Ambrosio C, et al. Consensus statement of the American Academy of Sleep Medicine on the recommended amount of sleep for healthy children: methodology and discussion. *J Clin Sleep Med*. 2016;12(11):1549–1561 PMID: 27707447 doi: 10.5664/jcsm.6288

58. Mahabee-Gittens EM, Ding L, Merianos AL, Khoury JC, Gordon JS. Examination of the "5-2-1-0" recommendations in racially diverse young children exposed to tobacco smoke. *Am J Health Promot*. 2021;35(7):966–972 PMID: 33641482 doi: 10.1177/0890117121995772

Chapter 4

Process for Stepwise Change

When families are experiencing toxic or intolerable levels of stress, the idea of doing anything differently may seem even more overwhelming than usual. Leaders often play a role in successful change, and having simple acronyms can help everyone remember what to do next under stressful circumstances.[1] As physicians, we are leaders and can support the children and families we care for in cocreating realistic, family-centered paths to reach their goals and implement changes they may not feel confident doing on their own, especially when they're experiencing stress. Living in poverty has been correlated with feeling overwhelmed by current stressors, being less able to focus on future goals, experiencing difficulty advocating for a child's educational needs, feeling decreased confidence in learning new skills and succeeding, struggling with a lower sense of agency to alter how one's life turns out, being less likely to take risks or try something new, and internalizing a sense of exclusion from society.[2] When we support families with a systematic approach to change, we can partner in addressing some of the barriers preventing them from shifting potentially toxic stress to tolerable.

Humans make changes in small, manageable, bite-size steps. By identifying what the family members want to change and then framing their goals with a stepwise process, we can address specific barriers to proven protective factors, foster resilience, and decrease the long-term mental health impact of the stress.

New Problem-Solving Skills

Plan-Do-Study-Act Cycles

Any meaningful change process starts with acceptance of the current moment. Just like any physical journey, if you don't know where you are, how can you know how to get where you want to go? Using the well-vetted change process of Plan-Do-Study-Act (PDSA) cycles, you can coach families to move toward new responses to any unpleasant experience or unwanted behaviors. These new responses facilitate connection and increase the child's ability to integrate

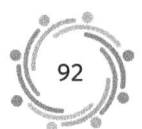

protective, positive childhood experiences (PCEs) and the parents' ability to put the affiliate response to use, even under high levels of stress.

Over time, my experience has been that as families internalize this process, they need less coaching and often initiate and implement cycles on their own. Yet in pediatricians' longitudinal relationship with children, we are readily available with support and ideas when new stress or trauma-related problems arise. Families can call on us to support them in addressing barriers to PCEs just like they can call on us for ideas about managing a persistent diaper rash.

Plan-Do-Study-Act cycles (**Figure 4–1**) are an ancient problem-solving strategy that helps operationalize intentional change. The approach for a PDSA cycle is the same whether you are trying to get your spouse to put their socks into the dirty clothes hamper or trying to make an automobile production line more efficient. The wonderful thing about teaching families this quality improvement strategy is they can apply it in any situation they find problematic and use the skills far beyond where you start with them.

There are 4 steps to a PDSA cycle:

1. **Plan:** Plan a change or test focused on improvement (eg, move the dirty clothes hamper).
2. **Do:** Carry out the change or test (preferably on a small scale, such as for 3 days).
3. **Study:** Study the results: What did we learn and what went wrong? (For example, did my spouse get their socks into the hamper more often?)
4. **Act:** Adopt the change, abandon it, or run through the cycle again (eg, things got worse, now their clothes and socks are on the floor so we will abandon this change and try something else).

Once you get the hang of using these steps in the clinical setting, it becomes a mix of continual quality improvement, active listening, and motivational interviewing (MI). The MI component is exploring with the family to identify one small, easily achievable change they could make to inch them in the direction of resilience. We do this by actively listening so we can coach families around barriers in the 4 building blocks of HOPE (Healthy Outcomes from Positive Experiences; as discussed in Chapter 3, Essential Toolkit) to promote safe, stable, nurturing connections and relational health.

For example, suppose the parents in a family coming to see you are having a hard time getting their child out of the house and into the car in the mornings when it is time to go to child care. They report they have tried everything, and it always ends in a meltdown. You highlight the strength of accessing care and reflect back what you hear. Next, you ask if they want to try something new. They say yes, and you inquire if they have tried singing with their child, which uses the vagus nerve to mitigate the stress response, to help their child transition into the car. The parents have not tried this and are grateful for a new technique. I like to use a validation sandwich—or the VIVA (Validate, Inform, Validate, Ask) approach (**Figure 4-2**)—with caregivers, which for these parents would sound like this: *It's totally normal to feel frustrated in this situation and as though you have tried everything already.* (Validate) *We know that singing with your child helps mitigate the stress response for both you and him.* (Inform) *Those meltdowns sound like they really derail the day and end up making you late for work, and that's not sustainable.* (Validate) *Do you want to try singing the ABCs with him as you head out the door, making the transition fun and seeing if he can be in his seat by the time you get to "Z"?* (Ask/offer to problem-solve). If the parents want to try it, you follow up with a plan to check in about how it went, either in person or by phone after the agreed-on amount of time, and support them with adopting this change or cocreating a new plan.

By way of this simple exchange, you have used a concise form of MI (see the Motivational Interviewing section in Chapter 3) to support a very basic, cocreated PDSA cycle. In this context, the 4 steps for the PDSA cycle reflect the resilience factors as follows (also illustrated in Appendix Q):

1. **Plan:** Identify which building block is involved, clarify what the family's goals are, honor strengths, and cocreate a plan to remove barriers or respond to an emotion/need.
2. **Do:** The family leaves your office to try a set of tools and strategies for a defined amount of time.
3. **Study:** Schedule a follow-up (in person or by phone) to check in and see how things are going: Could they integrate the coping skills and connect to the resources? If not, what do they think was happening?
4. **Act:** Discuss with the family if this is helping or not; validate frustration; if not helping, start over and cocreate a new plan, where you act as an "emotion coach" for the family, embracing family-directed goals with you supporting their next plan for change in small, manageable bites.

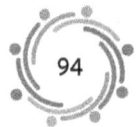
Figure 4-1.

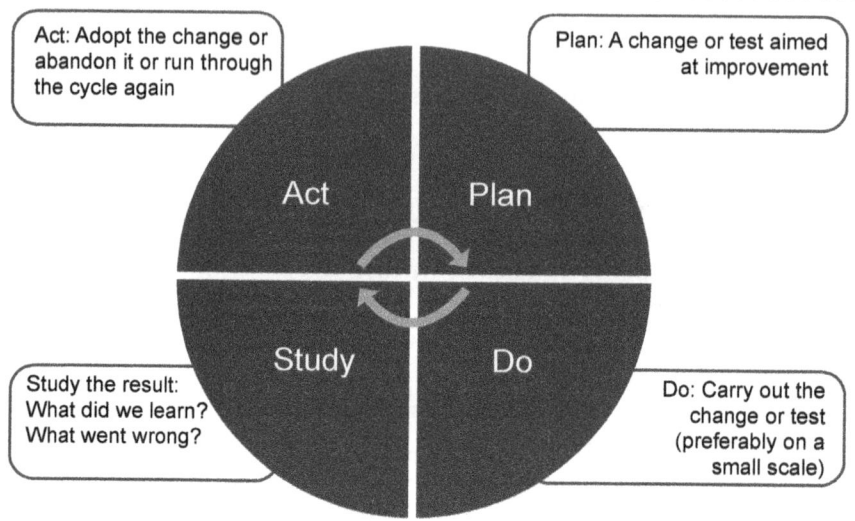

The Plan-Do-Study-Act cycle.

Figure 4-2.

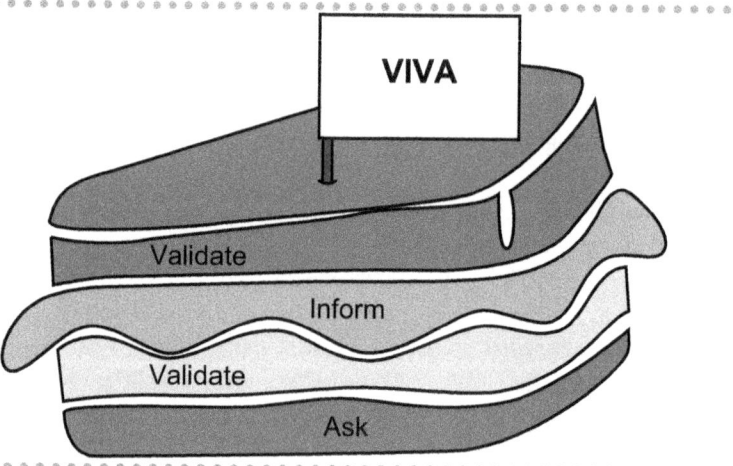

A validation sandwich, or the VIVA (Validate, Inform, Validate, Ask) approach, supports parental regulation and ability to foster trust.

Defining Success

"Success" can be an elusive goal when you are working with families, especially when everyone is under stress. As with anything else in medicine, my experience has been that families will sometimes come back and express that whatever you

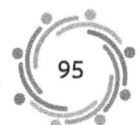

recommended from the last visit isn't working. When we see these experiences not as a failure of our recommendations but rather as a part of the change process, it helps us stay open and unguarded as we cocreate a new path. What has often happened is that the approach *did* work but only on the original issue, and now the parents have shifted their focus to another problem. It's easy for all of us to forget where we started. Parenting is a long-distance event, and when parents are still having struggles, it can feel like whatever they tried last must not have worked. Honoring success stories with families while holding space for the newer concerns is an important part of these Resilience University (RU) PDSA cycles. I find it is often helpful to write down what the parents are saying is happening, in their own words, in your note so you can reflect it back to them later.

Another possibility is that families may experience initially invisible barriers to implementing the change or recommendation after they leave our office. Parents and children may have varying levels of awareness about what these barriers are and how they can be addressed. Chapter 6, Using Relationship-Based and Trauma-Informed Anticipatory Guidance, is devoted to how this variability applies to our standard anticipatory guidance. To sustainably integrate a recommendation made in the office, families may need a bridge strategy if experiencing social drivers of health or other barriers.

Historically, resources for parents and caregivers to support resilience factors for children require that the adult be regulated and able to stay somewhat calm and connected. Sometimes, however, in families experiencing toxic stress, we have "perfect storm" moments where both adults and children are in fight, flight, or freeze mode. This multigenerational neurohormonal stress response may appear as mutual dysregulation and yelling (fight), disengagement of a parent and/or child (freeze), or poor follow-up or participation (flight). Some of these families may need specialized parenting instruction or Department of Health and Human Services (DHHS) interventions, while other families may respond well to a brief stress-mitigating strategy in the primary care setting. The key here is to identify who can participate and learn in the encounter: Parent? Child? Or both? Chances are, this will vary from one encounter to the next. Remember, use these strategies not in place of a referral or intervention you would normally do but rather in parallel.

Case Example: When the Caregiver(s) Is Engaged

A 5-year-old foster child, Emily, was constantly having "fits." These disrupted the day, and at night she would throw a fit about bedtime. Her behaviors included hitting people and walls and throwing things. The foster mom brought Emily to my office because she was worried Emily might hurt her 3-year-old little brother, Joey, who was also in this foster mom's care. The DHHS workers had witnessed these fits and told the foster mom she needed to be stricter and put Emily in

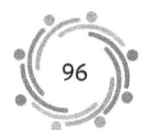

time-out every time they happened. The foster mom reported that when she put Emily in time-out, Emily's emotions escalated even more, and Emily had hurt herself hitting things. Emily didn't seem to be able to calm down in the time-out space. The foster mom had tried time-ins, but Emily just hit her instead. This foster mom was looking for help and an alternative strategy to respond to these fits.

We talked about how with Emily's trauma history, it's likely that the separation created by the time-out intensified her stress response and worsened her behaviors. The foster mom was experiencing lots of anxiety about whether she was doing the time-ins correctly. We reviewed how she was doing it and decided this wasn't an option because Emily's emotions were still escalating to violence. I taught the foster mom to use SUNBEAM for her own feelings and shared the NICER parenting strategy for the children (we'll talk about both these strategies in detail later in this chapter, in the Trauma-Informed Positive Parenting and Trauma-Informed Parenting Self-Care sections). We made a glitter jar for each child in their favorite color and talked about the time-versus-emotion curve. I taught both Emily and Joey how to meditate with their glitter jars and how to do toes-to-nose at bedtime. At each subsequent session, the foster mom reported seeing progress in how Emily was able to choose a healthy coping skill, express how she was feeling, and/or ask for help. By the end of the 4 sessions, the foster mom said she had stopped seeing these fits, and she was excited to see Joey beginning to use the same strategies too.

Case Example: When the Caregiver(s) Is Temporarily Disengaged

A 9-year-old boy, Liam, was constantly getting into fights with his brother and sister. He had threatened to stab himself and had an attention-deficit/hyperactivity disorder (ADHD) diagnosis but was not responding to medications. His mother had her own complex mental health history, and the family lived in an overcrowded apartment with no real room for Liam to take a break from his siblings when fights would start. When the family came to me, Mom had taken away everything, including Christmas, because the boy was acting up constantly. I started the visit with attempting to engage Mom but could not draw her attention away from her phone. So I talked with Liam directly about how his angry/frustrated/annoyed feelings started out. I asked if they started out small and then got bigger and bigger, before he hit his brother and got into trouble. He nodded, immediately relating to what I was talking about. We worked together to write a list of 10 things he could do when he felt "yucky" (see Appendix U), including meditating with a glitter jar, which I taught him during the session after Mom stepped out into the hall for a call. I gave Mom brief instructions on SUNBEAM and NICER parenting. She left the handouts on the chair when they left. I gave Liam his specific "homework": to try to notice that yucky feeling when it was still small and implement one of the ideas on the list of self-care strategies.

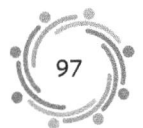

At the second session, I asked Mom how things were going with the fighting and aggression. She had moved on to another set of unwanted behaviors, but when I asked Liam how things were going, he proudly reported that he was noticing the annoyed feeling before it got too big and would hold his hands up in the air and do his breathing to keep from hitting his brother. Mom somewhat reluctantly agreed that Liam had actually stopped hitting his brother.

At the next session, I asked Liam if he was using his glitter jar. He shook his head and looked at his mom. She shook her head and said, *Why don't you tell her what happened?* Liam just looked down at his feet. Mom shrugged and said she had to take it away because of his bad behavior. I reinforced the importance of her modeling self-care and coaching him through his emotions but began to worry that in this situation, her stress level might make emotion coaching and coregulation impossible. Mom reiterated that her main goal was to see Liam behave differently, and she was not interested in coaching or modeling self-care at that point. I worked more with Liam on healthy coping skills and made sure Mom did not need any additional resources for herself. She declined referrals to community support resources, reiterating how she just needed me to make him stop misbehaving and she thought he needed medication.

At the last session, I asked Liam which strategies were helping when he had big unpleasant emotions. He told me everything had still been taken away. But his eyes lit up when he told me that now, when Mom was angry with him, he could do his deep breathing and then tell her how he was feeling instead of just yelling back. He said he knew his feelings were going to come and go and he was supposed to take care of himself while they were there. At his 10-year health supervision visit the following year, they shared with me that they had gotten their own house. Mom expressed how stressful that time had been and shared how she was not feeling as stressed now. She remembered some parenting handouts I had offered her before and that if I still had them, she wanted them now.

Timing Is Everything

As you can see from the second example, stress is just too overwhelming to take a whole-family approach all the time, yet we can still offer tools and strategies to mitigate the impact on the children. The right time to offer these varies from family to family and within families over time, so this process has to be fluid. Sometimes parents are stuck in old routines or habitual patterns and have not yet mastered the timing of using the tools and strategies, so they don't seem to be "working." Sharing the strategy of habit stacking, as defined in the Resilience University in Action section of Chapter 2, Overview of Resilience University, can help parents set themselves up for success when they want to make a change.

Many families I work with are aware of the importance of supporting the emotional development and regulation skills of their children. We can support parents

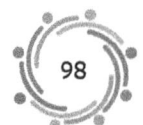
in how they operationalize this at home. For example, if a child is engaging in an unwanted behavior, caregivers may be very aware that identifying the emotion behind the behavior is important. But what often happens is that well-meaning adults approach a dysregulated child and ask them to use their words to explain what is going on so they can help. I explain it to families like this: *When a child is dysregulated, they can't use their words until their "fire-truck brain"* (see the Applied Mindfulness: Mitigating a Multigenerational Neurohormonal Stress Response section in Chapter 3) *is no longer in charge. So the first step is actually not using language but instead supporting the child in practicing some form of self-care to allow the prefrontal cortex to come back "online," and then the child will be able to better express what they are feeling. If we push children to use their words when they are unable to think clearly, we are poking the bear, so to speak, and that's likely to make things harder.* Depending on the age and developmental trajectory of the individual child, we can also ensure that we discuss with the caregivers what reasonable expectations are so they aren't expecting something the child is unable to do.

We can share a habit-stacking approach with parents to support them in modeling a moment of self-care, increasing the chance of coregulation. This can be very fluid since the parent just has to catch when they would normally ask their child to "use your words" and start with a moment of self-care. It sounds something like this when I am talking with families: *You already notice when he is having a meltdown, so when you notice that, model a form of self-care. If he starts getting upset because he can't do something, you respond with a big deep breath and a long exhalation as you validate his experience with your body language. The modeling may take a minute, but he is watching you and will likely imitate you while learning that this is a way to respond to that feeling.*

One common obstacle parents report is that their child is "refusing" to do whatever self-care strategy we were planning on for the PDSA cycle. The key part here is *refusing*. In this scenario, usually the parents are "strongly suggesting" (aka, "telling") their child to meditate or breathe, and to the child, it doesn't feel any different from when the parents were previously telling them to "stop it" or "calm down" or "use your words." When parents understand this difference, they can focus on staying regulated themselves instead of *making* their child do something. When parents can do this, it supports the ideal framework to mitigate the child's stress response. A dysregulated child can still put their mirror neurons and affiliate response to use, helping their nervous system respond to the parent's calm state through coregulation.[3]

Part of the PDSA cycle includes highlighting how and when defiance arises from a child's neurohormonal stress response. A parent who is stressed may jump to the conclusion that their child's defiance is willful and intentional. This situates child and parent as adversaries, and the parent may see their child as part of the danger,

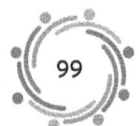

akin to the saber-toothed tiger. When parents view their child as the source of the danger, it inhibits their ability to put the affiliate response to use. We can help the parent reframe these moments, fostering an understanding that children want to feel better and are not intentionally setting out to ruin the day. Then parents are more able to see that they are in this difficult situation *with* their children and the focus can shift to how they will support each other through this difficult time.

Increased resilience arises when families can fluidly repair natural ruptures in their safe, stable, nurturing relationships. Shame can limit a parent's ability to change how they respond when ruptures happen. Parents often respond to relational health ruptures in a way similar to how their own parents reacted, or they may swing in the opposite direction to try to protect their children from their own childhood pain. All too often, these moments inadvertently lead to the perpetuation of intergenerational trauma and pain. To normalize these experiences, share with parents that "good enough" parenting is a constant dance of attuning and mis-attuning. Unless it's a true parenting emergency, cocreating a path where parents know they have permission to pause and take care of themselves so they can thoughtfully respond rather than instinctively react to their child's behaviors fosters a dynamic strength. This strength is at the core of the intergenerational resilience parents deeply want to pass on to their children.

If timing is important, so is tailoring specific coping skills to the situation at hand. Parents may need support classifying these as well as reminders that there are both high- and low-energy forms of self-care to soothe a frazzled nervous system. A 4-year-old with ADHD who never sits still may primarily rely on a fundamentally different set of self-care strategies than an 8-year-old who is studious, just because of their baseline level of energy. Similarly, for parents, one set of tools may work well when they are tired after a long day of work, while an entirely different set is needed when they are late and rushing out the door in the morning.

Resisting Rigidity

We can also normalize how it will not always be possible to use the same coping skill or stress-relieving strategy because of situational factors. Sometimes, only 1 or 2 strategies may be realistically accessible, and that may be enough to keep big emotions from derailing the day. I use Nadine Burke Harris' stress-buster wheel (**Figure 4-3**) to depict all the options, reminding families that not all of them will be on the table at any given moment.

If families are having a hard time identifying options for each of the stress-buster pie pieces, you can use ideas from **Figure 4-3** and **Box 4-1** to start a conversation with a family if they are not sure what might be accessible for self-care. I encourage them to have an initial go-to in each area as well as a second and third option just in case the preferred one is unavailable. I include what

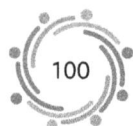

I consider "low-hanging fruit," or the things that are easier for the family to accomplish, even if this includes screen time or apps at first.

Figure 4-3.

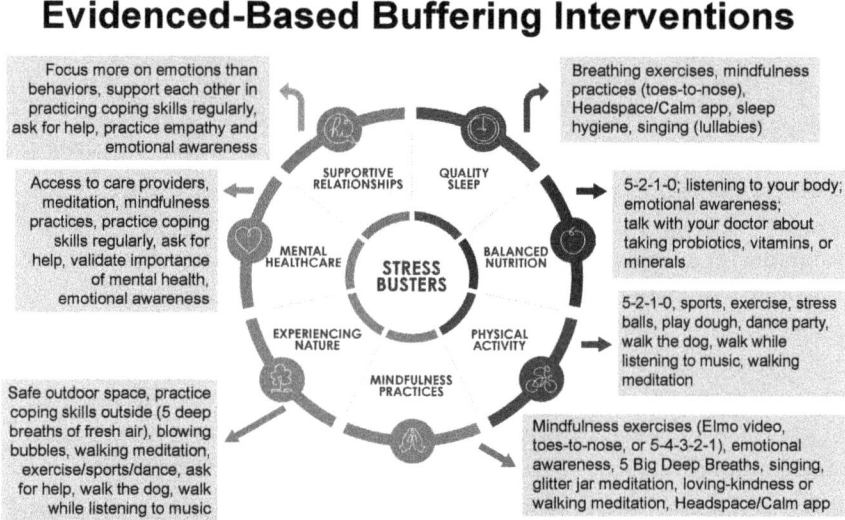

Combination of Nadine Burke Harris' stress-buster wheel with strategies from Resilience University.

Adapted from Office of the California Surgeon General. *The California Surgeon General's Playbook for Stress.* 2022. Accessed October 30, 2024. https://osg.ca.gov/wp-content/uploads/sites/266/2022/05/california-surgeon-general_stress-busting-playbook.pdf.

Box 4-1.

Stress-Buster Strategies

Mental Health Care
- Seek care from clinicians.
- Use meditation or mindfulness practices.
- Practice coping skills regularly.
- Ask for help.
- Validate the importance of mental health.
- Practice emotional awareness.

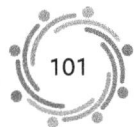

Box 4-1 (*continued*)

Supportive Relationships

- Focus more on emotions than behaviors.
- Support each other in practicing coping skills regularly.
- Ask for help.
- Practice empathy and emotional awareness.

Quality Sleep

- Do breathing exercises.
- Use mindfulness practices (eg, toes-to-nose).
- Use the Headspace/Calm app.
- Improve sleep hygiene.
- Sing (eg, lullabies).

Balanced Nutrition

- Listen to the body.
- Practice emotional awareness.
- Talk with your doctor about taking probiotics, vitamins, or minerals.
- Follow 5-2-1-0.[4]

Physical Activity

- Follow 5-2-1-0.
- Play sports, exercise, squeeze a stress ball or play dough, or have a dance party.
- Walk the dog, or walk while listening to music.
- Use walking meditation.

Mindfulness Practices

- Do mindfulness exercises (eg, Elmo video at https://youtu.be/yhRWpowOLyo, toes-to-nose, 5-4-3-2-1).
- Practice emotional awareness.
- Do 5 Big Deep Breaths, or sing.
- Use glitter jar meditation, loving-kindness meditation, or walking meditation.
- Use the Headspace/Calm app.

Access to Nature

- If feasible, enjoy a safe outdoor space.
- Take 5 deep breaths of fresh air.
- Practice coping skills outside (eg, walking meditation).
- Blow bubbles outside.
- Exercise, play sports, or dance outside.
- Walk the dog, or walk while listening to music.
- Ask for help.

Retrospectively Backing the Bus Up

One core problem-solving strategy I always offer is what I call "backing the bus up." Families living in poverty or under potentially toxic levels of stress may feel like they have little control or agency over how things turn out in their lives. When parents are trying to make a change and something goes wrong, it can feel demoralizing and as though nothing will ever change. For example, when we cocreate a PDSA cycle around self-care but in the moment, any healthy coping skills seem out of reach, I ask parents to metaphorically "back the bus up." I am amazed at how often parents will share that they actually knew this meltdown was coming; they just felt unable to change the course of the day. Often it is this dread combined with an inability to change what is coming next that heightens the parents' stress levels.

Encouraging the parents to look at the precursor, to be curious and investigate what might be contributing to this difficult moment, helps them stop recreating the same miserable-feeling parenting cycles over and over, day after day. This process is the same for parents and children.

I often use the handout shown in Appendix R, but you can also just draw a timeline on the exam table paper (**Figure 4-4**). With the parents and the child, identify the triggering moments that resulted in the subsequent disaster, going backward in time. What else was potentially going on? What other feeling(s) contributed to that moment of lower resilience? I like to use the child's language whenever I can, to help them feel heard. Using "hangry" as a descriptive example often engages the family in a relatable way as a universally accepted situation where big unpleasant feelings (hungry) result in big unwanted behaviors (displays of anger). Was the child hungry, tired, cold, hot, bored, frustrated...? Had they slept poorly, skipped a snack, just been told to relinquish a favorite toy or seat or coveted connection with a caregiver...?

Write these things down on a timeline, then try to identify if there were any precursor moments that were missed opportunities for self-care. Then remind parents that the ideal outcome here is to shift the locus of control and awareness inward, into the child, so that as they grow up, they understand how to work with all their different feelings. Emphasize how all these feelings are a completely normal part of being human; some are just more pleasant than others, and it is the unpleasant ones we are not prepared for that tend to derail our day.

Figure 4-4.

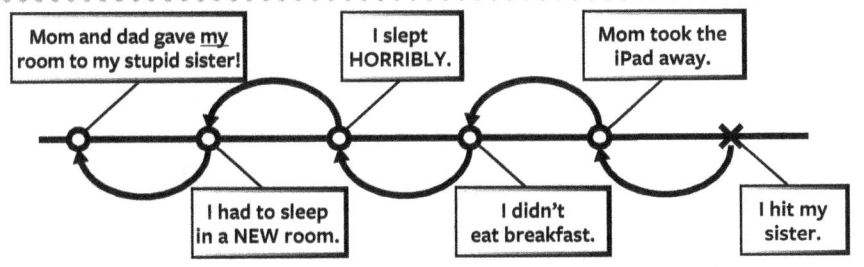

Sample "back the bus up" timeline; you can handwrite it on the exam table paper.

Proactively Integrating Healthy Coping Skills

When describing for caregivers why it is important to plan ahead and integrate healthy coping skills, access to resources, and self-care into the plan for the day, I begin with an analogy like this: *If you were going to drive your kids from Maine to Montana, you would never leave the house without a plan for sleeping, eating, bathroom breaks, entertainment, and other important activities. So why is it that we load the kids up in the car and head to the store, somehow expecting things to not fall apart the way they always do?* When parents can plan ahead recognizing that the family might all need stress-mitigating strategies throughout the most mundane of days, they can be primed for self-care and decrease the likelihood that everyone will end up mutually dysregulated in the checkout line at the grocery store.

So many activities parents already do with their children have a polyvagal component that can help a child regulate big emotions. When parents harness this awareness, they can integrate taking a break to go outside, blow bubbles (big deep breaths and prolonged exhalations), or squeeze play dough[5] to intentionally lower stress. Celebrating a family-strengths approach to this means we ask them what they have already found that helps when people in the family are having big emotions. Perhaps the kids take a break and cuddle the family pet or go outside to run around with the dog. The soothing power of pets has been thought to be related to a release of oxytocin, although more recent studies question whether this is actually the primary mechanism.[6] Whatever the precise biochemical process ends up being, families commonly identify spending time with family pets as soothing to a frazzled nervous system.

Singing involves deep breaths and prolonged exhalation, which, as noted in the Other Ways to Use the Breath section of Chapter 3, has been repeatedly proven to lower stress and promote calm. New caregivers often sing to their babies. Early childhood educators harness the calming powers of singing all the time. And you don't have to be singing to reap nervous system benefits from music. Listening to music as well as singing along has actual health benefits, such as lowering one's heart rate and cortisol levels, releasing endorphins, and reducing stress-related symptoms.[7]

Fostering Change

An important part of any new endeavor is celebrating when we can apply the new skill or tools. Families experiencing potentially toxic levels of stress can feel so overwhelmed by their current stressors that making changes to increase access to PCEs may feel out of reach. Traditional sticker charts to reward a child for behaving in a way that the parent commands (eg, obeying instructions) have fallen out of favor. Families are familiar with this idea of a sticker chart, so we can repurpose it as a celebration chart (**Figure 4-5**; also reproduced in Appendix S), since the technique of using stickers and a chart to celebrate change can be helpful in the setting of navigating family dynamics and integrating healthy coping skills. These sticker charts can help families start conversations about how they feel and how they can support each other through hard times. These charts can be as narrow or broad as you need them to be and are easy to tailor to the family's individual goals and needs.

Figure 4-5.

When I feel bored, I can... 😊	I did it!	RESILIENCE
Draw or write in my journal		
Use 5-4-3-2-1		
Listen to music		
Go for a walk or play with the dog		

Feelings sticker chart to encourage emotional awareness and celebrate self-care.

The core purpose of the sticker charts is to encourage everyone in the household to identify, normalize, and talk about feelings as a way to address barriers to this specific PCE. Start by having them put a family feelings chart (**Figure 4-6**; also reproduced in Appendix T) on the refrigerator or in a location where all family members will see it as a visual reminder for families that are not used to talking

about feelings, so they can practice. Add a few feelings to the list that are what I call "low-hanging fruit," such as *hungry*, *tired*, or *cold*. These are the feelings that families are often used to communicating and that we develop the ability to care for implicitly as we grow up. Caregivers don't think, *Hmmm, how do I teach my child how to take care of themselves when they are cold?* They just get them a jacket or a blanket, and the child learns to do so themselves through repetition and with their mirror neurons. I also add some feelings that may be more "taboo," that may not be talked about or cared for openly, such as *sad*, *bored*, *angry*, *lonely*, *left out*, or *overwhelmed*.

Figure 4-6.

Family Feelings Chart		Add a sticker, a check mark, or a comment when you notice you are feeling a certain way. Have each person in the family use a different sticker or color. See if you can start talking with each other about your feelings.
Angry Mad Frustrated Annoyed Irritated		
Sad Lonely Left out		
Hungry Famished Starving		
Confused Worried Scared Overwhelmed		
Cold Freezing		
Tired Sleepy Exhausted		
Happy Joyful Loved		
Overwhelmed Stressed Freaking out		

Family feelings chart to normalize talking about feelings.

Once families are talking about feelings and practicing healthy coping skills, they begin to normalize asking for help and identifying any obstacles to meeting unmet needs. A stepwise approach to start this process, one that parents can coach their child through, sounds something like this:

- *What feeling is it that I am experiencing?*
- *What does my body need me to do to take care of myself while this feeling is here?*

- *What is this feeling trying to tell me?*
- *Is this feeling connected to something important that I need or want to change in my life? Or is this just one of those feelings that comes and goes with its own rhythm, like an ocean wave, and my job is to take care of myself while it is here so it doesn't wash me out to sea?*

Parents often express concern that if they give their child attention around the emotion, then related behaviors will worsen. Illuminating the preexisting patterns for families can help alleviate this concern. For example, consider a child who isn't feeling good and is used to behaving in a certain way to get their caregiver's attention. A traditional behaviorist approach to this behavior would be to try to extinguish it by withholding the attention that the child is seeking. I explain to parents that this behaviorist approach predated the emerging literature on PCEs. We now understand that children who are supported in discerning what they are feeling and how they can respond to that feeling are more likely to grow up to be mentally healthy adults than children who are left alone to work out their unpleasant feelings. We can counsel families to be curious about the feelings behind the behaviors, and parents can feel prepared to offer helpful strategies.

As mentioned earlier in this chapter, the concise MI technique I use to help parents see why a change meant to promote health might be worth trying is offering a validation sandwich. When parents bring a behavioral or emotional concern to me, I respond with the mnemonic VIVA: Validate, Inform, Validate, Ask. This approach relies on you having already engaged the family and created the nonjudgmental space for their concern and allows you to focus on what is important, validating what you are hearing, evoking why change might be important for health, and summarizing the plan. We can validate the experience of the patient and/or parent both before and after we leverage our expertise as their pediatrician to provide information and guidance. Ending with asking for the patient and parent's input promotes family-centered care. For example, a parent says their child is misbehaving whenever the family has company over so they can "get all the attention" and "ruin the gathering." Parents are often stuck on a specific interpretation of their child's motivation for certain behaviors and can feel despondent, as if "nothing will work" or "we've already tried everything."

The VIVA response helps them get out of this stuck spot and could sound something like this: *That sounds frustrating. I totally get how it feels like he is trying to ruin your evening.* (Validate) AND *We know that when kids are acting out, often it is a bid for connection and they may be feeling left out.* (Inform) *I get how you would worry that giving him your attention might actually make things worse!* (Validate) *How about we go through some possible scenarios for balancing his need for attention with your concerns?* (Ask/offer to problem-solve). And the problem-solving segues into the first cocreated PDSA cycle.

When parents themselves have rarely had anyone respond in a helpful manner to their own emotions, they tend to respond to their kids with what they have heard from their own parents or others: "There's nothing to be sad about," or "Stop being angry," or "Don't be such a scaredy-cat," or "Stop crying or I'll give you something to cry about." These reflexive responses generally arise from the parent's frustration and can be shifted with tools and strategies. Preparing parents with curious, constructive language and a set of helpful, easily accessible tools allows them to effectively respond when their children are struggling. For example, they can help the child identify a troubling feeling or, if that seems out of reach, just start with the fact that what the child is currently feeling feels "difficult" or "yucky." I always point out to parents that at times, they will need to hold space for their child's big unpleasant feeling and take care of themselves with breathing or meditation/mindfulness strategies to hold that space of coregulation until their child comes out the other side. Ideally, if the big feeling is identified early enough, the parents will be able to offer connection and care that may shift the yucky feeling to something that feels more manageable or less overwhelming. For example, a child may be used to having meltdowns when they can't do something. As they begin to feel frustrated, they learn how it is important to ask for help early, and the caregiver has learned the importance of responding with something like a comforting and reassuring hug—promoting the affiliate response, mitigating the child's stress, and averting a meltdown.

Validating the feelings does not mean that the parents give up on boundaries or abandon the idea of consequences. It simply means that instead of focusing on punishing unwanted behaviors, parents are given permission and tools to focus on practicing self-care for big emotions. Parents can still allow for natural consequences to arise in response to a child's big behaviors. For example, *When you were feeling frustrated, you threw your favorite toy and it broke. Now you can't play with it anymore.* Parents can maintain the guardrails for their children to illustrate what is safe and unsafe behavior without unnecessarily punishing them.

A helpful strategy is another visual reminder: to make an actual list of 10 specific things they can do to take care of themselves (see Appendix U) when these yucky feelings happen and put it on the fridge or on the wall in the child's room. I use a chalkboard wall in my exam room with a sample list to get the conversation moving during my visits.

New Parenting Skills

Validate, Validate, Validate

Promoting resilience requires a multigenerational approach,[8] and we may refer families for therapies with this model, including Parent-Child Interaction Therapy and family-focused therapy. But in many areas, the resources to actually

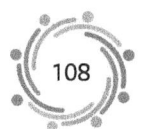

offer these services to families do not meet the need. As pediatric clinicians, we are already used to this framework, and when we add a few core trauma-informed parenting tools, we can serve as a bridge.

For parents, validating is a simple, easy-to-learn response they can work toward using, in any stressful moment, without having to harness too much prefrontal cortex input in the moment. Parents also need easily accessible language they can use, even when they are feeling stressed themselves, to shift their responses from invalidating or disapproving to validating and nurturing. Regulation of emotional states is key with people who have borderline personality disorder, so when we are looking for strategies to help a family begin to develop validation skills, I've borrowed a few fundamental techniques from dialectical behavioral therapy (DBT). The simple tool of validation, in the context of DBT, has been shown to increase positive affect states and decrease negative affect states in patients with borderline personality disorder.[9] **Box 4-2** models a concise way to explain the tool of validation to parents and caregivers; the accompanying handout is in Appendix V.

Box 4-2.

Validate, Validate, Validate: An Easy-to-Learn Tool for Caregivers

One of the most powerful tools we have as parents is to validate our child's emotions. You don't have to agree with your child to validate what they are feeling. Even if what they are saying or how they are behaving is not what you would like to hear or see, remember: validate first. Once they have returned to a calm baseline, you can problem-solve.

The following 3-sentence framework can help your child feel heard, understood, and as though you care about their feelings; remember to use this language:

- "I get..."
- "I totally understand..."
- "Anyone would feel..."

Example: Johnny comes home from school and throws his backpack onto the floor. You ask how his day was. He yells that he hates you and hates the school and hates his teachers and he never wants to go to school again! Then he stomps up to his room.

You can validate the feeling (even though you are not agreeing with everything he just said or giving him a free pass for his behavior) by saying

- "I get that you are angry."
- "I totally understand being frustrated with your teachers and the school."
- "Anyone who had a frustrating day like that would feel like they don't want to go back to school."

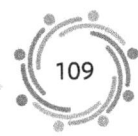

Box 4-2 (*continued*)

and

- "When you say you hate me, I feel sad and I'm wondering how you are feeling. Is now a good time to talk about how you feel, or do you need some time to take care of yourself first?"

Then, pivot back to the list of "10 Things I Can Do When I Feel Yucky." Once the big feeling has come and gone, you can start problem-solving about what happened to make Johnny feel that way.

Trauma-Informed Positive Parenting: NICER Parenting

Research indicates that certain parenting styles are more likely to result in children who have a healthy response to unpleasant emotions as they enter school.[10] Positive parenting (warm, supportive, and responsive) has been promoted as a healthier response to unwanted behaviors than other, more negative parenting styles (harsh discipline, inconsistent availability, and dismissive behavior and attitude). Most parents know that spanking is frowned on and in some states is illegal. Without other tools at their disposal, however, parents often resort to yelling and sometimes even shaming or insulting their children in a desperate attempt to get them to behave. An alternative, NICER parenting, involves a set of self-care strategies that work for both parents and children, coupled with a method for responding (instead of reacting) to children when they are behaving in an unwanted way. **Box 4-3** provides a real-life example of this approach in action.

Box 4-3.

Composite Example of Parenting Skills Shifting Problematic Behaviors

A mom called to make an appointment because her 8-year-old son had started being aggressive with his 4-year-old sister. Aggression had been an issue for him for years. He had a diagnosis of attention-deficit/hyperactivity disorder, but Mom didn't want to put him on medication. During the COVID-19 pandemic, his "bubble" included the kids next door. He would routinely go over there to play but then get into physical fights and be sent back home. Mom was watching this behavior, but what worried her even more was the boy's aggression toward his sister. Mom was putting him in time-out and taking away his games and privileges. His dad even tried spanking him. Nothing was helping, and they were at their wits' end.

I began working with the family on Resilience University sessions. I taught the boy to notice when he was feeling "yucky" and, instead of taking it out on his sister or his friends, to try taking a break and taking care of himself with breathing exercises or the glitter jar meditation. I coached Mom in not waiting until things got

Box 4-3 (continued)

so bad that he was in trouble but rather trying to help him notice when these yucky feelings were small, so he could work through them. The boy "graduated," and I saw him a few months later for his health supervision visit. He proudly told me that now, when he got frustrated at the neighbors, he would take a break, come back home to do his breathing, and then go back to play when he felt better. He had also stopped hurting his sister. A year later, he was still using his breathing, and Mom referred to the work we had done as "transformational."

Parenting is exhausting, and without a simplified approach, it can feel completely overwhelming to integrate any new strategies into one's approach. Positive parenting sounds good in theory, but often when parents try to shift what they are doing and how they respond, negative behaviors increase in the short term because the children are not used to that response. When parents feel frustrated, they often give up and resort to their original tactics. NICER parenting (handout in Appendix W) is the acronym I developed to help parents remember the plot when things get hairy so they can work through the process of change and actually integrate healthy strategies to improve family health.

Notice: Notice that your child is having a big feeling, emotion, or unmet need. They are not just behaving poorly.

Identify: Try to identify what that feeling, emotion, or unmet need might be. Are they hungry? Tired? Hot? Bored? Sad? Angry? Frustrated? Or perhaps that is too complicated in the moment; if it is, you can just go with yucky.

Connect/coregulate: Connect with your child around one strategy that might help. If you are at a loss, use empathy. Think of yourself feeling the way they do: What might help you? What would definitely not help you? It would generally not help to be told to "stop it" or "get over it." Would a hug feel helpful? A break? A walk? A few big deep breaths? Model the response for them if you need to. Once they get used to having a different response to big feelings, they will do this automatically. Hold on to the idea that no one intends to become dysregulated. Kids need guidance from adults to learn how to respond to their own emotions. And a dysregulated adult cannot help a child regulate.

After this step, wait until the big emotion has come and gone. Then, when both you and your child feel calm, proceed to the final 2 steps.

Explore: Sit down with your child and talk about what happened. For example, "Wow. When you were feeling angry, you threw your favorite toy at your sister. That could have really hurt her." Problem-solve for the next time that big feeling arises: "What could we do differently to try to help you sooner?"

"What options for self-care can you identify for that feeling so you don't end up throwing the toy?" "What makes it hard to use those self-care strategies?"

Review/repair: Did anyone or anything get hurt? Do you need to help your child with a relational health rupture? This is where natural consequences can be discussed, such as "Now that favorite toy doesn't work anymore. Do you feel sad? I feel sad."

Trauma-Informed Parenting Self-Care: SUNBEAM

Parenting is a long-distance sport. We often start out with so much energy when we're new parents and we want to do everything just right. But inevitably, we get tired and develop decision fatigue. We stop feeling as though we have got this and we are knocking it out of the park. Maybe we just feel like we don't care as much anymore, or perhaps we even start to feel like we're the worst parents ever. As a family's pediatrician, you can normalize these feelings and encourage parents to shift their lens from perfection to self-care and radical acceptance. And you can be poised to offer new skills to meet this moment, just like you do when the child refuses to eat their vegetables or use the potty.

Parental stress, defined as an aversive psychological reaction resulting from a mismatch between perceived parenting demands and available parenting resources,[11] affects child development and wellness.[12] High levels of parental stress have been correlated with more externalizing behaviors beginning in young children[13] and continuing on into adolescence.[14] Helping parents notice when they are feeling stress and then sharing realistic strategies to help decrease the impact of this stress on their child's behaviors enables them to problem-solve and change course to reduce the negative impact.

SUNBEAM is a mnemonic to help parents remember that taking care of themselves first is essential. Without this step, they will likely continue to repeat the very moments from their own childhood they wished they would never create for their own children. This very simple and powerful tool simply reminds parents that they have to put on their own proverbial oxygen mask first. When they care for their own neurohormonal stress response, they can better put the affiliate response to use and increase the chance of having a nurturing response to their child in that moment.

The best part about SUNBEAM is it reminds parents to use the exact same set of tools we are teaching the children. There's not one set of rules for parents and a different one for the kids. We're not saying that there is some imaginary moment when suddenly being a human becomes easier—not when we turn 21 and definitely not when we become parents ourselves. Normalizing this struggle and validating the parents' wish to not re-create their least favorite moments from their own childhood is a powerful stress-mitigating, preventive health care intervention.

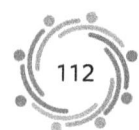

Offering SUNBEAM to parents follows 3 steps (see Appendix X for a handout):

1. **See:** See that you are having your own big emotion in response to your child's behaviors.
2. **Unhook:** You've been here before. This is nothing new, and you've probably ended up sounding like your own parents. Unhook from your traditional response, whatever it is. Don't do it. Don't take the bait!
3. **Nurture:** Instead, pause to nurture yourself. Remember, there are very few true parenting emergencies. Unless a child is running into traffic or wielding a weapon, you have the luxury of pausing to take care of yourself with one of the same nurturing strategies we are teaching the kids, as follows:
   - **Breathe:** Use a technique like 5 Big Deep Breaths, relaxation breathing, "box" or "square" breathing, singing, or blowing bubbles.
   - Be **Emotionally Aware:** Know that this feeling will come and go. It will not last forever. Your job is to take care of yourself while it is here so it doesn't wash you out to sea.
   - Be **Mindful:** Take a moment to do a body scan: check in from your toes to your nose. Use your senses to ground you in the moment (find the alphabet on the walls, 5 things that are blue, 3 things you can hear, etc).
   - Practice **Meditation:** Use your breath and your gaze to calm your stress response. Just a few moments of lightly placing your gaze onto the shadows of a tree or some other nearby object and breathing in and out 5 times can bring your stress level down a notch or two and allow you to practice NICER parenting.

I refer to SUNBEAM as the "antidote to meltdowns." If a parent doesn't have the antidote, both child and parent end up dysregulated. **Box 4-4** illustrates this antidote in action.

Box 4-4.

SUNBEAM: Stopping Mutual Dysregulation Before It Starts

A 5-year-old little sister with an older autistic brother was starting to have behavioral problems. Mom was worried because if the older brother didn't play with his sister exactly the way she wanted, she would become aggressive. The primary care physician who referred her to me thought she was imitating her brother. When I commented to Mom that her daughter's emotions might be driving this behavior and she wasn't trying to ruin the day, Mom replied, "Oh no. You don't know her. She actually is trying to ruin the day. Trust me."

Box 4-4 (*continued*)

After the next Resilience University session, Mom started to pause for her own moment of self-care when she noticed that her daughter was starting to get frustrated with her brother. This helped her see how her daughter might be feeling lonely, bored, or frustrated and that those feelings might require some self-care strategies. Mom then started suggesting singing a favorite song or taking a few deep breaths. When her daughter couldn't practice self-care, Mom modeled it by singing the ABCs, and her daughter would imitate her.

SUNBEAM:

- **See:** Mom could see that she was feeling angry when her daughter's behavior became aggressive.
- **Unhook:** Mom tried pausing instead of reflexively yelling.
- **Nurture (Breathe/Emotionally Aware/Mindful/Meditation):** Mom took a minute to breathe, aware this was her own feeling, and then she was able to recommend or model self-care for her daughter, realizing that singing worked well for both of them.

Emotion Coaching

Emotion coaching refers to how caregivers can see all emotions as an opportunity for teaching and connection, even when it is their own big unpleasant emotion. Emotion coaching is the opposite of dismissing emotions, part of what led to the complex scenario in the "When the Caregiver(s) Is Temporarily Disengaged" example earlier in this chapter. Routinely dismissing a child's unpleasant emotions correlates with poorer emotional regulation and more behavioral problems on the child's part.[15] Children whose parents use an "emotion coaching" approach experience lower rates of anxiety disorders in their teen years.[16] Emotion coaching also has been shown to buffer the internalizing symptoms of children (emotional reactivity, anxiety or depressive symptoms, somatization, and social withdrawal behaviors) from high levels of family stress and supports resilience.[17]

This well-respected approach arose from John Gottman's longitudinal research into factors that protected children from being negatively affected during their parents' divorces or marital discord. Gottman's seminal 1995 study[18] evaluated 56 children at age 5 years and again at age 8 years and compared parenting styles for responding to the children's emotions. Children of parents who used an emotion coaching style had greater math abilities, better health, and fewer behavioral problems at age 8 than children who had parents with non–emotion coaching styles. With this strategy, parents take on a proactive role in recognizing emotions and teaching their children how to manage them. Gottman outlines the other parenting responses to unpleasant emotions as

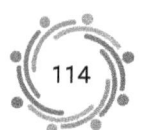

laissez-faire (allows/notices emotions but doesn't help the child work through them), disapproving (criticizes them for having emotions and portrays it is a sign of weakness), and dismissive (avoids emotions and tries to get over them quickly with distraction or immediate problem-solving).[19]

Emotion coaching is a fundamental component of RU. The way I explain it to parents sounds something like this: *If you wanted your child to become a soccer player, you wouldn't expect them to become Abby Wambach overnight. You would take them outside into the backyard and kick a soccer ball around, probably starting when they were too young to really understand what they were doing. If the ball accidentally ended up going through the neighbor's living room window, you would apologize and perhaps pivot to a new location or strategy, but you wouldn't give up entirely on soccer just because something didn't go as planned.*

Just as the parent can coach their child through the mistakes and pitfalls of soccer, they can apply the same problem-solving approach to helping the child understand their emotions. The basic concepts of emotion coaching are as follows (see Appendix Y for a handout):

- Kids need help and modeling to learn how to identify their emotions and take care of themselves when they feel unpleasant emotions.
- When parents lean in, listen, and validate their children's feelings, they help their children learn these important skills.
- There are no bad or trivial emotions. Children can learn not to ignore or dismiss the unpleasant ones. Parents can separate unwanted behaviors from preceding emotions and not punish their children for having emotions.
- Your patients' parents may not have gotten this help from their parents; and their parents may not have gotten it from their own parents and so on. This is where you help by coaching them so they can start now and change the family culture.
- Parents can help their children learn something new, even if no one in their family has learned it before, by taking an interest, learning about it, working on it with their children, and not giving up when something goes wrong.
- Just like when a soccer ball gets kicked through a neighbor's window, things may sometimes go sideways and parents may wish they'd done something differently. These are not times to give up! They are opportunities for do-overs: talk about what happened, pivot, and try again.

Parents want to raise children who are healthy emotionally and who can identify and respond to all their own feelings—not just the pleasant ones or the easy ones to "fix" but all the messiness of being a human. This is hard and requires practice. Normalizing how hard this is involves not trying to pretend it comes easily for them as parents. Parents may worry that their children will feel

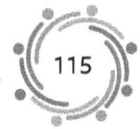

insecure if they don't think their parents are 100% capable at every moment and in any situation. But it is essential to model for children how to respond when they feel yucky rather than to keep that process hidden behind the proverbial curtain, so they have no idea how anyone else does it and just think it comes naturally once you become a grown-up.

We are the default emotion "coaches" for our patients' parents. We can support parents as they develop their own skills by temporarily coaching the family in addition to problem-solving barriers to other proven protective factors.

References

1. Walk M. Leaders as change executors: the impact of leader attitudes to change and change-specific support on followers. *Eur Manage J.* 2023;41(1):154–163 doi: 10.1016/j.emj.2022.01.002

2. Sheehy-Skeffington J, Rea J. *How Poverty Affects People's Decision-Making Processes.* Joseph Rowntree Foundation; 2017

3. Rosanbalm KD, Murray DW. *Co-Regulation From Birth Through Young Adulthood: A Practice Brief.* Office of Planning, Research, and Evaluation; Administration for Children & Families; US Dept of Health and Human Services; 2017. OPRE brief 2017-80

4. Rogers VW, Hart PH, Motyka E, Rines EN, Vine J, Deatrick DA. Impact of Let's Go! 5-2-1-0: a community-based, multisetting childhood obesity prevention program. *J Pediatr Psychol.* 2013;38(9):1010–1020 PMID: 23933841 doi: 10.1093/jpepsy/jst057

5. Uvnäs-Moberg K, Handlin L, Petersson M. Self-soothing behaviors with particular reference to oxytocin release induced by non-noxious sensory stimulation. *Front Psychol.* 2015;5:1529 PMID: 25628581 doi: 10.3389/fpsyg.2014.01529

6. Marshall-Pescini S, Schaebs FS, Gaugg A, Meinert A, Deschner T, Range F. The role of oxytocin in the dog-owner relationship. *Animals (Basel).* 2019;9(10):792 PMID: 31614747 doi: 10.3390/ani9100792

7. de Witte M, Pinho ADS, Stams GJ, Moonen X, Bos AER, van Hooren S. Music therapy for stress reduction: a systematic review and meta-analysis. *Health Psychol Rev.* 2022;16(1):134–159 PMID: 33176590 doi: 10.1080/17437199.2020.1846580

8. Howell KH, Miller-Graff LE, Martinez-Torteya C, Napier TR, Carney JR. Charting a course towards resilience following adverse childhood experiences: addressing intergenerational trauma via strengths-based intervention. *Children (Basel).* 2021;8(10):844 PMID: 34682109 doi: 10.3390/children8100844

9. Carson-Wong A, Hughes CD, Rizvi SL. The effect of therapist use of validation strategies on change in client emotion in individual DBT treatment sessions. *Pers Disord.* 2018;9(2):165–171 PMID: 27918168 doi: 10.1037/per0000229

10. Neppl TK, Jeon S, Diggs O, Donnellan MB. Positive parenting, effortful control, and developmental outcomes across early childhood. *Dev Psychol.* 2020;56(3):444–457 PMID: 32077716 doi: 10.1037/dev0000874

11. Deater-Deckard K. Parenting stress and child adjustment: some old hypotheses and new questions. *Clin Psychol Sci Pract.* 1998;5(3):314–332 doi: 10.1111/j.1468-2850.1998.tb00152.x

12. Păsărelu CR, Dobrean A, Florean IS, Predescu E. Parental stress and child mental health: a network analysis of Romanian parents. *Curr Psychol*. 2022;1–13 PMID: 35967498 doi: 10.1007/s12144-022-03520-1

13. Stone LL, Mares SH, Otten R, Engels RC, Janssens JM. The co-development of parenting stress and childhood internalizing and externalizing problems. *J Psychopathol Behav Assess*. 2016;38(1):76–86 PMID: 27069304 doi: 10.1007/s10862-015-9500-3

14. Kochanova K, Pittman LD, Pabis JM. Parenting stress, parenting, and adolescent externalizing problems. *J Child Fam Stud*. 2021;30(9):2141–2154 doi: 10.1007/s10826-021-01996-2

15. Lunkenheimer ES, Shields AM, Cortina KS. Parental emotion coaching and dismissing in family interaction. *Soc Dev*. 2007;16(2):232–248 doi: 10.1111/j.1467-9507.2007.00382.x

16. Hurrell KE, Houwing FL, Hudson JL. Parental meta-emotion philosophy and emotion coaching in families of children and adolescents with an anxiety disorder. *J Abnorm Child Psychol*. 2017;45(3):569–582 PMID: 27370681 doi: 10.1007/s10802-016-0180-6

17. Lobo FM, Lunkenheimer E, Lucas-Thompson RG, Seiter NS. Parental emotion coaching moderates the effects of family stress on internalizing symptoms in middle childhood and adolescence. *Soc Dev*. 2021;30(4):1023–1039 PMID: 36158116 doi: 10.1111/sode.12519

18. Hooven C, Gottman JM, Katz LF. Parental meta-emotion structure predicts family and child outcomes. *Cogn Emotion*. 1995;9(2–3):229–264 doi: 10.1080/02699939508409010

19. Gottman J, DeClaire J. *Raising an Emotionally Intelligent Child: The Heart of Parenting*. Simon & Schuster; 1998

Chapter 5

A Structured Approach to Resilience Coaching

This chapter will walk you through a stepwise approach to fluidly respond to any stressful situation your families ask for help with in a way that fosters resilience. This involves a deepening and broadening of the existing resilience parenting advice you are providing, as well as additional opportunities for touchpoints with families to serve as a bridge while they are awaiting other necessary services or supports or if the family declines referrals. Mitigating stress can reduce the impact of adversity while our families are awaiting additional interventions, evaluations, referrals, and community support.

After asking us for help with a stressful situation, a family may still have to wait for months until their child has a neuropsychological evaluation, gets in with a counselor, or sees a psychiatrist. During that waiting time, behavioral problems and relational health issues can worsen, becoming barriers to resilience. Additionally, harm can arise in the form of harsh discipline and unrepaired relational health ruptures. Without a bridge, families may arrive a year later for their next health supervision visit and we find out no one ever called them back about our referral(s), and the original problem has compounded over time. Arranging for a family to participate in a community program or a local initiative sometimes doesn't result in real help if the program runs out of funding or the family can't get there because of transportation issues. We can decrease the frequency of these frustrating scenarios by making sure our offices have a closed-loop referral process and begin building bridges between the moment we have the family in our office and the moment they obtain the desired service or intervention.

The stepwise approach outlined in this chapter helps you introduce tools and strategies to cocreate this proverbial bridge with families, including trauma-informed parenting skills that promote the affiliate response. In a post-pandemic world where resources are spread thin, the approach described in this chapter, which I call Resilience University (RU), became my way of responding to potentially toxic levels of stress in my day-to-day practice. A licensed clinical

social worker embedded in my practice would refer patients to RU before, after, or alongside traditional counseling for coping skills and positive parenting support. I've found myself integrating the RU approach, resources, and tools routinely outside of formal RU sessions. These days, it is rare for me to complete any patient encounter without offering or reinforcing at least one of these stress-reducing, connection-promoting, problem-solving skills. You will learn more about this universal integration in Chapters 6, Using Relationship-Based and Trauma-Informed Anticipatory Guidance, and 8, Universal Integration in Practice. Here, we are going to focus on what to do if you want to work closely with a family for a series of sessions so you can support them in making a change to foster resilience in response to a specific concern (ie, behavioral or mental health issues).

Who Can Benefit From Resilience University

Almost all families could learn a few new skills and strategies if they completed the formal 4-session course, but certain patient-parent dyads become mutually dysregulated more often than others, which can prevent protective, positive childhood experiences (PCEs) from arising. Often this pattern is related to a history of trauma and/or toxic stress, and both parent and child are simultaneously having a neurohormonal stress response. For some families, the idea of going to counseling or undergoing a more thorough evaluation feels even more stressful; with these sessions, you can work more intensely as you continue to encourage the family to obtain services. You can offer this multigenerational, trauma-informed approach in the context of your existing care structure, folded in with medication follow-up visits or as separate visits to increase equitable access to PCEs.

The age range I designed the tools in this book for is 4 to 11 years, although the language and handouts can be modified for older children and teens. Younger children can learn by imitating the older siblings and parents. Depending on the maturity of the children you are working with, you can modify the language as appropriate. You'll of course need parent or caregiver participation in the 4 sessions since RU uses a multigenerational approach. The more caregivers or parents who can be involved, the better. For example, when a child goes between households, it is important to send a second copy of the handouts so there is awareness of the strategies in both places. Because of the nature of the approach, however, children can still use the strategies in the other guardian's or co-parent's home even if the other caregiver is not engaged in the sessions. Involved caregivers can celebrate the child's abilities, and over time, the other parents/caregivers may request sessions or resources as well.

The families I prioritize for the series of formal RU sessions include

1. Children who have experienced or are experiencing any of the following adversities:
   - Physical abuse, verbal abuse, sexual abuse, physical neglect, or emotional neglect
   - Having a parent/caregiver with a substance use disorder, a caregiver who has experienced domestic violence, a family member who is incarcerated, or a family member who has been diagnosed with a mental illness, or experiencing divorce of parents
   - Losing a caregiver (eg, grandmother, mother, grandfather) or beloved family pet
   - Current or past homelessness
   - Surviving and recovering from a severe injury, illness, or emergency
   - Witnessing a loved one (including animals) being abused or mistreated
   - Witnessing a grandparent abusing a parent
   - Involvement with the foster care system
   - Involvement with the juvenile justice system
2. Children with a diagnosis of
   - Behavioral problems
   - Sleep disorder
   - Mood changes
   - Anxiety
   - Depression (including suicidal thoughts)
   - Aggression
   - Attention-deficit/hyperactivity disorder
   - Oppositional defiant disorder

Ideally, we hope caregivers will be able to respond to children when they are in distress and in need of coregulation, yet we know that even in the best of times, this attuned response occurs about 30% of the time.[1] For the remaining 70% of the time, having accessible self-care strategies fosters a sense of self-efficacy for children. Parents may become more able to attune as they understand the process of emotion coaching and more able to reconnect after relational health ruptures with tools and skills to facilitate repairs.

Resilience University is designed to be offered in parallel with all other necessary reporting obligations, interventions, prescriptions, referrals, and evaluations. If you are concerned for an emerging mental health problem, refer as you would normally for psychiatry, counseling, a neuropsychological evaluation, etc.

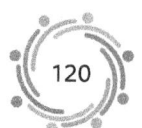

Parent-Child Interaction Therapy, play therapy, trauma-focused cognitive behavioral therapy, eye movement desensitization and reprocessing, Circle of Security parenting, and dialectical behavioral therapy are all potential options for therapeutic referrals, and you can still work with the family while they are waiting to become established with one of these therapists.

If you are concerned about abuse or neglect, report as you would normally to the appropriate person in your state. Being open about how hard a Department of Health and Human Services (DHHS) report can be may mitigate the potential for this to damage the trust and connection you have worked so hard to establish with the patient and family. Reporting concerns for abuse or neglect to the DHHS often feels unpleasant for us and terrifying for families. We can use language with the family that helps normalize the process and maximize the chance of us maintaining our trusted role in their lives. Remember the validation sandwich—or VIVA (Validate, Inform, Validate, Ask) approach—from Chapter 4, Process for Stepwise Change. For example, your discussion might sound something like this: *Thank you so much for bringing Mary in today so I could look at these bruises the child care provider is worried about. It is often really scary and difficult for families when something like this is happening.* (Validate) *My role is to report anything that could be a sign that Mary is in harm's way, and since the lab test results were all normal, I need to report my findings to the DHHS.* (Inform) *Any parent would feel stressed in this situation.* (Validate) *What questions do you have for me? How are you holding up?* (Ask). You can also ask if the parent has any self-care strategies for these tough times, such as breathing, mindfulness, meditation, or social supports or resources they can connect to. You can offer SUNBEAM (See, Unhook, Nurture, Breathe, Emotionally Aware, Mindful, Meditation) and make glitter jars with the family at the end of the same visit. I often add another validation sandwich around the PCE study,[2] pointing out that even if something is happening to put Mary in harm's way, feeling protected by one adult at home and being able to talk about feelings help offset any long-term impact.

Launching the Resilience University Process

I recommend dovetailing RU with existing visits for behavioral or mental health concerns whenever possible. You can also start by using one tool here or there, as we will discuss in Chapters 6, Using Relationship-Based and Trauma-Informed Anticipatory Guidance, and 8, Universal Integration in Practice. Asking for chunks of time to be reserved in our schedule for a set number of these visits per day or week, just as we do for newborns, facilitates launching the process. In the Appendix, you'll find patient- and family-facing handouts for many of the tools discussed throughout this book, as well as information on how to access downloadable versions and electronic resources.

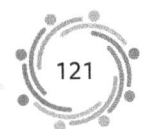

If you are screening for food insecurity, housing insecurity, or trauma symptoms, you may identify factors that affect family health. Instead of just referring out or categorizing a patient or family as high-risk for long-term problems from historical adverse childhood experiences (ACEs) reported on a screening form, you can immediately offer evidence-informed interventions that support neuroplasticity and PCEs and help foster and repair essential safe, stable, nurturing relationships.

With these strategies, you can be prepared to cocreate a path forward as you respond to anything stressful affecting family health. You will often notice that all 4 building blocks of HOPE (Healthy Outcomes from Positive Experiences) are involved when a family is experiencing potentially toxic levels of stress. Highlighting how you have seen them do hard things in the past and offering to work with them as they face this challenge, just like you do with any other health-related challenge, can help normalize their journey and ensure they don't feel judged or alone.

Stressful situations, such as a death in the family, divorce, or the incarceration of a loved one, are often shared in the context of regular clinical care. These stressors can affect the living environment, engagement, emotional growth, and relational health. Preparing families with strategies to address barriers to PCEs when new stressors arise can promote more equitable access to protective factors.

Beginning RU during a visit for behavioral or mental health issues means that in the process of clarifying the concerns and cocreating a plan with the family, you also offer handouts and supplies. Consider storing these in your exam room cabinets for ease of access. By starting the sessions immediately, the caregiver and child have easily accessible healthy coping skills and stress-lowering strategies to use while they are waiting for the other things to start helping (ie, medications, counseling, community supports, evaluations). This inherently provides one additional PCE—you!—as you become one of the nonparent adults who genuinely take an interest in the child.

Scheduling Resilience University Sessions

In the context of a busy primary care practice, it can be challenging to figure out how to create space for four 30-minute sessions over a few months. But once RU becomes part of your practice, you can identify how much time you want reserved for these visits, just as you would for acute care visits and follow-ups. Often this is already time you would be spending caring for this family, just with a different focus. For example, consider the child who isn't sleeping and appears on your schedule almost weekly with the parents requesting medication; once you help the family identify the relational health component of the sleep issues,

you can address it with a series of Plan-Do-Study-Act (PDSA) cycles that promote nurturing relationships and improved sleep hygiene.

Another situation where RU is helpful is when you have already referred a child for a neuropsychological evaluation and the caregivers were hoping for medication to improve behaviors, but the report doesn't align with medication as part of the plan. Many times, these reports list resources and counseling options that will support the family, although often these are not readily available to or swiftly actionable for families. You can work on RU with the family and mitigate stress while you simultaneously address barriers to any needed services or supports.

Normalizing both the stress of waiting for referrals and the fear parents may feel about their child's well-being can alleviate the impact on the family's health. For a child with multiple referrals that may take time, the skills provided in RU allow parents and children to have something to work on while everything else is getting set up. Anecdotal reports from counselors who have seen children after they have completed RU reflect that the skills learned there are helpful and allow the counselor and family to get to what they need to work on sooner. It's sort of like having the constipation talk and getting a child on a regular toilet routine and stool softener before they go see a gastroenterology (GI) doctor. That way, the GI doctor can start farther down the road with what is really going on.

Core Components

Structure

Each session builds on the previous one(s) as you work with the family to cocreate PDSA cycles that support their goals and promote resilience (see Chapter 4, Stepwise Process for Change). Together, these 4 sessions form a base for future family PDSA cycles, preparing families with a stepwise process for responding to stress and making change. Beginning the visits with open-ended questions about how things are going allows the family to drive the focus of the next PDSA cycle. Using an abbreviated motivational interviewing (MI) approach, you can get to the heart of what the family feels is important to work on, while promoting resilience-building relational habits between family members.

Supplies

A breakdown of the supplies needed for RU is listed in **Table 5-1**. It is possible to offer RU with just exam table paper and a pen, but these supplies can help it

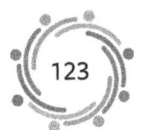

feel more interactive and engaging. You will also appreciate having access to a printer, printer paper, color markers and/or crayons, and a stapler.

Table 5-1. Resilience University Supplies (Costs are estimated at the time of publishing and may change over time)

Item	No. Needed per Patient	Estimated Cost Total, $	Cost per Patient, $
Voss still water bottle (plastic)	1	33.10 for 24-pack (1.38 ea)	1.38
Glitter glue tubes	2	29.02 for 72-pack (0.40 ea)	0.80
Glitter packets	2	5.99 for 48-pack (0.12 ea)	0.24
Stress ball	1	15.99 for 24-pack (0.67 ea)	0.67
Bubbles	1	18.99 for 24-pack (0.80 ea)	0.80
Small stickers	100	5.99 for 1,200-pack (0.005 ea)	0.50
Emoji/facial expression stickers	10	8.99 for 200-pack (0.05 ea)	0.45
Cardstock for charts	3	17.44 for 100-pack (0.17 ea)	0.52
Glitter jar reminder stickers	1	0.60 (on Canva)	0.60
Total per patient	121	Not applicable	5.96

Abbreviation: ea, each.

If you work within a larger hospital system, administration may want you to complete a pro forma process and map out the costs with the potential revenue generated. Revenue varies drastically depending on facilities and payers, but in an attempt to outline whether this program is financially feasible, I offer some estimates for reimbursement (**Table 5-2**). You can also check with local agencies to see if you can get a grant or a local charity organization to cover the cost of the program.

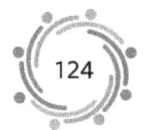

Table 5-2. Potential Revenue[a] From Resilience University (Reimbursement varies over time and by region; these are estimates at the time of publishing meant for planning purposes only)

Visit Code	Visit Description	Approximate Per-Visit Estimate, $	At the End of Resilience University (×4), $
99214	Established patient office or other outpatient visit, 30–39 minutes	97.60–156.02	390.40–624.08 per patient
99215	Established patient office or other outpatient visit, 40–54 minutes	143.34–233.27	573.36–933.08 per patient
99417	Prolonged office or other outpatient evaluation and management service(s), add one for each additional 15 minutes	32.00[b] each	Variable

[a] Centers for Medicare & Medicaid Services. Physician Fee Schedule. Accessed November 11, 2024. https://www.cms.gov/medicaremedicare-fee-service-paymentphysicianfeeschedpfs-federal-regulation-notices/cms-1770-p.

[b] American College of Allergy, Asthma & Immunology. Billing, coding & payments. New prolonged service *CPT* code for 2021. September 21, 2020. Accessed November 11, 2024. https://college.acaai.org/new-prolonged-service-cpt-code-for-2021.

I developed the curriculum as four 30-minute sessions (**99214**), but some of the sessions may end up being coded as **99215** if you spend longer with the family or end up calling a co-parent or another caregiver at the end of the day to discuss the plan you cocreated in the office. **Table 5-2** represents a low estimate to ensure that even with poor reimbursement, any additional supply costs will be more than covered. **99417** can be added to account for any time spent on the day of the visit preparing for/documenting care provided or discussing the patient's care with counselors, other clinicians, or other caregivers (eg, child care providers, grandparents, babysitters).

Curriculum

The families I've worked with have taught me what works and helped me clarify in what order the skills are most helpfully learned. Initially, I was working mainly on instinct, but over time, with family feedback, I structured the sessions more consistently. **Table 5-3** represents my standard schedule of interventions. You can start with this organized approach, and then, once you are familiar with the process and the tools, you can apply them in different clinical encounters. Or you can start by using individual tools as needed (see Chapters 6, Using Relationship-Based and Trauma-Informed Anticipatory Guidance, and 8, Universal Integration in Practice) and then dive deeper with families once you are more comfortable with each individual tool and strategy.

Table 5-3. Formal 4-Session Resilience University Curriculum/Schedule of Interventions

Intervention	Visit 1	Visit 2	Visit 3	Visit 4	Location in This Book
No. of days between visits	Not applicable	At least 7 days after 1st session	At least 7 days after 2nd session	At least 7 days after 3rd session	
Enrollment form	X (beginning of 1st session)				Appendix Z
Glitter jar meditation	X	O		O	Chapter 3, Appendix E
Family feelings chart	X				Chapter 4, Appendix T
Time-versus-emotion curve	X	O	O	O	Chapter 3
Emotional awareness	X		O		Chapter 3, Appendix F
"Fire-truck brain" analogy	X		O	O	Chapter 3, Appendix L
Emotion coaching	X	O		O	Chapter 4, Appendix Y
Validate, Validate, Validate	X	O	O		Chapter 4, Appendix V
Self-care nook	X		O	O	Chapter 2, Appendix CC
"Box" or "square" breathing	X	O		O	Chapter 3, Appendix B
Toes-to-nose	X	O	O	O	Chapter 3, Appendix K
5-4-3-2-1	X	O	O		Chapter 3, Appendix J
"10 Things I Can Do When I Feel Yucky" list or stress reduction plan	X	O	O	O	Chapter 4, Appendix U; Chapter 3, Appendix O
Self-care sticker chart		X			Chapter 4, Appendix S
"Back the bus up" approach		X	O		Chapter 4, Appendix R

(continues)

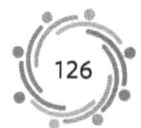

Table 5-3 (*continued*)

Intervention	Visit 1	Visit 2	Visit 3	Visit 4	Location in This Book
NICER parenting		X	O	O	Chapter 4, Appendix W
SUNBEAM		X	O	O	Chapter 4, Appendix X
Loving-kindness meditation		X		O	Chapter 3, Appendixes G and H
Walking meditation		X		O	Chapter 3, Appendix I
5 Big Deep Breaths		X	O		Chapter 3, Appendix A
Using the breath (blowing bubbles/ singing)		X	O		Chapter 3, Appendix D
Stress balls		X	O		Chapter 5 (this chapter)
Strengths-based (HOPE) building blocks			X	O	Chapter 3, Appendixes M and N
Relaxation breathing			X	O	Chapter 3, Appendix C
My Little Book of Big Feelings			X	O	Chapter 2
Stress-buster wheel				X	Chapter 4
9-5-2-1-0 checklist				X	Chapter 3, Appendix P
Self-care super-powers sticker chart				X	Chapter 5 (this chapter)
"Graduation" certificate				X	Appendix AA

Abbreviations: HOPE, Healthy Outcomes from Positive Experiences; NICER, Notice, Identify, Connect/coregulate, Explore, Review/repair; SUNBEAM, See, Unhook, Nurture, Breathe, Emotionally Aware, Mindful, Meditation.

X indicates introduce; O, reinforce.

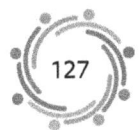

Session Format

Start each session with a check-in and review of how things are going. End each session with some "homework" around a cocreated plan. I will outline the components, general content, and language I use when I am working with families at each session. Remember, this is an interactive, dynamic coaching process, not just telling a patient and parent to do something. It requires that we arrive authentically as humans in the exam room with our families, not assuming that we know what they need or don't need until they've explained what is going on to us. For that to happen, you may need to integrate your own self-care strategies into your day. An example may be something like using habit stacking to add one self-care strategy (5 Big Deep Breaths or walking meditation) between each patient visit.

VIVA is the abbreviated MI approach (see Chapter 4, Process for Stepwise Change) you will use regularly. Specific tools and strategies will be offered as unmet needs or big emotions are jointly identified; in these moments, you will take a more didactic role. When parents or children ask for help with a problem, you start with celebrating at least one strength and then cocreate problem-solving cycles with them (PDSA cycles), often using habit stacking to find opportunities to integrate new tools and skills. Families appreciate knowing that the system you are sharing with them is evidence based, but sometimes they may find scientific terminology to be dense and overwhelming. Your role is to highlight how change is possible when addressing a stubborn problem and build their capacity to feel confident that, whatever arises, together you will figure out a path forward.

Session 1

Rooming and Scheduling

Have your medical assistant (MA) or nurse ask for the child's favorite color when rooming the patient and give the parent or guardian an enrollment form to fill out.

Supplies and Handouts

Bring in supplies to make a glitter jar in the child's favorite color with the reminder sticker (if you are planning to use that; **Figure 5-1**, explained later in this session breakdown): plastic bottle of Voss still water, 2 tubes of nontoxic glitter glue, and a small packet of glitter. Some of the glitter packets can be torn open and others require scissors, so check to see which kind you have and plan ahead!

Handouts for this session include "Glitter Jar Meditation: Your Body Will Thank You" (see Appendix E); "Box Breathing" (Appendix B); "Emotions Are Like Ocean Waves" (Appendix F); "Time-Versus-Emotion Curve" (Figure 3-3); "Fire-Truck Brain" (Appendix L); "Resilience University Emotion Coaching" (Appendix Y); "Self-Care Nook: A Cozy Spot Where Everyone Can Pause to Take

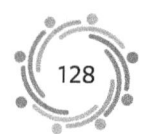
Care of Big Feelings" (Appendix CC); "Validate, Validate, Validate" (Appendix V); "Feeling Nervous? Worried? Bored? Try Toes-to-Nose!" (Appendix K); "5-4-3-2-1 Grounding With Your Senses" (Appendix J); "Family Feelings Chart" (Appendix T); and "10 Things I Can Do When I Feel Yucky" (Appendix U; younger child) or "Stress Reduction Plan" (Appendix O; older child).

Check-In

Start by sitting down and rolling your chair over to the kid(s) and, at their eye level, letting them know this is a different kind of doctor's appointment than they are used to: *Don't worry, there are no shots and I'm not even going to use my stethoscope! People come to the doctor's office when they are sick or they don't feel good. What we are going to do in these sessions is work on different ways you can take care of yourself when you don't feel good, like when you feel frustrated or angry or annoyed, so that you feel better* [or *stop getting in so much trouble, have an easier time at school,* etc].

Often you have a reason for why they are there, either an identified source of childhood adversity or a specific behavioral or emotional concern. Validate that you know things are hard or changing, depending on what brings them in, and clarify something they would really like help with first: *What is one situation where things routinely go sideways and everything is really hard?* For younger children, I start by asking the parents what is hardest, but you can direct this question to the child if it seems developmentally appropriate. If the parent and child appear to have different ideas about what is hardest, you can address both in parallel.

After they share what the hardest thing is, take a minute to reflect back what you heard and validate how things are challenging: *There is a lot going on, isn't there? Sounds like things have been really hard.* Then, you can normalize how behaviors arise when things are challenging: *You know, it's OK to not be OK when you are going through hard times. Any family going through this would be experiencing similar things.*

Frame With Strengths

Remind the family of how you have seen them do hard things in the past. Highlight a specific family strength or historical success. This helps you set the tone for why you are the right person to help: *Just like when you had pneumonia and things were stressful but together we figured it out, we are going to do the same thing with this too, OK? And the cool thing is, Mom and Dad are going to learn exactly the same thing you are so everyone can work together when things get hard.*

Cocreate a Plan

For this first session, the parents and child bring in their specific concerns and goals and they are asking for help with something concrete. Your focus in cocreating this first PDSA cycle with them is to ensure that they are more able to practice healthy coping skills and increase the capacity to welcome and talk about feelings as a family.

Tools and Skills

The family may identify healthy coping strategies that are family specific (eg, cuddling the pet bunny, sitting with Grandpa in the living room, asking an auntie for help), and you can start by celebrating these strengths. It is often quickly apparent that specific healthy coping skills are not always available, so having a bunch to choose from can help. Once the family engages and we have cocreated a goal, I shift into a more didactic mode to cocreate a few options for a new path. I make a glitter jar with the child's help and teach everyone how to use it to meditate.

I add a circular sticker on top of the glitter jar (**Figure 5-1**; see Appendix DD for a printable sheet sized to fit the lid) so they can easily remember how to use it later. I've found it important to remind parents that this is not a time-out timer and should not be taken away as a consequence for unwanted behaviors. Instead, remind parents that it is a tool for their child to take care of themselves and practice a form of meditation.

Figure 5-1.

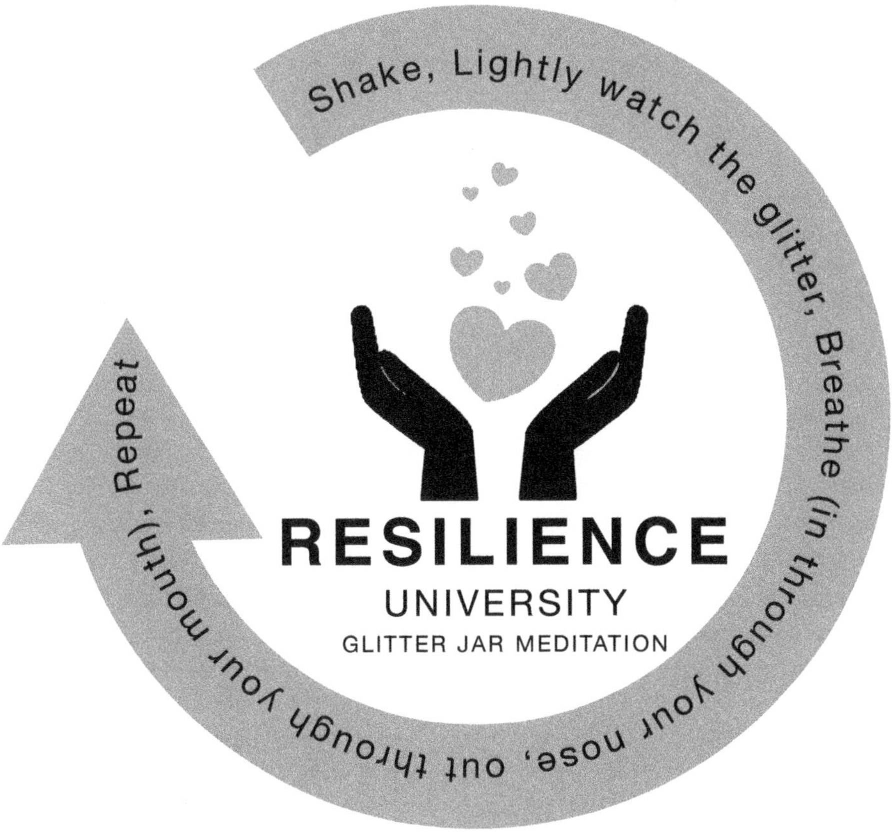

Shake, Lightly watch the glitter, Breathe (in through your nose, out through your mouth), Repeat

RESILIENCE
UNIVERSITY
GLITTER JAR MEDITATION

Resilience University glitter jar reminder sticker.

While you're making the glitter jar, talk with the parent and child about what has brought them here and how everyone has been feeling (eg, getting into trouble a lot, hitting a friend or sibling, getting suspended, getting kicked off the bus). I have the children squeeze the glitter into the bottle and add the packet of glitter. Ask the parent how they tend to respond to the child's behaviors and what they would like to see change, reflecting back what they say and validating how difficult this can be. Also ask what tools and strategies they have found helpful so far and how they currently are coping.

Draw on the exam table paper or share the "Time-Versus-Emotion Curve" handout and then ask if the day currently feels like a constant series of "zero to screech" moments; explain how self-care strategies can help make it feel more manageable.

Next, ask the child the following questions, pausing in between for them to answer:

- *How do you take care of yourself when you are hungry?*
- *How do you take care of yourself when you are tired?*
- *How do you take care of yourself when you are cold?*

I celebrate each answer as a strength. Point out to the parents that *You didn't specifically sit them down and teach them these things, right? It happened over time because you modeled it for them. You brought them a blanket or food until they could do it for themselves. You reminded them it was bedtime or nap time. Just like you taught them to respond to those feelings, you can help them learn how to respond and care for themselves with other unpleasant feelings or difficult emotions. Often we don't do that naturally because our parents didn't do it for us and their parents didn't do it for them and so on for generations before us.*

Point out to both parents and kids how it is everyone's job to figure out how to care for themselves when they don't feel good and how to ask for help with what they need. Parents begin to see how the behaviors they want to see less of are related to underlying unmanageable physical and/or emotional states. Remind parents that a child's ability to understand what they need and take care of themselves will change over time, and much of this is learned by emulating what the parents do.

Continue by explaining the next steps: *OK, so now we are going to work on how you can take care of yourself when you are sad, worried, or angry, so it's just as easy as when you're hungry, tired, or cold, OK?* Briefly discuss emotional awareness and give them the "Emotions Are Like Ocean Waves" handout: *Emotions are like ocean waves. They can be big or small, and they kind of have their own rhythm. Even when they feel big, remember that they won't last forever. Your job is to take care of yourself while the waves are there so they don't wash you out to sea.*

Point out how glitter jar meditation helps us take care of ourselves with any "yucky" feeling: *Just shake it up and breathe in through your nose and out through your mouth while you watch the glitter settle. If you're still feeling yucky when the glitter has settled, you can shake the jar up and start over again.* Ensure that you complete at least one round of glitter jar meditation before they leave so both parent and child can experience how they feel before and after.

Explain how sometimes, we just suddenly don't feel good and a big emotion takes over. Share the "fire-truck brain" analogy, giving them the "Fire-Truck Brain" handout to take home. With the handout, you can explain that *The good-thinking part of your brain has a fancy name; we call it the* prefrontal cortex. *But it goes "offline" and can't work when you have a really big emotion. When that happens, another part of your brain, which has another fancy name, the* amygdala, *takes over. I like to call this your "fire-truck brain." It likes to show up sirens blaring and hoses ready. But it can't do math, answer Mom's questions, or figure out how to solve a problem. Using the glitter jar or another one of these self-care and coping strategies can help calm your nervous system so that good-thinking part of your brain comes back "online." Then you can figure out how to finish your homework or clean your room.*

Next, return everyone's focus to the time-versus-emotion curve to explain how these simple self-care strategies can improve a frustrating day. Make note of how our big unpleasant feelings are easier to care for if we notice them early, when they are still small, and if we have practiced the healthy coping skills before we actually need them. Sometimes this means proactively scheduling little self-care breaks throughout the busy day.

After this guidance, introduce the concept of emotion coaching and the importance of validating big feelings to the caregiver(s) or parent(s). Parents can coach their child in how to respond to big emotions just like they help coach their child in sports. Point out how validating is not the same as just letting the child get away with everything; the parents will still have a functional way of helping their child with behavior modification. One of the essential first steps to shift to a validating, coaching response is for the parents to accept that the unpleasant feelings are happening. Parents who are used to dismissing difficult emotions or responding in a disapproving manner will probably need new language to use. Even parents who can acknowledge that an unpleasant feeling is there may feel frustrated and that they don't have a meaningful response to offer or that the feeling is lasting for too long, which can result in the parents' own emotion(s) becoming the central focus. Ask the parents how they are currently responding to their child's big unpleasant emotions and if they are frequently frustrated by them. This can help clarify what their starting point is. Even if the parents are routinely responding with yelling, reassure them that with tiny, step-wise changes, these habitual responses can shift over time.

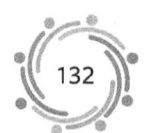

Provide parents with language to validate big unpleasant feelings by introducing a set of starter phrases they can finish to suit the specific situation. This is explained in the "Validate, Validate, Validate" handout: *Of course you are* [eg, *angry*]. *Anyone would feel* [*angry*] *if* [*they lost their favorite toy*]. *It's totally normal to feel* [*angry*]. Make sure the parents know they can add a sentence after that to clarify the boundaries if behaviors have gone off the rails: *AND it's not OK to throw your shoes at your sister.* They also can add a sentence to invite a conversation about feelings. Give them the validation handout and encourage them to use this language. Remind them that any new skill is easier to master when we're not having a big emotion ourselves. If they can practice this script when they feel calm, it will be easier to use when they feel tense and overwhelmed.

Point out how it is a good idea for the family to have a few other tools and skills they can use along with the glitter jar (or instead of it, if it's not readily available) so they can figure out what works in different settings and for different family members. Honor how only each individual person will know what kind of self-care strategy works best for each big unpleasant feeling. If they are interested, explain the role of breathing exercises and the role of the vagus nerve (see the 5 Big Deep Breaths section in Chapter 3, Essential Toolkit). Give them the "Box Breathing" handout and practice tracing the box with the child. Point out to the child that this technique can be used anytime, anywhere—even when they're riding on the bus or when they're stuck in the back seat on a long car ride with a sibling they find annoying. Encourage them to trace the outline of the box on the back of the car or bus seat in front of them. I often bring up the reference to the Navy SEALs (see the Box Breathing section in Chapter 3) and point out that they have to be able to take care of their big feelings in any situation and keep going with the mission.

Introduce briefly what mindfulness is and review the 2 core mindfulness strategies (5-4-3-2-1 and toes-to-nose). I describe mindfulness as *using your body to ground yourself when you're experiencing a big unpleasant or yucky feeling.* Explain toes-to-nose as a way to check in with their body at any time: *Just like you could use your breathing, and no one has to know what you're doing, you could be sitting at your desk in school and feel a wave of worry about a test and use toes-to-nose to ground yourself in your body.* Or, *You might be waiting in the exam room at the doctor's office and feel a wave of fear or nervousness, and you can use your senses to ground yourself.*

I walk them through it as described in the Body Scan for Kids: Toes-to-Nose section of Chapter 3. If they want to, suggest that they put their hand onto their chest and try to feel their heartbeat. Have them thank each part of their body, if they want to, as they go. Remember, you can have them combine gratitude with the body scan for a different twist.

The last healthy coping skill for this session is 5-4-3-2-1, or the sensory grounding exercise, from Chapter 3; you walk them through how to do this as described in that chapter.

Strategies for Change

New tools and skills are good, but you also have to have a plan for how to integrate them. This is where you introduce the idea of habit stacking within a PDSA cycle to the family. Cocreate some ideas that might work for at least one PDSA cycle they can try when they get home, incorporating one or more of the self-care skills into the day. Encourage the family to create a self-care nook (by using the relatable "hangry" kitchen analogy introduced in Chapter 2, Overview of Resilience University) and reinforce the concept of taking care of yourself so your fire-truck brain can go back into its garage and you can think straight again.

Send them home with 2 additional strategies to try: a family feelings chart and a list of 10 things the child can do when they feel yucky. A family feelings chart is just a prop to get the family talking about feelings. Talking about feelings with one's family is one of the 7 studied PCEs that offsets the long-term mental and physical health impacts of childhood adversity.[2,3] Many aspects of family dynamics influence whether this is happening at home or not. One is the way parents respond to emotions in general.[4] If they use an "emotion coaching" approach or something similar, they are probably already talking about feelings to some degree. On the other hand, if they are routinely dismissing emotions, perhaps no one can talk about them. Similarly, if the routine response is disapproving, children will quickly learn to not express their feelings. Finally, parents who fall into the laissez-faire category may allow kids to talk about feelings but not be prepared with helpful strategies for the kids to care for themselves while the emotion is present. Encourage parents to simply start with validating unpleasant feelings, starting with the language provided.

These are both strategies to support habit stacking. For example, when family members come into the kitchen to get food or drinks, they can stop to notice their feelings and mark those on the feelings chart. For children who are getting into trouble often, the child can be encouraged routinely to try one self-care strategy from the "10 Things I Can Do When I Feel Yucky" list. For older children, you can use the stress reduction plan instead. For parents, they can try one coping skill before they speak with their child about the child's behavior.

Homework

Have the caregiver put the family feelings chart onto the fridge and either give them stickers or tell them they can use a pen or highlighter to make a note when each person in the family notices they are feeling a certain way. Let the kids and parents guide which feelings to put on the chart, but make sure you include some of the "low-hanging fruit" that everyone already knows what to do with (eg, *hungry, tired, cold*). Also include

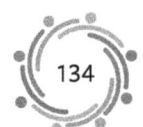

a few of the harder ones the family is going to learn more about with these sessions. Tell them to add a sticker, a check mark, or a comment when each person in the family notices they are feeling a certain way. Sometimes it's fun to have each person use a different sticker or color so everyone else knows how they are feeling. Encourage the family to start talking with each other about everyone's feelings. It's important to remind people not to take other people's feelings personally: *This is not an exercise in blaming other family members for making you feel a certain way. Instead, it is a chance to listen to each other and offer strategies that may help you when you feel that same way.*

If time allows, start creating the "10 Things I Can Do When I Feel Yucky" list, including anything the child has already been doing at home. Then, you can add the glitter jar, breathing exercises, and mindfulness exercises. This facilitates the discussion about other things that might help them feel better, like taking a break to blow bubbles or snuggling with the family pet. Steer them away from things that are more distractions (eg, watching TikTok) and toward things that have a biological basis for lowering stress and improving health (eg, mindfulness, breathing exercises, physical exercise, connection). The stress reduction plan is a tool for older children. Have them keep this plan in a central location to help remind everyone to try self-care for big emotions.

On the way out, ask the parents to continue to notice any specific scenarios that are most difficult and bring those back to the next session.

Session 2

Rooming and Scheduling

Sessions should be scheduled at least a week apart, although it may be longer, depending on the family's schedule and yours. Involve the family with the interval they think would give them time to work on what they want to do. This session has no specific rooming instructions for the MA or nurse.

Supplies and Handouts

Bring in supplies to make a self-care superpowers sticker chart (**Figures 5-2** and **5-3**, explained later in this session breakdown) and a stress ball (also explained later). If you have them, you can also bring in a small container of bubbles with a wand. Bring in the "Back the Bus Up: A Parenting Problem-Solving Approach" (see Appendix R), "NICER Parenting" (Appendix W), "SUNBEAM: A Parent's Antidote to Meltdowns" (Appendix X), "Loving-Kindness Meditation" (Appendix G for caregivers and Appendix H for older kids/teens), "Walking Meditation" (Appendix I), "5 Big Deep Breaths" (Appendix A), and "Use Your Breath" (Appendix D) handouts.

Check-In

Begin the second session with open-ended questions: *How is everything going?* Some families will bring their homework sheets with them and some won't. I've noticed

many times that the children are so proud of their new tools and skills that they want to bring the glitter jar back to subsequent visits to show you how they are using it. If you want to, you can provide them with a sturdy gift bag to carry things in and as a temporary storage container for home. There is enough material to cover at each session, so this is not necessary, but if the kids want to, it is a powerful part of the process to enjoy celebrating their successes and honoring what they are proud of.

Frame With Strengths

Ask the parents and child to share anything they feel is going well: *What are some things you are proud of? Were you able to notice any new feelings? Talk about feelings more? Were you able to use any new ways of taking care of yourself when you didn't feel good?*

In my experience, kids are always ready to answer some or all of these questions. Parents will usually have multiple new concerns to ask for help with, now that they understand what these sessions are about. Once everyone has shared, we can celebrate successes and validate challenges.

Cocreate a Plan

For this second session, the parents and child may have new concerns and goals. Your focus in cocreating this second PDSA cycle with them is to help identify barriers to integrating PCEs and to using healthy coping skills. In this session, you expand the idea of self-care for yucky feelings to the caregivers as well as reinforce it for the children.

Tools and Skills

Starting with the child, I ask about ongoing challenges: *Anything hard you specifically wanted help with for this session?* Identify any specific struggles or concerns the child has before you pivot back to the parents and ask them how they feel things are going: *Were you able to notice and anticipate when things were about to get hard? What was particularly challenging for you?* The parents' and child's concerns will be used to cocreate the next PDSA cycle.

Have the child start working on their project for this session, making a self-care superpowers sticker chart (**Figures 5-2** and **5-3**) with different feelings they find challenging. Bring in emoji/facial expression stickers or draw some faces for the kids, then let them decorate the chart. You can also print the PDF (from the Appendix) and use the feelings and self-care strategies listed. Making their own chart allows kids to start pairing the things they have figured out they can do when they feel yucky with different feelings. You can draw a chart on the exam table paper with a pen if you don't have a printer or access to the templates (see Appendix BB). Emphasize that the child can put their own sticker or star onto the chart for any ability they've shown to recognize a feeling or any attempt they've made to practice one of the self-care strategies. Point out that the parents are not rewarding "good" behavior like in a traditional sticker chart. Rather, everyone is celebrating any attempt at trying new coping skills.

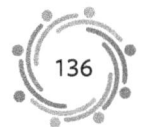

Lack of check marks, stickers, or stars should never be used to shame the child but rather be framed as an open opportunity to try something new. Kids develop their own "superpowers" and are more able to use healthy coping skills in times of stress.

Almost all the families I work with have at least one family member who loves the glitter jar, but for some people, it is not a primary tool. As you work with families, remember that you are cocreating new strategies to manage stress, and the last thing you want them to do is stress about using a coping strategy!

Figure 5-2.

My Self-Care Chart

When I feel...	I can...	I did it!
Mad	• Use my squishy ball • Take a break • Do 5 big breaths	
Sad	• Cuddle the dog • Ask Mom for a hug • Use my glitter jar	
Tired	• Take a break • Rest • Toes-to-nose	
Bored	• Box breathing • 5-4-3-2-1 • Sing	

Self-care sticker chart on exam table paper.

Figure 5-3.

How I feel...	What I can do...	I did it!	RESILIENCE UNIVERSITY
Angry Mad Frustrated Annoyed Irritated	• Squishy ball • Run outside • Take a break • 5 big breaths	★ ★ ★	
Sad Lonely Left out	• Cuddle pets/stuffies • Hug Mom/Dad • Glitter jar • Listen to music	★ ★	
Confused Worried Scared Overwhelmed	• Glitter jar • 5 big breaths • Sing • Blow bubbles	★ ★	
Tired Sleepy Exhausted	• Take a break • Toes-to-nose • Rest • Sleep	★ ★ ★	

Self-care sticker chart example PDF.

Strategies for Change

While the kids are decorating the sticker chart with markers/crayons and stickers, introduce the caregivers or parents to 2 of their own core strategies: NICER (Notice, Identify, Connect/coregulate, Explore, Review/repair) parenting and SUNBEAM. By this point, parents understand that it is the big emotions that lead to the big unwanted behaviors. Explain to them that just like for their children, the self-care skills are simple but powerful and they can use these as well to take care of themselves so they don't say or do something they promised themselves they wouldn't and end up with a "parenting hangover." Explain NICER parenting and SUNBEAM as described in Chapter 4, adding in the loving-kindness and walking meditation options for parents.

Next, help the family identify any barriers to using healthy coping skills and integrating PCEs. I start with saying, OK, *so if you have your glitter jar and your stuffies, you'll probably be OK. But what about when you don't have them? Like if you're stuck in the car?* Introduce one tool that is always available: 5 Big Deep Breaths. *By breathing in through your nose and blowing out slowly through your mouth, you are using your breath to tell your nervous system that you are safe and not being chased by saber-toothed tigers.* By this point, the kids and parents understand that there are ways they can work with their own nervous systems to help return to a lower stress level and a calmer, "rest and digest" state sooner. Offer the "Use Your Breath" handout here and celebrate any times when the family identifies already using these techniques.

Timing is another common barrier to being able to regulate emotions or integrate healthy coping strategies. Here is an example of how to address this type of barrier in a stepwise fashion. Let's say the parents are coming to you for help because their daughter is routinely "falling apart" every morning before she leaves the house for school. They have "tried everything" and are about to do homeschooling even though they would rather keep her in public school. You can suggest that before taking drastic steps, *Why don't we "back the bus up" and see if we can figure out a way the day could go differently?* This is a different way to approach the time-versus-emotion curve, starting with the problematic behavior and investigating what may have contributed. Draw a timeline on the exam table paper, starting with the unpleasant event—in this case, the daughter's behavior before school. Then, work backward in time with the family to see what experiences or emotions might be related to this event and when there could be opportunities for self-care (**Figure 5-4**).

Perhaps she hasn't been sleeping well. Maybe her parents' well-intended "healthy breakfast" is unappealing, so she doesn't eat much and is still hungry when it's time to leave for school. You can also take into account that her little brother always wants her to play with him in the morning when she is still tired,

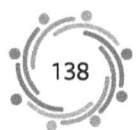
which she finds frustrating. By the time everyone is trying to get out of the house for school, the daughter is already in tears and is in no place to learn.

To address the lack of sleep, encourage the parents to work on getting the child to bed earlier and emphasize sleep hygiene. If they are already following all the recommended sleep routine guidelines, when you are trying to help them shift to an earlier bedtime, you can discuss if using melatonin following the American Academy of Sleep Medicine guidelines (endorsed by the American Academy of Pediatrics) may help.[5] Another strategy for bedtime struggles can be making a "bedtime pass." While not officially part of RU, this tried-and-true parenting trick can often help kids stay sleeping in their own rooms. A bedtime pass is a "ticket" families can make out of cardboard or wood and decorate together while they talk about the plan for nighttime. The bedtime pass allows the child to visit Mom and Dad (or another caregiver) once through the night if they need them. Then, the parent/guardian takes the bedtime pass, and the child gets it back the next night at bedtime. The pass serves as a transitional item: because it provides a sense of connection, kids will hold on to it and not want to use (and let go of) it, which facilitates independent sleep.

Cocreating a plan to address other barriers may look something like this: For breakfast, discuss a compromise to include food with healthy ingredients that the child would actually eat. Move her breakfast spot away from her brothers, perhaps to the screened-in porch, where she can blow bubbles and have space to herself (make this fun, not punitive, and call this her "bubble breakfast"), so she can have a little space from her brother.

Figure 5-4 provides another example to illustrate this process and the way I draw it out for families, either on the exam table paper or on a piece of printer paper. You can also print a blank "Back the Bus Up" template (see Appendix R) and fill it in with them.

Anger is one of the most challenging emotions for children and families to learn to work with. It tends to arise quickly and is a layered composite of other, more vulnerable emotions like fear, sadness, and loneliness. So often, children act out when they feel angry and parents react to the behavior and, as a result, the underlying emotion goes uncared for. The parents' response becomes part of the barrier to being able to talk about the feeling or feel supported through hard times. When helping a family with anger, first of all, remind them that feeling angry is a normal part of being human and bring in the emotion coaching concept for the parents: *The angry feeling is probably trying to tell you something, but you don't want to hurt yourself, anyone else, or anything else while it is there.*

Figure 5-4.

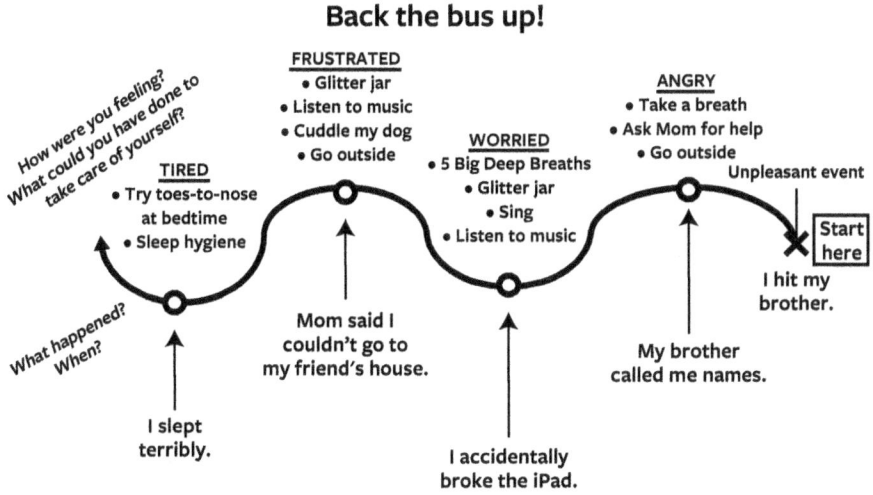

Back the bus up!

"Back the bus up" exercise for families, which can be drawn on exam table paper or printer paper. In this scenario, the parents bring their daughter in because she keeps hitting her brother. The pediatrician asks permission to back the bus up and figure out how the day could have gone differently, drawing the time-line backward on the exam table paper, starting with the unpleasant event. The inquiry begins with *How were you [the daughter] feeling? What could you have done to take care of yourself while that feeling was there?* It proceeds backward through the rest of the day, asking, *What happened next? How were you feeling then? What could you have done to take care of yourself while that feeling was there?* You can also use the "Back the Bus Up: A Parenting Problem-Solving Approach" handout from Appendix R.

You can give the child a squishy stress ball and ask them to practice giving it a really good squeeze while remembering what the angry feeling is like. Explain how sometimes, that big angry feeling ends up taking over their body; then they act in a way that later means they get into trouble, and they might have even accidentally hurt someone. The squishy balls don't mind being squished; that is what they are made for. When children are tired of getting into trouble all the time, they can be quite open to the idea of trying something different to see if they can stop losing privileges and playdates. Parents appreciate understanding that there is nothing wrong with the fact that their child feels angry and they can begin that process of coaching their child about taking care of themselves during those big feelings. Remind parents that they can model healthy responses to anger in the context of NICER parenting and they can care for their own anger with SUNBEAM before responding to their child.

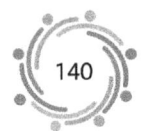

Homework

Send the family home with the sticker chart as homework for the child to work on by using any strategies they can think of for those big yucky feelings. Remind them they can use the "10 Things I Can Do When I Feel Yucky" list at home to come up with ideas for the yucky feelings. Make sure they have at least 1 or 2 strategies listed for each challenging feeling and know it's their job to figure out what works best for each feeling. The parents have their own homework this time too—to work on NICER parenting and practice SUNBEAM. If a caregiver or co-parent is not present, I recommend sending a second set of handouts for that person and offering to call them to review the plan and answer any questions. I will also often invite caregivers or co-parents to attend different sessions if they are not comfortable attending sessions together.

Session 3

Rooming and Scheduling

This session should be at least a week from the previous session. Since a large part of this work is for the caregivers, make sure all involved adults have an opportunity to practice the NICER parenting and SUNBEAM before the follow-up. This may mean that the time between appointments is longer, depending on relevant visitation schedules.

Supplies and Handouts

Bring in a small stapled booklet, markers and/or crayons, and face/emoji stickers to make *My Little Book of Big Feelings*. The handouts for this session include the 4 building blocks of HOPE worksheets (see Appendixes M and N) and "Relaxation Breathing" (Appendix C). You will be reinforcing many of the topics covered in prior sessions, so it sometimes helps to have extra copies of the other handouts readily available if the family is struggling with one in particular. It is always useful to either have a "Back the Bus Up" handout (Appendix R) with you or be prepared to draw it on the exam table paper.

Check-In

Begin this session similarly to the previous one, with open-ended questions like *How have things been going since I saw you last?* Stay with open-ended questions and affirm anything they report as a strength or success. Even if it *felt* like a failure, they were able to *try* something new! Review their homework: *How was the feelings sticker chart? Was it easy or hard to try self-care? If hard, what got in the way? Have you figured out a place to keep your self-care tools? Are you noticing anything different around talking about feelings? Tell me what you have noticed about behaviors.*

Frame With Strengths

Ask what the family is proud of. What was hard and they figured out how to do it anyway? What have the parents been proud of?

Cocreate a Plan

Asking what was particularly challenging since the previous session helps you identify where more multilayered barriers exist to integrating PCEs and mitigating the impact of stress on family health.

Tools and Skills

Emotional awareness is a key concept to reinforce for this session. Highlight how, many times, the feeling that this unpleasant emotion will last forever combines with the idea that we are not OK. This combination drives our actions to try to get the unwanted emotion to stop as soon as possible. For example, it is culturally acceptable and common in many families to blame one's anger on someone else: *He made me mad.* This leads us to feel as though if we "let him have it," we will feel better. Point out that if instead, we focus on helping everyone understand that no one can actually *make someone else* feel any way, we can use our energy to each take care of our own big feelings. Once we've taken care of ourselves while the angry feeling is there and our fire-truck brain is no longer calling the shots, we can think through what happened and develop a conscious, thoughtful response.

Because our brains are often trying to tell us that *It is someone else's fault I feel this way*, it helps to have a breathing exercise with a mantra to drown out the brain's rather unhelpful narrative. I call this tool "Relaxation Breathing," and it is the only new skill you teach at this session. You will spend time reviewing what has worked so far, problem-solving what hasn't worked, and identifying not only barriers that have arisen but also the barriers to addressing the barriers.

Strategies for Change

This session tends to be about barriers to change. Following is a list of common barriers with some simple next steps. Cocreating the next PDSA cycle around addressing these can help support PCEs and mitigate stress. Remember, you may need to reach out to co-parents or caregivers who are unable to be present and share the ideas for addressing barriers over the phone or in a subsequent visit.

- **Being unable to catch emotions when they are small, before they get too big:** Support parents in identifying what always happens before the "meltdown" or before their children fight; work to integrate healthy coping skills before that.
- **Parents' awareness of fire-truck brain:** Parents may need to first use validation and self-care to return their child to a calmer nervous system state *before* the parent expects the child to be able to use their words to explain themselves or do their chores or another wanted behavior (NICER parenting).
- **Doing breathing exercises, for both child and parent(s):** When we are still in fight-or-flight mode, it may be difficult for us to use our breath; using toes-to-nose or 5-4-3-2-1 *first*, before trying to do breathing exercises, can help.

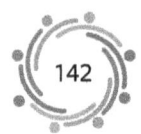

- **Using the stress ball for angry feelings or glitter jar for worried feelings:** Some kids will just throw the ball when they are angry or refuse to use the glitter jar when they are nervous; giving options to the child for what is available to them for self-care for this feeling in this moment, as well as parents modeling the strategies, can help.
- **Parents become frustrated with their child:** If the child's lack of follow-through or defiance is causing embarrassing situations for the parent, they may be stuck in fight-or-flight mode and actually be seeing their child consciously or subconsciously as the source of danger; review the neurohormonal stress response and how SUNBEAM can help parents put the affiliate response to use, which can help them remember they are in this together with their child.
- **Being unable to improve sleep hygiene:** Parents will often say they are trying everything but their child is still not sleeping; practice the bedtime version of toes-to-nose in the office. Have the child lie on the exam table and pretend they are going to bed, then walk them through putting their body to sleep, starting with their toes and working their way up to their nose, eyes, and head. The Public Broadcasting Service has an Elmo version of toes-to-nose (https://youtu.be/yhRWp0wOLyo), which may engage children and facilitate improved sleep hygiene over time.
- **Parents become dysregulated with their child's "whining" or high energy:** Recommend that they use toes-to-nose with their child to calm a hyperactive body or distract from minor aches and pains. High-energy kids may need high-energy coping skills, like running around the backyard 5 times or doing 50 jumping jacks.

In addition, the 4 building blocks of HOPE worksheets help you review confounding stressful factors to more broadly mitigate stress. These building blocks include relational health and emotional growth but also extend to environment and engagement. Ask permission to explore how these areas are going for them through a resilience lens, and celebrate sources of support and strength they already have in place. Give the kids and parents a building blocks worksheet and encourage the child to fill it out, if that is age appropriate (or the parent can write answers). If neither parent nor child wants to do the writing, you can have a verbal discussion and take notes on the worksheet for them. Depending on time considerations, you can either work on it during the session or invite them to work on it at home and bring it back to discuss at the next session. When you review it, celebrate anything they have identified and explain it as noted in Chapter 3. If the child lives in multiple households, you can send copies home for the child to do with their other caregivers.

Next, help the child make a *My Little Book of Big Feelings* (see Figure 2-4). Take 5 sheets of plain printer paper, fold them in half lengthwise, and then cut them in the center, creating 2 small, almost square 10-page booklets. Staple each along the

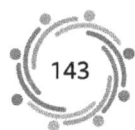

folded edge to make a little book. Bring in markers and start with writing *My Little Book of Big Feelings* on the cover. You can also write the child's name (eg, *Joey's Little Book of Big Feelings*) and then start filling it in together with the child.

Ask them to pick the feeling they are struggling the most with. For example, if they pick "sad," draw a sad face on one of the pages, then write the words that go with that feeling (start with *sad*, ask the child if there are any other words they would use for that face, and write them too). Next ask the child what helps them when they feel like that, writing that list below the drawing and descriptors. Then, open to a new page, ask for another feeling, draw an image, and write all the words the child uses to describe that feeling. Then, ask them for self-care strategies that help and note them below. If they are struggling with self-care strategies, it is OK to celebrate the use of media in their self-care plan. For example, if they find the Daniel Tiger "When You Feel So Mad" song (www.pbs.org/video/daniel-tigers-neighborhood-when-you-feel-so-mad-song) helpful, that might be a good starting place.

Leave a page after each feeling and tell the kids that this is their own reference book for themselves, like an encyclopedia all about their feelings. They can add to it later and go back and use it as needed. You can start with a 10-page book, which can hold 4 or 5 feelings. If you want to, you can use 10 pieces of paper initially to make a 20-page book, which gives the child more opportunities to add their own ideas later, over time.

Homework

For homework, cocreate a plan for what the family wants to work on. If they filled out a building blocks worksheet, is there a specific resource you can offer to help support them in strengthening one of the 4 building blocks? You can cocreate a PDSA cycle to try to connect to this resource. From the questions you asked at the beginning of the session, identify a few things the parents want to work on between now and the final session. Choose one and cocreate a PDSA cycle for it; perhaps it's remembering to use validation. They may need you to reassure again that it is OK to validate feelings even when they don't want to see the same behaviors. They could use a habit-stacking approach to validate the feelings behind the behaviors before they speak with their child about how the child is behaving. If the parents identified issues with implementing NICER parenting or SUNBEAM, cocreate a plan with 1 or 2 strategies they can try in the form of habit stacking with a PDSA cycle to address barriers to implementing those strategies. For example, if they tend to still try to discipline in the heat of the moment, have them just try to pause for 5 Big Deep Breaths before they do any discipline as they check in with their own emotional state. Encourage the child to keep working on their *My Little Book of Big Feelings* when they get home. Ask the child and the parents to watch for areas where things are still consistently hard and bring them to the final session.

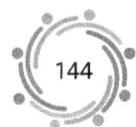
Session 4

Rooming and Scheduling

For this final session, I like to print and sign a "graduation" certificate for the child (**Figure 5-5**; also available in Appendix AA), so print and fill this in ahead of time. The scheduling of this last session should be at least the same as the distance between sessions 2 to 3 to account for any visitation schedules and allow for all caregivers to try new cycles of change. There are no specific MA instructions for this session.

Figure 5-5.

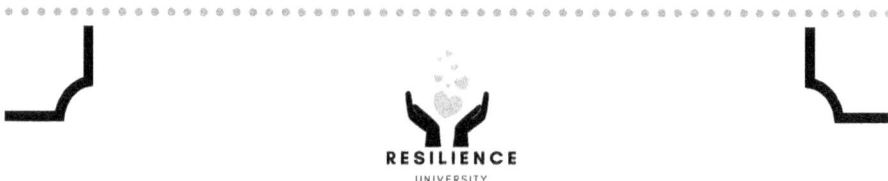

CERTIFICATE OF COMPLETION

This certifies that on this   day in the month of
in the year

has satisfactorily completed
Resilience University
and now has
emotional agility superpowers!

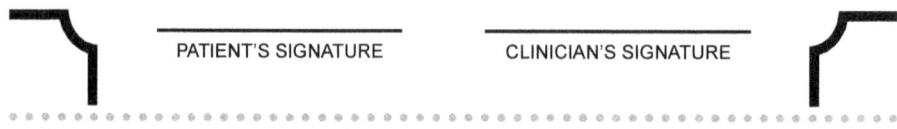

PATIENT'S SIGNATURE   CLINICIAN'S SIGNATURE

Resilience University "graduation" certificate.

Supplies and Handouts

Bring in the certificate of completion, as well as the stress-buster wheel diagram (see Figure 1-10), a 9-5-2-1-0 checklist (Appendix P), and the self-care super-powers sticker chart (Appendix BB). Bring in paper and color markers and/or crayons. If you have starter stickers to provide for the charts, bring those in as well. You will be reinforcing many of the prior tools at this session, so you may want to have additional handouts available if needed.

Check-In

When I welcome the family back for the last session, I open with the same questions as always: *How have things been going since I saw you last?*

Frame With Strengths

Honor how much work they have been doing and how exciting it has been for you to work with them. Ask about what they are noticing. Ask, *What are you proud of? What has worked well? Not so well? New concerns since the previous visit?* Were there any family strengths or connections restored from completing a building blocks worksheet?

Review

Review their homework with them. From the building blocks worksheet, ask the parents, *Do you need any other resources?* Ask the child, *How has your* My Little Book of Big Feelings *come out?*

Reflect and Celebrate

This session encompasses plenty of time for reflection and celebration, giving the family a chance to distill what they have learned and have been able to do into a fluid, adaptable strategy going forward. Give them a printed copy of either Nadine Burke Harris' stress-buster wheel or a stress reduction plan (see Appendix O) and review how each of the areas can help offset stress and foster wellness. I remind them that this, just like the building blocks and PCEs, is a dynamic array of strategies. No family is expected to have all of these all the time. Again, I use the equalizer or music app analogy and reinforce that life is a symphony, not a grocery list. I have them write at least a few strategies they can usually apply from each piece of the pie and celebrate the new tools and skills. If they are struggling to think of things, you can use the template in Chapter 4 (see Figure 4-3). Make sure they have the thing that they would normally do and then at least 1 to 2 backups in each area. For example, *If your exercise is usually going to the park, how would you exercise if it were pouring rain?*

As you are filling these out with them, you can explore and reinforce the strategies they've already learned: *Do you feel confident using the building block framework not only to know what might be needed but also to celebrate what is going well? Do you feel confident using at least one of the mindfulness strategies? Have you tried/do you think you can use toes-to-nose for sleep* [or *aches and pains* or *to calm a hyperactive/anxious body*]*? Do you feel like everyone is starting to talk about feelings? How are you* [parent] *doing with pausing for 5 breaths and taking a minute for self-care when you feel like you might yell or "lose your cool"? As a family, do you feel like everyone is focusing more on emotions and connection instead of punishment and discipline?* Using the 9-5-2-1-0 checklist on the fridge can be a useful tool to continue with

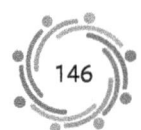

general good health recommendations around nutrition, exercise, sleep, screen time moderation, and hydration.

Make sure everyone is comfortable using at least one breathing exercise and one mindfulness technique. Ask if they are beginning to know which type of self-care strategy works best in each scenario and for each feeling. Revisit again the idea of catching emotions when they are small and taking a break for self-care. Ask how this is going. Check in about the self-care nook and if this was helpful. If they haven't set one up, be curious about why. Ask if they need help problem-solving where to put the self-care nook or how to set it up; you can walk them through a PDSA cycle. Maybe it seemed too loud to have it in the living room, but no one wanted to create a shared space in their own bedroom, so you could work with them to find a cozy spot elsewhere in the house or encourage each person to create their own spot in their own space.

Have the kids make a self-care superpowers sticker chart. If you aren't feeling artistic, you can just use one of the printed templates (see Appendix BB). You can explain it to them like this: *Just like you don't even think about getting food when you're hungry or a blanket when you're cold, over time you will be able to use these healthy coping skills without even having to think about using them. Think of these as your superpowers. Meditation, breathing exercises, and mindfulness are things you can take with you anywhere and do anytime, no matter what.*

For the chart, pick one or more feelings that seem to still be derailing the day. Encourage the child to practice self-care and healthy coping skills, and remind the parents to celebrate *any* attempt. They can decorate it and use stickers, check marks, *x*'s, stars, or anything they want to document an attempt at self-care when the child has that feeling. Remind them that they are not waiting for perfection but working on skill building, and the idea of the chart is to celebrate *any* attempt, even if in the end it felt unsuccessful. Use the analogy of learning a new sport, if that feels helpful here. Reinforce the importance of emotion coaching and how parenting is a long-distance event, not a sprint.

Remind the kids that it's OK to not be OK when things are hard. Things won't always be this hard. Taking care of ourselves and each other is really important.

Graduation

Check in with the parents and ask them what other services or referrals they may still want or need. If there are any recommendations you have for further therapy or services/support, explain what benefit they might bring and offer to make connections. Ask if they want to do a follow-up in a month or after they have had more time to work on these strategies. Make sure they have enough copies of any helpful handouts if the school or child care providers need them. Before they leave, give the kids a signed graduation certificate (see **Figure 5-5**).

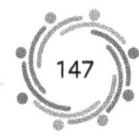
References

1. Tronick E, Gold CM. *The Power of Discord: Why the Ups and Downs of Relationships Are the Secret to Building Intimacy, Resilience, and Trust.* Little, Brown Spark; 2020

2. Bethell C, Jones J, Gombojav N, Linkenbach J, Sege R. Positive childhood experiences and adult mental and relational health in a statewide sample: associations across adverse childhood experiences levels. *JAMA Pediatr.* 2019;173(11):e193007 PMID: 31498386 doi: 10.1001/jamapediatrics.2019.3007

3. Huang CX, Halfon N, Sastry N, Chung PJ, Schickedanz A. Positive childhood experiences and adult health outcomes. *Pediatrics.* 2023;152(1):e2022060951 PMID: 37337829 doi: 10.1542/peds.2022-060951

4. Hooven C, Gottman JM, Katz LF. Parental meta-emotion structure predicts family and child outcomes. *Cogn Emotion.* 1995;9(2–3):229–264 doi: 10.1080/02699939508409010

5. Paruthi S, Brooks LJ, D'Ambrosio C, et al. Recommended amount of sleep for pediatric populations: a consensus statement of the American Academy of Sleep Medicine. *J Clin Sleep Med.* 2016;12(6):785–786 PMID: 27250809 doi: 10.5664/jcsm.5866

Using Relationship-Based and Trauma-Informed Anticipatory Guidance

American Academy of Pediatrics (AAP) policy statements and Bright Futures guidelines[1] help clinicians prioritize what guidance to offer for each developmental stage at routine health supervision visits. Anticipatory guidance is designed to help caregivers anticipate what needs may arise regarding the child's growth development between this visit and the next. Yet we may notice barriers families face when trying to operationalize our anticipatory guidance recommendations. For example, we routinely recommend that school-aged children participate in activities or sports. For some families, making this happen is a relatively simple process; it may be stressful at times, but participating ends up being a form of positive stress. For other families, the barriers are compounded and may be prohibitive (eg, lack of transportation, inability to get a sports physical in time, costly equipment) and feel overwhelming.

This chapter provides a way to integrate the tools and strategies you have already learned from this book into an expanded Plan-Do-Study-Act (PDSA) cycle (**Figure 6-1**) to tailor anticipatory guidance accounting for the diversity of families we serve. The first step is to honor family strengths. Second, identify a barrier to integrating the anticipatory guidance recommendations. Third, take a moment for self-care since many of these barriers can feel overwhelming and seem insurmountable at first. The fourth step is to clarify the barrier and choose an area to address. The fifth step is to cocreate a plan with the family. And the sixth step is to plan to follow up and see how the plan worked. If it did not work, you cocreate a new plan and follow up within a short interval after the family has tried it in the form of another brief PDSA cycle.

Figure 6-1.

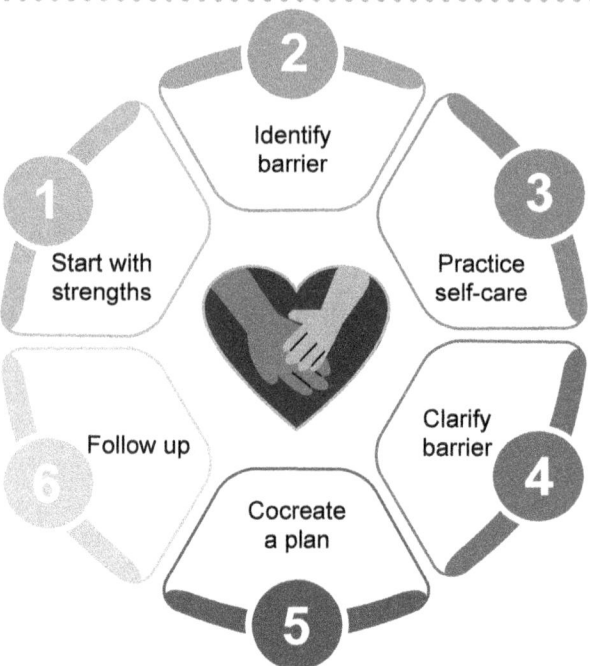

A 6-step, family-centered approach to relationship-based, trauma-informed anticipatory guidance.

Adapting how we offer anticipatory guidance to support families experiencing high levels of stress and trauma, as well as complex social drivers of health (SDOH), increases access to these valuable recommendations. Trauma-informed anticipatory guidance allows us to embrace the diversity of our families' experiences, and integrates the cocreation of plans to address barriers, through a lens that supports positive childhood experiences (PCEs) and the repair of relationship ruptures.

Establishing Trust

We live in a world flooded by information sources, many of which are not grounded in evidence-based research. Since you are a pediatrician, families look to you for knowledge, and the relationship you establish with parents as a trusted source of information is a form of *epistemic trust* or "the willingness to accept new information from another person as trustworthy, generalizable, and relevant."[2] Epistemic trust is key in human development, fostering an "openness to social learning and thus constitut[ing] a source of resilience through increasing the individual's capacity to benefit from social relationships."[3] In modern health care settings, the advice provided by a clinician may not immediately be trusted by parents or caregivers. Our health care encounters often involve a dance of the caregiver questioning the clinician's advice (referred to as "epistemic vigilance") and the clinician diligently answering questions and addressing the parent's or caregiver's concerns to reach a space of trust.[4] Parents are increasingly trusting of non-research–based sources of advice, such as influencers on social media. In a parallel process to providing trauma-informed care, we need to maintain our ability to stay open-minded, resist judgments, and continue with active listening as we negotiate the trust needed for parents to accept our anticipatory guidance. Especially when families have experienced trauma, engagement moves only at the speed of trust.[5]

It's completely normal to sometimes feel exhausted by this dance, so remember how important it is for you to practice your own self-care throughout your busy day. If you reframe feeling challenged as modeling how to be a trusted source of information, you as the clinician are also modeling steps the caregiver will hopefully re-create when they are providing advice to their growing child. This epistemic dance, from vigilance to trust, may resonate with parents of teenagers, and normalizing this process can promote an enhanced understanding of this dynamic when it arises within the relationship between caregiver and child. By honoring the lived experienced of parents and caregivers and responding to their concerns, we enhance trust as we model that we can listen and consider different points of view and reflect back to the family how their concerns fit within our professional experience and the research-based literature. Using a validation sandwich, which I call the VIVA (Validate, Inform, Validate, Ask) approach, provides you with a framework for this process (see Chapter 4, Process for Stepwise Change, and Figure 4-2).

Acknowledging Trauma

Trauma can be a barrier to integrating many of the standard anticipatory guidance recommendations. Bruce Perry's neurosequential model highlights how neural networks change both with traumatic experiences and in the absence of safe, stable, nurturing caregiver responses. A child's brain architecture develops differently depending on the environment, biology, and developmental stage.[6] For example, a "delay" in milestones may be related to not only the child's environment and biological structure but also the relational health between the primary caregiver and the child. For example, families experiencing trauma may be more apt to find themselves in a frustrating cycle of mutual dysregulation when trying to implement changes we recommend at routine health supervision visits.

Healthy coping skills and a stepwise response to problems can reduce the frequency of mutual dysregulation and support caregiver coregulation. Supporting

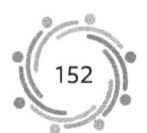

relational health by modeling self-care tools and problem-solving strategies can support relational health repairs in this crucial dyad. SUNBEAM (See, Unhook, Nurture, Breathe, Emotionally Aware, Mindful, Meditation) and NICER (Notice, Identify, Connect/coregulate, Explore, Review/repair) parenting help you walk parents and caregivers through the steps of Perry's sequential engagement and processing "Regulate [Reflect], Relate, Reason."[7] They're detailed in Chapter 4, Process for Stepwise Change (see the Trauma-Informed Positive Parenting and Trauma-Informed Parenting Self-Care sections). As clinicians, we can offer support on a multigenerational level, responding to the needs of both parents and children.[8] Clarifying the family's concerns, sharing your concerns and expertise, and then cocreating a plan by using active listening and encouragement results in a process parallel to trauma-informed, research-based interventions for behavioral problems.[8]

The "back the bus up" approach, also detailed in Chapter 4 (see the Retrospectively Backing the Bus Up section), helps parents see that behaviors aren't inherently "bad"; rather, they are a bid for connection and often a normal response to a difficult situation. Parents can learn new change processes to work toward offering a coregulation space more consistently and to respond in a predictable, moderate, and controlled manner. We can also support parents in recognizing when they are in a dysfunctional relational pattern with their child and the child repeats unwanted behaviors to get a predictable response from their parents, even if it is unpleasant, because predictability is reassuring.

Trauma-informed parenting tools (like NICER parenting and SUNBEAM) support a parent's ability to provide coregulation, see behaviors as a symptom of something else, and foster an understanding of the developmental stage and needs of their child. By viewing our anticipatory guidance through this dynamic lens, we support a growth mindset for our patients and their caregivers. A *growth mindset* refers to the belief that one's talents and abilities can be developed (through effort, strategies, and feedback) over time.[9] If families are used to a fixed mindset, where individuals believe their talents and abilities are innate, they may feel like change is futile or lack a sense of agency that anything they do will result in an improvement. As we have explored in previous chapters, SDOH and lived experiences of poverty and toxic stress can reify this sense that nothing can ever change. Having a growth mindset in the context of anticipatory guidance means we prepare families with tools and skills to try small tests of change so they can work toward our recommendations, rather than simply expect them to be able to do what we say. Normalizing this within the context of parent-child relationships, we can address barriers to repairing relational health ruptures: ruptures are normal, and repairs (especially when families have experienced trauma) may take some trial and error.

Toxic levels of stress can lead both parents and children to feel like they need to barter for essentials, including connection. Yet in this setting, everything becomes

transactional rather than relational. When parents literally need more support and resources than they have, it is understandable that they may expect more from their child than is developmentally appropriate. When children need more connection and coregulation than parents feel they can give, it's normal for children to behave in a manner that attracts attention (positive or negative). Part of shifting toxic stress to tolerable is honoring this perceived need for a child to always behave appropriately. Framing the parent's understanding of behaviors through an "anatomy of a meltdown" lens, detailed in the Anticipatory Guidance Tools section later in this chapter, can help them put the affiliate response to use and adopt a "we can do this together" approach. Teaching parents SUNBEAM can support shifting away from a frustrating, transactional, often adversarial stance to a more nurturing dyadic dance. We can emphasize from Tronick's research that parents who have experienced low levels of stress and trauma are attuned to their kids about 30% of the time and can normalize that the bulk of caregiver-child interactions will be a mixture of mis-attunements, disconnections, and subsequent repairs.[10]

When our intention is to provide universal trauma-informed care, our anticipatory guidance can feel more meaningful in every encounter. The Rutgers University behavioral health program[11] lists 5 core principles for providing universal trauma-informed precautions:

1. Take into consideration the impact of pervasive crises (eg, the COVID-19 pandemic).
2. Use therapeutic communication.
3. No room for judgments.
4. Create a healing environment.
5. Practice self-care.

These principles, within the context of providing guidance, support families in integrating evidence-based recommendations. Using active listening, honoring pervasive stressors such as racism and violence, and catching yourself when you are judging all foster a healing environment. In addition, supporting each other as clinicians in doing this work includes peer support practices as well as consistent, regular self-care.

By *self-care* here, I am referring to the same type of coping skills we are sharing with patients and parents, not a weekend at the spa or a Wednesday night yoga class. Those things are great, but here, I'm referring to how you take care of your own stress in the moment, while you are providing care. **Figure 6-2** outlines what providing universal trauma-informed care might look in the course of your day. Universal trauma-informed precautions also apply to us as clinicians. Remember, try to avoid judging yourself! If you catch yourself judging how you handled something, just notice it and practice self-care as instructed in Chapter 3,

Essential Toolkit (eg, 5 Big Deep Breaths, toes-to-nose body scan, 5-4-3-2-1 sensory grounding, loving-kindness meditation); ask open-ended questions; and keep going. We're learning these tools and strategies alongside the families we care for.

Figure 6-2.

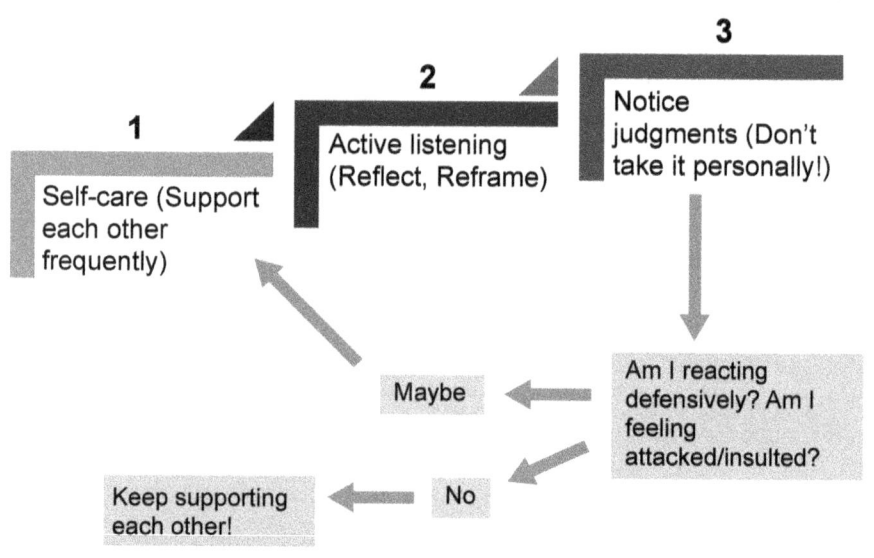

A stepwise approach to offering universal trauma-informed care precautions.

Identifying Barriers

Elements of our anticipatory guidance, while designed to be universal, can feel out of reach for many families. The barriers to equitable access tend to involve stress, trauma history, and SDOH. Having a stepwise approach to promote equitable access begins with curiosity. Think of how many times one of your mentors in residency talked through breastfeeding issues. You heard different approaches from many different experienced clinicians. In any clinical scenario, you had a depth and breadth of recommendations based on a myriad of your mentors' clinical experience. As long as you remain curious about what the barriers to breastfeeding are, you can dig into your memory bank and offer ideas to address them. For many of us, we simply haven't had that same level of depth and breadth in addressing relational health ruptures and obstacles to resilience factors.

Anticipatory guidance includes parenting advice to promote healthy physical and mental development. In a Zero to Three[12] National Parent Survey, parents

gave primary care providers a "D" for the usefulness of our parenting advice. Tronick's research has shown that blanket advice not only is unhelpful but can be harmful when it doesn't take into account the complex, dynamic nature of relationships between caregivers and children.[13] When we view anticipatory guidance as a dynamic area that requires a trauma-informed approach, our parenting advice is less rote and more accessible, tangible, and useful.

It's also crucial that we're aware of when and how intergenerational transmission of trauma may occur within families. Neuroplasticity and epigenetic regulation create an opportunity for families to shift this process with new family routines, behavioral patterns, and environmental factors. We know that parents who have a history of trauma are more likely to interpret natural, mismatched interactions with their children in a negative way.[14] Our dynamic parenting advice can include self-care practices that support "neuroceptive safety,"[15] making mutual dysregulation less likely.

Parenting guidance supporting natural mismatches and repairs also puts the affiliate response to work by reminding caregivers that their child is not the proverbial saber-toothed tiger. Rather, their child may be struggling to tie their shoes and slowing down the exodus from the house, but the child and the caregiver are inherently in this experience together. When parents feel stressed and notice that they are seeing their child as the cause of this stress, they're able to take a minute to breathe deeply and regulate their own nervous system first. If they are then less entrenched in fight-or-flight mode, there is a better chance they will be able to restore a felt sense of safety for the child and be available physically and emotionally for the upcoming repair. The families I work with share vast differences in how each generation views apologizing to their kids.

For many parents, this is an entirely new concept. Many of us as pediatricians have not been coached in how to support relationship repairs. We can start with coaching parents on how to identify things from their childhood that they want to re-create for their kids, as well as what they definitely don't want to re-create. Each caregiver has their own relational health dance with a child, so ensure that any tips or strategies you offer are also available to caregivers who don't attend the office visits. For example, send home extra copies of any handouts you provide, specifically the trauma-informed parenting ones (ie, "NICER Parenting" and "SUNBEAM: A Parent's Antidote to Meltdowns"; see Appendixes W and X) and the problem-solving strategies (ie, "Fire-Truck Brain" and "Back the Bus Up: A Parent Problem-Solving Approach"; see Appendixes L and R).

Many families experiencing toxic stress are simultaneously experiencing poverty. Using poverty as a marker for potentially toxic stress, we can extrapolate impacts on psychological, social, and cultural decision-making. Some or all of

the following factors can affect both parents and children as an adaptive shift in their processing in response to overwhelming stress[16]:

- Overwhelmed by current stressors and less able to focus on future goals
- Difficulty advocating for their own educational needs or their child's
- Decreased confidence in learning new skills and succeeding
- Lower sense of agency that they can alter how their lives turn out
- Being less likely to take risks or try something new
- Sense of exclusion from society

Blanket parenting advice and recommendations may feel unrealistic to families living in this space. Providing dynamic, tailored, trauma-sensitive guidance with stepwise problem-solving strategies can be encouraging for families and support their agency. When a parent is presenting to us as overwhelmed and stressed, we need to know how to immediately shift into Heather Forkey's "building the buffering" strategy while remaining mindful that if a parent's choices don't appear to us to be in line with our recommendations, it may be related to modifiable barriers and be a consequence of this adaptive shift in processing. This chapter will help you identify shared goals and cocreate a safe, effective path forward.

Barriers can come in many forms but universally include the natural neuro-hormonal stress responses: "fight," "flight," or "freeze" (**Table 6-1**). Fighting is generally not tolerated in the clinical setting and, without a trauma-informed response, may limit access to care. Similarly, a flight response may result in no-shows and decrease access. Freezing may be hard to identify, as families may be stuck in frustrating patterns or appear to be understanding but not be in a space where they can process or act on new information. Also, when power dynamics exist between a physician and a parent or caregiver, families may feel like they have to appease us or we might report them to child protective services or somehow threaten their relationship with their children. Remaining mindful of these responses, along with the 5 principles of universal trauma-informed precautions, allows us to better understand the needs of our families and what may be preventing access to protective factors, PCEs, and standard anticipatory guidance recommendations.

Barriers can be a stressful concept for us. We tend to see barriers as concrete and immovable when we've not had practice responding to them. Once we've named a barrier, we can begin a series of change cycles to support the family in addressing it. While sometimes we may be unable to fundamentally "move" this barrier, we may be able to decrease the impact it is having on the developing child either through mitigating the stress it causes or via an alternative route to the recommendation. For example, perhaps a child cannot play sports because they have to babysit their little sibling after school. We can use VIVA to invite the parents to cocreate an alternative

way for the child to be involved in an activity where they feel they matter and will have nonparent adults who take a genuine interest in them as well as an opportunity to feel supported by friends. Perhaps this ends up being a Sunday school group or a Girl Scout troop where another parent can bring them at times that don't overlap with babysitting responsibilities.

Table 6-1. Potential Barriers to Implementing Anticipatory Guidance

Potential Barrier	Examples
Relational stressors	Interpersonal violence, yelling, unrepaired relational health ruptures, mutual dysregulation, viewing behaviors as an intentional affront, unfamiliar with how to play
Practical stressors	Insecurity around employment, food, housing, transportation, diapers, and/or child care; unmet mental and physical health needs; lack of safe places to play
Parental relationship with their own parents (including parents' adverse childhood experiences)	Intergenerational trauma, learned response patterns, suboptimal coping strategies, familiar only with harsh discipline responses to behaviors
Misaligned developmental expectations	Expecting a child to regulate before they are developmentally ready or without consistent coregulation from a parent, expecting language beyond capabilities, delayed development arising from trauma history
The child's temperament	Sensory sensitivity, developmental and neurological variation, impulsivity, oppositionality, anger, anxiousness
School difficulties	Impulsivity, defiance, oppositional behaviors, inattentiveness, trouble making friends, bullying framed as the child overreacting
Exposure to racism and/or community violence	Inequitable access to protective factors; inequitable impact of stress; power dynamic affecting the ability to connect to necessary resources or supports; inequitable access to safe, child-friendly activities
Lack of agency	Lived experience of things being static even if change is desired, sense of outcomes being out of one's control, inability to afford or connect to essential resources or supports
Inexperience with effective change strategies	Lived experience of being unable to change circumstances and outcomes, history of incomplete attempts to make a change in the past, inequitable access to resources and supports needed for successful change
Educational disempowerment	Barriers to getting an education feeling impossible to change, parental stress and an adversarial relationship with the school amplifying disempowerment, inequitable access to understanding the educational process (ie, cultural or language barriers)
Inequitable access to protective factors	Talking about feelings not part of the family culture, seeing each other as causes of stress, isolation, household factors affecting friendships, financial constraints for activities

Cocreating a Plan

Diving Deeper

We rely on honesty from our families, but sometimes without meaning to, we don't authentically welcome it. Again, curiosity is key. For example, parents may not tell you they smoke inside because they know you will just tell them not to. Instead of listing dos and don'ts, stay curious about what challenges families face when working toward your recommendations. For example, if an adult consistently becomes angry with the other when asked to smoke outside, it may be safer to have the family create a smoking room where the kids don't play, rather than continue to expect the adults to be able to create an entirely smoke-free home. Useful anticipatory guidance has to be dynamic and applicable within the context of a realistic relational health lens. Instead of trying to make families fit within narrow, prescriptive guidelines, we can make our guidelines flexible and adaptable to each family's unique experience, recognizing the role stress plays.

As I've noted before, stressed parents commonly interpret their child as a source of their stress, perhaps seeing them as intentionally trying to bother, upset, or manipulate them. Then they're likely to share this view with others. As people label a baby a "drama queen," this affects how everyone responds to the infant. Patterns can persist as the child grows, changing the arena within which future relational health repairs will occur. Parents who had insecure attachments in their own childhood may be unable to see how a crying child is using a developmentally appropriate form of communication. Sharing a nonjudgmental response to these expressions supports parents in letting go of their childhood narratives and fostering safe, stable, nurturing relationships. Try using VIVA to respond in these scenarios:

> Validate: *Of course you feel like she is trying to ruin the day when she has a tantrum as you're leaving the house! A lot of parents feel that way.*
>
> Inform: *Oftentimes, crying is a bid for connection and a sign that the child might have an unmet need or big emotion they are struggling with.*
>
> Validate: *It's totally normal to interpret this as intentional.*
>
> Ask: *Would you like to explore different ways to respond in those moments that might help you develop trust and strengthen your relationship with your daughter?*

One aspect of anticipatory guidance is asking what parents enjoy about their child in order to celebrate strengths and support nurturing relationships. But when a family is enduring potentially toxic levels of stress, it can be difficult to enjoy *anything*, including the child. Asking this type of question can bring up feelings of shame and guilt, especially if parents are experiencing burnout. Research has shown that "exhausted parents disengage emotionally rather than physically, i.e., they provide practical care such as feeding or sleeping but [become] less emotionally involved, sensitive and responsive to their offspring."[17] Instead of asking this

question, we may want to lean in with curiosity and ask about how they connect with their child when it feels like things are unraveling. Maybe they all watch a movie or eat ice cream; ask and celebrate it as a strength.

Did you learn in medical school that about 1 in 7 parents regrets having children?[18] I didn't. Research from Poland suggests that this may be even more common among parents who have experienced high levels of adversity themselves,[19] which aligns with what we know about how trauma can affect a caregiver's interpretation of a child's behaviors.[20] When we can witness honest expressions of how difficult it can be to raise a child, we can also decrease isolation, identify strengths, and connect families with needed coping skills, support, and resources. Normalizing parental exhaustion and stress welcomes vulnerability and a chance for us to honor their journey. Instead of pathologizing caregivers for typical stress responses, we can work closely with them, offering relational health strategies to support them just like we would medical strategies for an asthma exacerbation. Tools for this include the 4 building blocks of HOPE (Healthy Outcomes from Positive Experiences) worksheets (see Appendixes M and N), NICER parenting (Appendix W), and SUNBEAM (Appendix X) to support access to healthy coping skills and necessary supports and resources.

Trauma-informed approaches to behavioral problems involve us coaching parents to focus less on control and more on understanding. This includes helping them identify unmet needs, including necessary emotional support, and holding space for the trauma that both parent and child may have experienced. Imagine Susie who has a "tantrum" every time she "doesn't get her way." Her parents may instinctively double down on limits and rules to try to extinguish this behavior. They may attribute her kicking and crying in the shopping cart to the fact that she didn't get a new toy when the family was out shopping at a big box store. Perhaps out of frustration, one parent may have called her a "spoiled brat." When coached to look deeper, her parents can understand that she was just tired, hungry, and making a bid for connection because her parents had been yelling in the car. Not getting the toy allowed for an emotional release and, as Tronick points out, presents the parents with an opportunity for meaning making and repair. We can give these parents "permission" to shift their focus from Susie's behaviors to her internal circumstances and the need for a relational health repair. We can offer them some language and structure to apologize (ie, Authentic Apologies, detailed in the Anticipatory Guidance Tools section later in this chapter) and support reconnection. When parents see unwanted behaviors as a normal part of a dynamic repairable relationship, the stressful behaviors can become more tolerable and less likely to be experienced as toxic stress by either parent or child. As families practice doing this routinely, "tantrums" become less frequent, the child's behaviors feel easier to manage, parents feel more confident in responding to their child's needs, and both connection and repair become more accessible.

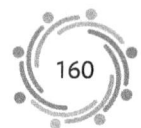

Observing Stress

Universal trauma-informed care means we must be mindful of the role that toxic stress and trauma play in our observations during clinical encounters. Consider a situation where a family is facing housing insecurity and the mother is not sure where she and her children are going to sleep that night and they happen to be in your office for a health supervision checkup. Mom may feel ashamed and that her lack of housing is her fault. She may worry that if she talks with you about it, you might report her to social services. She's in fight-or-flight mode while she is in your office and may be holding both her baby and her toddler close since she is used to keeping them near her. She may not be used to being in a safe, childproofed environment, so she isn't accustomed to letting them run free. She may appear tense and controlling. But none of this represents pathology; it is simply an adaptive response for uncertain times.

In other scenarios, we may see caregivers responding dismissively to their children or a child acting disrespectfully to their parents. Think for a moment about whether you acknowledge these interactions when you see them in the exam room. And if you do acknowledge them, what do you say? For years, the best thing I felt I had to offer in these scenarios was to refer out for family counseling. All too often, the family would decline and I'd leave the encounter with a heavy heart, observing relational health issues but being unable to offer anything. Now, I routinely offer PCE and relational health support. For example, being able to talk about your feelings with your family (a PCE) is grounded in the family's relational health. When asked, children will often share that they don't have anyone in their family they can talk about their feelings with. Many parents habitually react negatively to expressions of unpleasant emotions, taking them personally and being unable to listen or be there for their child, especially if rules have been broken. When parents become more adept at routinely regulating their own stressed nervous systems (SUNBEAM), they can better understand their child's need to talk about feelings (NICER parenting, "backing the bus up") and can validate their child's experiences.

Part of our role as primary care clinicians is to observe the interactions between parent and child. Being mindful that behaviors can either worsen or improve during a clinical encounter helps us take our observations lightly and stay curious. The way the family behaves in the office may not reflect what is going on at home but rather just be a stress response (or vice versa). If you see a caregiver harshly disciplining a child (eg, calling them names or yelling at them), lean in with curiosity and invite them to try backing the bus up for both caregiver and child. Maybe you identify that they couldn't find a parking spot outside the clinic and that the stress this created was the last straw. Conversely, a calm-appearing parent with children who follow every request may be a reflection of the child's fear of harsh discipline if they don't do exactly what the parent expects of them. You won't know if you don't ask.

Using VIVA to frame behaviors helps us request permission to explore what may be underneath the surface and ask parents if they are interested in shifting their interactions to support relational health and offset the long-term impact of adversity in childhood. If parents have asked you for help with behaviors before and it's been either unhelpful or ineffective (hence our "D" grade), they may not initiate asking for help again. Imagine a caregiver with a child who refuses to sit down and is banging the cupboards shut in the exam room. When you walk in, the caregiver is yelling at the child to "cut it out or else." VIVA would sound something like this:

> Validate: *It can be so hard to manage behaviors when you're in public with your kids and they act out.*

> Inform: *We know that behaviors often reflect an underlying unmet need or big emotion.*

> Validate: *It's totally normal to feel overwhelmed by the behavior itself, and sometimes that means we end up yelling or doing something we later wish we hadn't done.*

> Ask: *Do you want to try some different responses to these behaviors that may help you navigate these moments and understand what is driving these behaviors?*

When parents express frustration with their child during an office visit, we can use similar language to introduce the parents to SUNBEAM. Caring for their own frustration first, before the child's, builds parents' capacity to get out of stuck cycles in the way they relate to their children. Once they are feeling regulated, they can respond to their child's needs and emotions rather than just act out of their own frustration and react to their child's behaviors. Defiant behavior such as breaking the rules, especially in public, can feel sudden, throwing any parent off track. It is easy to take these kinds of behaviors personally, and many caregivers will frame them as the child intentionally trying to "ruin the day." Using the VIVA stepwise process, we can model and teach parents a trauma-informed response to their children's behaviors.

Family stress can make it difficult for children to follow rules and meet expectations. Stressed parents' emotions may escalate to harsh discipline (ie, name-calling or threatening) when the kids aren't responding to calmer tactics. While rules can help the parents regain a sense of control and may be particularly important when families are feeling unsafe, reconnecting and repair are the ultimate goal. Normalizing that big behaviors are so often bids for connection, not a sign that the parents are doing something wrong, can help. We can also frame how our responses to unwanted behaviors can align with the longer-term goal of establishing an internal locus of control for the child. Reviewing the "fire-truck brain" analogy (see the Applied Mindfulness: Mitigating a Multigenerational

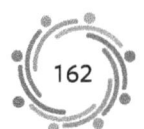

Neurohormonal Stress Response section in Chapter 3, Essential Toolkit) in the context of emotion coaching reminds parents that discipline is about teaching their child, not punishing them, and that parents need to have their prefrontal cortex "online" to teach (using SUNBEAM).

Reviewing developmental expectations can help parents understand where behaviors may be coming from and how not to take them personally. Parents may be reluctant to share that they routinely use harsh discipline tactics. Open a dialogue by validating how frustrating it can be when a child doesn't behave and how often this is developmentally appropriate. When parents can anticipate regressions during times of stress and transitions, they are less likely to take these personally. Adopting this coaching approach allows for flexibility in your anticipatory guidance and supports parental understanding of the dynamic emotional interplay between parents and their children.

Avoiding Judgment and Pathologizing

We are trained to label things as "healthy" or "unhealthy," "good" or "bad," or "positive" or "negative," but this habit can lead us to jump to unhelpful judgments. For many families experiencing potentially toxic levels of stress, we want to honor self-identified coping mechanisms as strengths. Over-pathologizing existing coping techniques like media use can be counterproductive and lead to an unnecessarily adversarial stance between you and the families you care for. Decades of research show that adults use screen time to help them lower stress.[21,22] During the COVID-19 pandemic, TV watching was a common adaptive, stress-reducing strategy.[23] We know that watching a favorite show can be extremely effective for managing a child's anxiety or stress.[24] Ask when, how, and why families rely on digital media, and ask if they're interested in adding in alternative stress-relieving strategies (eg, walking, singing, or loving-kindness meditation) to give everyone's nervous system a break from screens.

Similarly, shame can arise quickly when families feel chastised for trying to use screens to promote their infant's development or even just to relieve their own stress. While we know that digital media in the early years isn't an alternative to parental speech for developing language skills,[25] a parent watching a show with their child can foster shared attention and be a meaningful relational health rupture repair strategy. Similarly, a dysregulated parent may be making a safe choice to use screens as a temporary "babysitter" if they need time for self-care, especially after a relational health rupture. Be curious about how those essential serve-and-return interactions occur around screens in the home, and support the parents in making those a conscious part of the family's media use plan.

We know that not all families prioritize child-directed speech, so having a culturally and socially sensitive way of approaching this is essential.[26] Social drivers of health, cultural norms, and linguistic differences all play a role. The

controversial "30-million–word gap" suggests that, by the age of 4 years, children from professional families hear an average of 45 million words compared to a child in poverty who hears an average of 13 million words.[27] As we operationalize recommending that parents "talk with your child," we need to take into account a myriad of factors. Parents trying to make do with insufficient resources may find that their mental bandwidth is consumed by the stress of trying to make ends meet and keep their children safe at the expense of other aspects of life.[28] Even if we demonstrate how to talk to an infant in the office, barriers may prevent this from happening at home. Explore barriers with caregivers and invite them to cocreate a plan to increase child-directed speech if their child appears to have delayed speech milestones and this hasn't been a priority for them.

Supporting a parent's awareness of their own coping strategies can make it less likely they will unintentionally pass along unwanted ones through the human mirror neuron system.[29] Instead of pathologizing parental responses to stress and less ideal coping strategies, we can embrace where a family is and what is currently working for the family. Strategies for coping with frustration, anger, and worry are unintentionally passed down from generation to generation. Make sure parents know that babies have the ability to observe and execute novel tasks before language develops, which means they can begin imitating unwanted behaviors from a very young age.[30] We can lean in with curiosity about what isn't working and use VIVA to set the stage for cocreating a new path.

Supporting Serve and Return

Play becomes even more important when facing toxic stress and adversity,[31] yet families under stress may feel like they have neither time or mental bandwidth to play with their children nor access to safe play resources (eg, physical space, toys). They also may not have experienced being played with when they were little and therefore have no personal experience to draw from. Modeling play and offering ideas for how to connect in a playful way with children at different ages[32] can be helpful when we also ask if and how these ideas might work for them at home. Cocreating PDSA cycles (see the Plan-Do-Study-Act Cycles section in Chapter 4, Process for Stepwise Change) to integrate play into the family dynamic may be a useful next step. If families find it challenging to start these new routines, you can offer them the Attachment, Regulation and Competency Five-Minute Connection activities for caregivers and their kids.[33]

For families who feel like they don't have time to play with their kids, encourage them to include a playful approach to things like cleaning up, brushing teeth, and cooking dinner. The essence of play is not the behavior itself but the "motivation and mental attitude"[34] associated with the behavior. A playful attitude can help parents connect with a child during stressful times when tasks and chores need to be completed, and we can help caregivers understand that

interactions with kids don't have to be either fun or functional, but both can be true simultaneously.

Bypassing Blanket Advice

We may have our own unawareness about what is actually consuming the mental bandwidth of parents, which makes our advice sound generic and out of reach. "Depend on your social networks" and "maintain social contacts" are unhelpful recommendations when these valuable assets are routinely disrupted by factors outside a family's control. Imagine a mom who has just left a violent home; she and the kids are living in a shelter. She may be getting tons of unwanted advice, have no time to herself, be unable to connect with friends and family, and feel unsupported. She's likely unrested and feeling frustrated by her children's big emotional expressions, sleep problems, and/or behavioral issues. Frame your questions with a strengths-based foundation. Start with validating the journey they have been through; you can use VIVA and the strengths-based building block worksheets to explore PCEs and family supports. Ask if Mom would like more support in any of the 4 building block areas, and be prepared with tangible resources (eg, local support groups or video chatting with distant relatives). If you aren't sure of what to offer, the building block worksheets come with a list of suggestions to start with (see Appendix N).

Being Mindful of Financial Constraints

Economic constraints may also curtail a family's ability to follow our recommendations. Child care is expensive yet essential for parents who work outside the home. Trying to balance rent, food, and child care may mean choosing a less than optimal child care situation. Similarly, food choices that appear unhealthy may be the only options the family can afford. In my master's of public health program, we were encouraged to try to do our family's grocery shopping for a week on what we would be eligible for if our family depended on Supplemental Nutrition Assistance Program benefits. If you have not experienced a limited food budget before, you may want to try doing this for your family or yourself (www.fns.usda.gov) and notice how it feels to experience the financial trade-offs many families face daily. For example, see if you could afford fresh fruits and vegetables in addition to good sources of calcium and protein on this limited budget. The foods that are most affordable are often also nutrient poor and processed. Be mindful that families who rely on food pantries may not have much choice in what they offer their kids at meal and snack times.

When families are working with minimal resources, we can help prioritize goals and discuss levels of risk, including what factors do the most to ensure a child's safety and well-being. Choosing from an array of less-than-ideal circumstances may be the only option. It may be safer to have a child stay in a safe home with an elderly grandparent who feeds them processed cake snacks and allows the

child to watch TV all day, if the only other realistic option is a neighbor with similar-aged children and no TV but a partner with a history of violence. Dynamic anticipatory guidance includes honoring that a safe and media-free play space may just not exist in their current living situation. Harm reduction can include encouraging all caregivers to watch kids' shows and interact with the kids.

Financial constraints can also affect the consistency of nonparent adults in a child's life. Ongoing disparities prevent many families from maintaining consistency, with research showing that families with lower incomes are more likely to experience child care disruptions,[35] averaging one change annually in the first 3 years after birth.[36] Child care instability can negatively affect family well-being[37] and is linked with behavioral problems. Ensure that parents know this is not their fault, identify other protective factors, and frame these changes with a HOPE-informed lens. Emphasize how other nonparent adults who take an interest in their child's well-being can offset disruption in the child care setting.

Supporting Educational Goals

A significant amount of anticipatory guidance involves helping children succeed in school. We can support parents in advocating for their child's educational needs before the child is even in kindergarten. Without support, children who have experienced trauma may act out and be less able to access their education. Child care centers and preschools will sometimes expel or suspend a child for behavioral problems. Preschool children are suspended 3 times more frequently than children in K through 12.[38] This is another area where ongoing disparities mean the burden of suspensions disproportionately and unjustly affects certain children. Boys make up 54% of preschool enrollments but 75% of preschool suspensions and 82% of repeated suspensions. African American children comprise 18% of preschool enrollments but almost 50% of suspensions. Native American and Native Alaskan children represent less than 1% of preschool enrollments but 3% of suspensions. The US Department of Health and Human Services[39] states that expulsions and suspensions are detrimental to a child's education, removing the child from the learning environment, delaying the identification of underlying issues (disabilities or mental health issues), delaying the provision of necessary services, and increasing family stress. And we know that early suspension is correlated with a 10-fold increase in the chance of dropping out of high school, experiencing academic failure, holding negative attitudes toward school, and facing incarceration.

We can help parents on an individual level with dynamic support and leverage our own experience with the educational system to promote the family's agency. Children who are tired, hungry, or frightened, or who have other unmet needs, are more likely to act out. We can write letters and share resources to support our patients and help child care and preschool providers understand what is and isn't expected in the typical development of a child at this age.

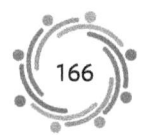
For example, in preschool, children are still learning to regulate their emotions, so expecting them to never become dysregulated is unreasonable developmentally. The tools and strategies you share with the family can also be shared with the school(s) to encourage positive discipline and respond to the needs underlying the behaviors. If your region has an early childhood consultation program, this is a great resource for a referral. Often, however, there is a delay in being able to connect to this resource as well as to early intervention services. The same trauma-informed behavioral approach with tools adapted for schools can help you bridge the gap between needs and availability of resources (eg, breathing, meditation, mindfulness, NICER parenting, SUNBEAM, fire-truck brain, backing the bus up).

When there's a concern for bullying, ensure that families are connected with the appropriate school officials. Before agreeing with anyone who may be saying the child is "overreacting," try to have a counselor observe the child's experience and assess the interactions. Trauma may affect the child's responses, and they may need coping skills. Unpleasant but age-appropriate interactions may trigger a child's trauma response, and they may need more support at school. In addition, consider using appropriate screening tools for mental health concerns and ensure that the parents know how to ask for a learning evaluation.

Schools may notice absenteeism rising or grades falling and note that the child has a conduct issue when it is actually more complex. Let's say a teen is experiencing toxic stress at home and has an undiagnosed processing disorder. They are getting failing grades and being yelled at by stressed parents that they're "ruining their future." They already feel like they are doing everything wrong and are telling themselves that no one wants to be around them, they can't do anything right, and they're unlovable. With SUNBEAM, we can help the parents calm their own nervous systems so they can see that the teen needs emotional support and validation of their experience, not a lecture on why they need to do more. We can teach the teen about how they don't have to believe everything they think (ie, "TikTok/YouTube brain"; see the Sensory Grounding section in Chapter 3) and prepare them with a few healthy coping skills (eg, relaxation breathing, 5-4-3-2-1; see those sections in Chapter 3) while we work with the parents to advocate in the school.

Familiarize yourself with the NICHQ Vanderbilt Assessment Scales packet for parents regarding educational rights. This educational rights parent/teacher packet was developed for kids with attention-deficit/hyperactivity disorder (ADHD) but can be applied to any mental health or physical diagnosis. Use the appropriate validated screening questionnaires such as the PHQ-9 Modified for Adolescents, Generalized Anxiety Disorder 7-item scale, and Vanderbilt parent/teacher forms to help you clarify any underlying diagnosis. Trauma symptoms can overlap with ADHD, depression, and anxiety symptoms, and our goal is to provide patient-centered trauma-informed care. Because someone has a trauma history does not mean they

shouldn't ever be treated for ADHD, anxiety, or depression; rather, these children should receive comanagement with mental health professionals and judicious use of medication.[40] Refer as you would normally for appropriate counseling, neuro-psychological testing, and/or psychiatry consultation, realizing that there could be a delay in obtaining these forms of care and that appropriate use of prescription medication may allow the child to have access to their education while awaiting referrals. If you are starting medication, you can combine "med check" appoint-ments with PDSA cycles to promote access to resources, supports, and healthy coping skills as a bridge to the referrals as discussed in the previous chapters.

Another place where we can help with supporting a child's educational access is in fully understanding the McKinney-Vento Homeless Assistance Act and the protec-tions it offers for students experiencing homelessness.[41] Many families experiencing poverty and toxic stress will also experience a period of homelessness. As noted in the Identifying Barriers section earlier in this chapter, poverty can affect a parent's agency in advocating for their child within the school system. We can support par-ents in identifying what their child might need in order to have equivalent access to their education and serve as a key player in ensuring all legal provisions are available to our patients. For example, McKinney-Vento–eligible students may be able to have access to additional funds that can be used for transportation, tutor-ing, and one-on-one support to catch up if they have missed substantial amounts of work because of the stress associated with becoming homeless. Another exam-ple of educational support is when a child has been referred for special education services. When neither parent is able to participate in the child's individualized education program or other school meetings, another adult can apply to be the homeless child's educational surrogate parent and sign forms and make educational decisions. If a homeless child is living with a friend or family member, their "house parent" may be interested in this role.

For patients who don't speak English, ask how they are translating material that comes home from school or other educational resources. Parents may feel like they are less able to be involved with their child's education if they are unable to read what gets sent home or emailed. Encourage the parents to ask for a translator within the school system and to use a translation tool such as Google Translate if they are without an interpreter and needing to communicate.

Anticipatory Guidance Tools

When I refer to "change/problem-solving strategies," "positive discipline," and "self-care/healthy coping skills" throughout this chapter, it refers to using the tools presented in this book. These are listed in **Table 6-2** in the categories where you may find them helpful.

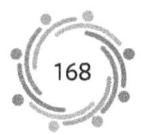

Table 6-2. Anticipatory Guidance and Resilience University Tools and Strategies

Tool or Strategy	Location in This Book
Positive Discipline	
SUNBEAM	Chapter 4, Appendix X
6 Steps to Connect	Chapter 6 (this chapter), Appendix EE
NICER parenting	Chapter 4, Appendix W
"Fire-truck brain" analogy	Chapter 3, Appendix L
Authentic Apologies	Chapter 6 (this chapter)
The Anatomy of a Meltdown	Chapter 6 (this chapter)
Leveling Up Your Container of Love	Chapter 6 (this chapter)
Emotion coaching	Chapter 4, Appendix Y
Validate, Validate, Validate	Chapter 4, Appendix V
Self-Care/Healthy Coping Skills	
5 Big Deep Breaths	Chapter 3, Appendix A
Relaxation breathing	Chapter 3, Appendix C
"Box" or "square" breathing	Chapter 3, Appendix B
Glitter jar meditation	Chapter 3, Appendix E
Walking meditation	Chapter 3, Appendix I
Loving-kindness meditation	Chapter 3, Appendixes G and H
Toes-to-nose	Chapter 3, Appendix K
5-4-3-2-1	Chapter 3, Appendix J
Using the breath (blowing bubbles/singing)	Chapter 3, Appendix D
Stress reduction plan	Chapter 3, Appendix O
Stress-buster wheel	Chapter 4
Change/Problem-Solving Strategies	
"Back the bus up" approach	Chapter 4, Appendix R
PDSA cycles	Chapter 4, Appendix Q
It's OK to Not Be OK	Chapter 6 (this chapter)
Time-versus-emotion curve	Chapter 3
Emotional awareness	Chapter 3, Appendix F
Strengths-based (HOPE) building blocks	Chapter 3, Appendixes M and N
VIVA	Chapter 4
Family feelings chart	Chapter 4, Appendix T
"10 Things I Can Do When I Feel Yucky" list	Chapter 4, Appendix U
My Little Book of Big Feelings	Chapter 2

Abbreviations: HOPE, Healthy Outcomes from Positive Experiences; NICER, Notice, Identify, Connect/coregulate, Explore, Review/repair; PDSA, Plan-Do-Study-Act; SUNBEAM, See, Unhook, Nurture, Breathe, Emotionally Aware, Mindful, Meditation; VIVA, Validate, Inform, Validate, Ask.

The following strategies are also useful when providing trauma-informed anticipatory guidance and tailored parenting advice:

Anatomy of a Meltdown

If a child is having a meltdown, this stepwise approach can help you and/or the caregiver understand what else is going on. Similarly, if 2 children are fighting, this can be a good place to start for each involved individual (children and caregivers). Validating feelings and planning for specific healthy coping skills can help prevent prolonged mutual dysregulation.

1. How is the child feeling?
2. How is the parent feeling?
3. How can the parent and child shift to tolerable stress and improve relational health?
4. How can they return to coregulation, away from mutual dysregulation?
    - Ahead of time, when they are in a calm state, have parents and children each make a list of things to do and self-care strategies for each feeling.
    - The parent notices the child's energy level and intensity of feelings and chooses their response accordingly.
    - Encourage the parent to address the child's underlying needs and feelings rather than focus only on their behavior.
    - Encourage the parent to practice self-care too, especially when they have a big emotional response themselves.

It's OK to Not Be OK

Instead of catastrophizing every time something goes "wrong," encourage parents and caregivers to try radically accepting the circumstances. We're not therapists, but we can offer key components to foster resilience and distress tolerance. For example, dialectical behavioral therapy[42] starts with radical acceptance of where we are in order to meaningfully change. By normalizing the parts of parenting that routinely feel abnormal to millions of parents, we can lower stress levels and promote bonding and nurturing.

Following is an example of how to talk with parents about these things:

It's not just "OK" to not be OK. It's normal! Take a minute to take care of yourself before responding to your child's behavior. Using walking meditation as you go upstairs to check on a crying baby helps you arrive calmer and more able to interpret your baby's needs. To do this, inhale and count a few steps while breathing in, then exhale and count the same number of steps while breathing out: breathe in 2, 3, 4 and breathe out 2, 3, 4; repeat.

Authentic Apologies

Apologies often aid in repairing relationship ruptures both within and outside the family. When parents haven't experienced sincere apologies themselves,

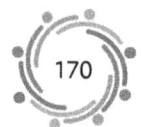

they may not know how to teach their child to apologize. Forcing an "I'm sorry" can be another source of conflict without a meaningful result. Instead, coach caregivers in a more meaningful response. For example, if a child threw a toy because they were angry and it hit another child, they may not want to apologize. Exploring the following 3 questions may lead to a more authentic repair:

1. What is one thing you can take full responsibility for? (I was angry and took it out on someone else instead of taking care of myself.)
2. What is one thing you are actually sorry for? (The other person got hurt.)
3. What can you do differently next time? (Ask for help from a grown-up when I start to feel frustrated.)

Leveling Up Your Container of Love

Kids need to be able to express their experiences and feelings and not worry about freaking out their parents. This may get harder as kids grow older. All parents can increase the strength of their emotional "container" using the following 3 simple steps (a fusion of Validate, Validate, Validate; NICER parenting; and SUNBEAM):

1. Validate whatever your child is expressing, even if you do not agree with how they are/were behaving.
2. Breathe. Take care of your own feelings so your child can take care of theirs.
3. Tell them you are right there loving them through this no matter what. You are prepared to support them even when things go sideways.

6 Steps to Connect

The AAP has 2 trauma-informed parenting resources, *The Three Rs: Ways to Support Your Child's Resilience*[43] and *Parenting Kids Who Have Experienced Trauma: Stop, Drop and Stay in Control*[44] to support parents in responding to their children after trauma. In my experience, these are useful when parents themselves are not also having some form of a neurohormonal stress response. When both child and parent have experienced trauma (synchronously or asynchronously), we can offer a concise combination of SUNBEAM and NICER parenting. This also is helpful for families in extremely stressful situations or when you yourself are overwhelmed with stress (eg, if you don't have materials in the language the parent speaks or are running behind on time). This simple 6-step process can be easily relayed to caregivers:

1. See that something has brought up big unpleasant feelings in you.
2. Unhook from your traditional response; try to be kind to yourself!
3. Nurture yourself with [*offer one specific strategy*] before you respond to your child.

4. Notice your child is also having a big feeling.

5. Identify what you think the feeling might be or just say *This is hard*.

6. Connect by doing [*choose a child-focused self-care strategy*] to create a coregulation space.

Once the parent's stress level is lower, encourage them to validate their child's experience. Invite them to think about hard things their child has accomplished recently. This can start with "low-hanging fruit," like getting out of bed. Help them model a way to share this with their child. It could sound something like "I notice things have been feeling really hard for you lately. I know it wasn't easy to get up and go to school this morning, and you did it anyway." If they want to add more, instead of saying, "I'm proud of you," which often ends up sounding to the child like it is all about the parents, they can say, "I have seen you overcome a lot of challenges while we have been going through a hard time as a family. I know it hasn't been easy, and I believe in you and your ability to do hard things."

Summary

In this chapter, we reviewed stepwise strategies to offering dynamic anticipatory guidance for families affected by toxic stress and trauma. Equipped with these approaches, you can help your patients and their families integrate the powerful protective effect of many of our standard anticipatory guidance recommendations even when they are experiencing potentially overwhelming stress. With this trauma-informed, relational health–based guidance, you can model a healthy stress response, consistently provide a coregulation space, and increase equitable access to anticipatory guidance for all families.

The next chapter presents a series of case vignettes illustrating how these strategies can be applied in daily practice.

References

1. Hagan JF Jr, Shaw JS, Duncan PM, eds. *Bright Futures: Guidelines for Health Supervision of Infants, Children, and Adolescents.* 4th ed. American Academy of Pediatrics; 2017 doi: 10.1542/9781610020237

2. Schröder-Pfeifer P, Talia A, Volkert J, Taubner S. Developing an assessment of epistemic trust: a research protocol. *Res Psychother.* 2018;21(3):330 PMID: 32913771 doi: 10.4081/ripppo.2018.330

3. Li E, Campbell C, Midgley N, Luyten P. Epistemic trust: a comprehensive review of empirical insights and implications for developmental psychopathology. *Res Psychother.* 2023;26(3):704 PMID: 38156560 doi: 10.4081/ripppo.2023.704

4. Caronia L, Ranzani F. Epistemic trust as an interactional accomplishment in pediatric well-child visits: parents' resistance to solicited advice as performing epistemic vigilance. *Health Commun.* 2024;39(4):838–851 PMID: 36967666 doi: 10.1080/10410236.2023.2189504

5. Covey SMR, Merrill RR. *The Speed of Trust: The One Thing That Changes Everything*. Free Press; 2008

6. Perry B. Examining child maltreatment through a neurodevelopmental lens: clinical applications of the neurosequential model of therapeutics. *J Loss Trauma.* 2009;14(4):240–255 doi: 10.1080/15325020903004350

7. Think:Kids. Insights: regulate, relate, reason. Massachusetts General Hospital. Accessed November 12, 2024. https://thinkkids.org/regulate-relate-reason

8. Perry BD, Ablon JS. CPS as a neurodevelopmentally sensitive and trauma-informed approach. In: Pollastri AR, Ablon JS, Hone MJG, eds. *Collaborative Problem Solving: An Evidence-Based Approach to Implementation and Practice*. Springer; 2019. Rosenbaum JF, ed. *Current Clinical Psychiatry* doi: 10.1007/978-3-030-12630-8_2

9. Dweck C. Managing yourself: what having a growth mindset actually means. Harvard Business Review. January 13, 2016. Accessed November 12, 2024. https://hbr.org/2016/01/what-having-a-growth-mindset-actually-means

10. Tronick EZ, Gianino AF. Interactive mismatch and repair: challenges to the coping infant. *Zero Three*. 1986;6(3):1–6

11. Department of Health, Division of Behavioral Health Services. Universal trauma informed care precautions. Rutgers University. Accessed November 12, 2024. https://sites.rutgers.edu/shp-shpri/trauma-informed-care-universal-precautions

12. *Tuning In: Parents of Young Children Tell Us What They Think, Know and Need*. Zero to Three, Bezos Family Foundation; 2016. Accessed November 12, 2024. https://www.zerotothree.org/resource/national-parent-survey-report

13. Tronick E, Gold CM. *The Power of Discord: Why the Ups and Downs of Relationships Are the Secret to Building Intimacy, Resilience, and Trust*. Little, Brown Spark; 2020

14. Forkey H, Griffin J, Szilagyi M. *Childhood Trauma and Resilience: A Practical Guide*. American Academy of Pediatrics; 2021 doi: 10.1542/9781610025072

15. Porges SW. Making the world safe for our children: down-regulating defence and up-regulating social engagement to "optimise" the human experience. *Child Aust.* 2015;40(2):114–123 doi: 10.1017/cha.2015.12

16. Sheehy-Skeffington J, Rea J. *How Poverty Affects People's Decision-Making Processes*. Joseph Rowntree Foundation; 2016. Accessed November 12, 2024. https://www.jrf.org.uk/report/how-poverty-affects-peoples-decision-making-processes

17. Roskam I, Raes ME, Mikolajczak M. Exhausted parents: development and preliminary validation of the parental burnout inventory. *Front Psychol.* 2017;8:163 PMID: 28232811 doi: 10.3389/fpsyg.2017.00163

18. Piotrowski K, Mikolajczak M, Roskam I. I should not have had a child: development and validation of the Parenthood Regret Scale. *J Fam Psychol.* 2023;37(8):1282–1293 PMID: 37796606 doi: 10.1037/fam0001158

19. Piotrowski K. How many parents regret having children and how it is linked to their personality and health: two studies with national samples in Poland. *PLoS One.* 2021;16(7):e0254163 PMID: 34288933 doi: 10.1371/journal.pone.0254163

20. Christie H, Hamilton-Giachritsis C, Alves-Costa F, Tomlinson M, Halligan SL. The impact of parental posttraumatic stress disorder on parenting: a systematic review. *Eur J Psychotraumatol.* 2019;10(1):1550345 PMID: 30693071 doi: 10.1080/20008198.2018.1550345

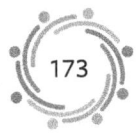
21. Eden AL, Johnson BK, Reinecke L, Grady SM. Media for coping during COVID-19 social distancing: stress, anxiety, and psychological well-being. *Front Psychol.* 2020;11:577639 PMID: 33391094 doi: 10.3389/fpsyg.2020.577639

22. Anderson DR, Collins PA, Schmitt KL, Jacobvitz RS. Stressful life events and television viewing. *Communic Res.* 1996;23(3):243–260 doi: 10.1177/009365096023003001

23. Boursier V, Musetti A, Gioia F, Flayelle M, Billieux J, Schimmenti A. Is watching TV series an adaptive coping strategy during the COVID-19 pandemic? insights from an Italian community sample. *Front Psychiatry.* 2021;12:599859 PMID: 33967845 doi: 10.3389/fpsyt.2021.599859

24. Trottier ED, Doré-Bergeron MJ, Chauvin-Kimoff L, Baerg K, Ali S. Managing pain and distress in children undergoing brief diagnostic and therapeutic procedures. *Paediatr Child Health.* 2019;24(8):509–535 PMID: 31844394 doi: 10.1093/pch/pxz026

25. Karani NF, Sher J, Mophosho M. The influence of screen time on children's language development: a scoping review. *S Afr J Commun Disord.* 2022;69(1):e1–e7 PMID: 35144436 doi: 10.4102/sajcd.v69i1.825

26. Schwab JF, Lew-Williams C. Language learning, socioeconomic status, and child-directed speech. *Wiley Interdiscip Rev Cogn Sci.* 2016;7(4):264–275 PMID: 27196418 doi: 10.1002/wcs.1393

27. Hart B, Risley TR. *Meaningful Differences in the Everyday Experience of Young American Children.* Paul H. Brookes Publishing; 1995

28. Mani A, Mullainathan S, Shafir E, Zhao J. Poverty impedes cognitive function. *Science.* 2013;341(6149):976–980 PMID: 23990553 doi: 10.1126/science.1238041

29. Thanikkal S. Mirror neurons and imitation learning in early motor development. *Asian J Appl Res.* 2019;5(1):37–42 doi: 10.20468/ajar/104654

30. Marshall PJ, Meltzoff AN. Neural mirroring mechanisms and imitation in human infants. *Philos Trans R Soc Lond B Biol Sci.* 2014;369(1644):20130620 PMID: 24778387 doi: 10.1098/rstb.2013.0620

31. Yogman M, Garner A, Hutchinson J, et al; American Academy of Pediatrics Committee on Psychosocial Aspects of Child and Family Health and Council on Communications and Media. The power of play: a pediatric role in enhancing development in young children. *Pediatrics.* 2018;142(3):e20182058 PMID: 30126932 doi: 10.1542/peds.2018-2058

32. Forkey H. The power of play: how fun & games help children thrive. HealthyChildren.org webinar. May 2, 2023. Accessed November 12, 2024. https://www.youtube.com/embed/figizs7ejKc

33. Attachment, Regulation and Competency. *Five-Minute Connection Activity Examples.* Accessed November 12, 2024. https://arcframework.org/wp-content/uploads/2020/03/Five-minute-connection-activities-updated.pdf

34. Gray P. *Free to Learn: Why Unleashing the Instinct to Play Will Make Our Children Happier, More Self-Reliant, and Better Students for Life.* Basic Books; 2013:160

35. Chaudry A. *Putting Children First: How Low-Wage Working Mothers Manage Child Care.* Russell Sage Foundation; 2004

36. Pilarz AR, Hill HD. Unstable and multiple child care arrangements and young children's behavior. *Early Child Res Q.* 2014;29(4):471–483 PMID: 25635158 doi: 10.1016/j.ecresq.2014.05.007

37. Pilarz AR, Sandstrom H, Henly JR. Making sense of childcare instability among families with low incomes: (un)desired and (un)planned reasons for changing childcare arrangements. *RSF*. 2022;8(5):120–142 doi: 10.7758/RSF.2022.8.5.06

38. Office for Civil Rights. *Civil Rights Data Collection: Data Snapshot; Early Childhood Education*. US Dept of Education; 2014

39. US Department of Education. *Policy Statement on Expulsion and Suspension Policies in Early Childhood Settings*. US Dept of Health and Human Services; 2016. Accessed November 12, 2024. https://www.acf.hhs.gov/sites/default/files/documents/ecd/expulsion_suspension_final.pdf

40. Keeshin B, Forkey HC, Fouras G, et al; American Academy of Pediatrics Council on Child Abuse and Neglect and Council on Foster Care, Adoption, and Kinship Care; American Academy of Child and Adolescent Psychiatry Committee on Child Maltreatment and Violence and Committee on Adoption and Foster Care. Children exposed to maltreatment: assessment and the role of psychotropic medication. *Pediatrics*. 2020;145(2):e20193751 PMID: 31964760 doi: 10.1542/peds.2019-3751

41. *The Most Frequently Asked Questions on the Educational Rights of Children & Youth in Homeless Situations*. National Association for the Education of Homeless Children and Youth, National Law Center on Homelessness & Poverty; 2017. Accessed November 12, 2024. https://naehcy.org/wp-content/uploads/2018/02/2017-10-16_NAEHCY-FAQs.pdf

42. Chapman AL. Dialectical behavior therapy: current indications and unique elements. *Psychiatry (Edgmont)*. 2006;3(9):62–68 PMID: 20975829

43. *The Three Rs: Ways to Support Your Child's Resilience*. Parent handout. American Academy of Pediatrics. Accessed December 2, 2024. https://downloads.aap.org/AAP/PDF/3%20Rs%20AAP.pdf%20FINAL.pdf

44. *Parenting Kids Who Have Experienced Trauma: Stop, Drop and Stay in Control*. Parent handout. American Academy of Pediatrics. Accessed December 2, 2024. https://downloads.aap.org/AAP/PDF/Responding-to-Trauma-English-Infographic_kids_trauma.pdf

Chapter 7

Examples of Tailored Anticipatory Guidance: Vignettes

The following vignettes are designed to bring to light specific strategies to make anticipatory guidance more accessible and relatable for families experiencing toxic or potentially toxic levels of stress. These approaches are designed to promote relational health and the affiliate stress response regardless of the context families find themselves in. I have intentionally used complex scenarios with multiple sources of stress to elucidate how you can still support families in integrating anticipatory guidance recommendations, even when they are facing multiple social drivers of health (SDOH) and prolonged relational health ruptures. In your practice, you may begin with addressing only one of these barriers at a visit. As this process becomes more fluid for you and your office, you may be able to address multiple barriers at a time.

Tailored anticipatory guidance becomes more of a 2-way process. You're not providing generic, blanket recommendations. Instead, you're modeling how to celebrate strengths and clarify unmet needs. You're offering healthy coping skills to mitigate stressors currently preventing the family from being able to experience the benefit of our standard recommendations. Families may need a series of Plan-Do-Study-Act (PDSA) cycles to address barriers, as these systems are complex and influenced by a multitude of factors. The goal is to prioritize needs and break them down into a stepwise process for change, cocreating a plan with one or more healthy coping skills and/or strategies for each issue the parents identify, and then follow up by phone or in person to see if the plan is helping or if they need support with developing a new plan.

Case 1: Mohamed's Newborn Visit

Mohamed is a new patient to your practice. He arrives late for his newborn visit with his mom, Hani, because their ride was late. Through an interpreter, you

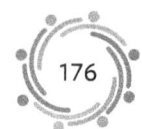

welcome her to your practice and ask about her support system and living situation. You have minimal newborn records, and in the visit, you learn she is an asylum seeker and the father is not involved. She recently arrived in the United States after a long and grueling journey with her other children, who are now 13 months, 5 years, and 8 years of age. They are all sheltered in a motel by the local public housing agency.

You're concerned that Hani may be at high risk for postpartum depression and ask her to complete a verified postnatal depression screening (eg, Edinburgh Postnatal Depression Scale). You talk with her about how stressful this journey must have been and how now she has a new baby. You explain how it's important for her to have the support she needs, and she appreciates your help scheduling an appointment with her obstetric clinician before they leave. As you give them a book for the baby, the older children start fighting over it. Hani appears nervous and apologizes for their behavior. She calmly redirects them and tells you it has been so hard for them. She shares that they fight over everything. Since they had to leave in such a hurry, they couldn't bring anything with them when they fled to the United States.

You observe poor eye contact between Hani and her kids. She leaves the baby on the exam table when you ask to examine him and sits back down to look at her phone. Although the baby is within the expected weight loss for a newborn at this age, you worry about the other children's sources of food. When you ask if she has the means to cook, Hani says no. All they have in the motel room is a microwave, and a family in a neighboring room recently got kicked out for bringing a blender into the room for food preparation. She says she doesn't know what to do but doesn't want to get into trouble and lose her shelter.

Addressing Food and Housing Insecurity

When you ask Hani if she has connected with the Special Supplemental Nutrition Program for Women, Infants, and Children (WIC) and the Supplemental Nutrition Assistance Program (SNAP), she appears irritated and says she has but these don't come close to covering her family's food needs. You notice how you feel a wave of empathy and frustration and take a minute to do 5 Big Deep Breaths before you validate how the system is not enough and give her a list of local food banks; if your clinic has community health workers, you can offer to have them help her connect with the most convenient food banks.

You can ask Mom if the older kids are already enrolled in school or if she has encountered barriers to enrollment. If you have a community health worker, they can help with this too. You can also ask if the older children are bringing home additional food from school and encourage her to ask for this if they aren't. You can help Mom connect with local places of worship and charities that may allow families to use their kitchens. Before they go, ask if she needs any

help with their application for more stable housing and connect her with local agencies or your community health worker. If you are feeling like you need more support as a clinician and practice with addressing SDOH, the Safe Environment for Every Kid program (https://seekwellbeing.org) can help you deepen and broaden your capacity to respond in a meaningful way.

The stepwise response centers on strengths (**Figure 7-1**). Ground every step in family strengths when you identify a barrier (eg, insufficient benefit coverage for the family's food needs). Next, use habit stacking to add a self-care strategy to your own frustrated or overwhelmed feeling (eg, 5 Big Deep Breaths, sensory grounding). Then, clarify the barrier or immediate need (more food). Next, cocreate a plan to address this barrier/need (community health worker outreach, school food bags, or local charities/food banks). Last, plan for follow-up (eg, have the nurse reach out in 1 week or schedule a follow-up with you in 2 weeks). With this approach, you can break down what may initially feel like insurmountable barriers into smaller, more manageable change cycles, preparing the family to attain what they need.

Figure 7-1.

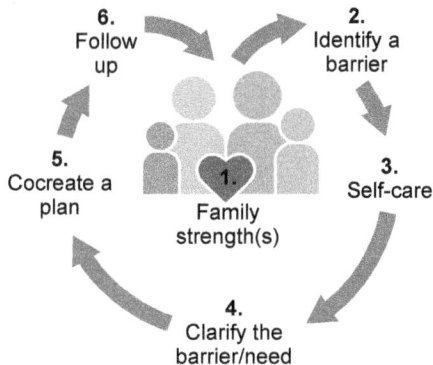

Strengths-centered, stepwise response when identifying barriers to integrating anticipatory guidance recommendations.

Supports and Routines

Connection

1. Family strength(s): The family's ability to navigate this journey.
2. Identify a barrier: Hani is feeling isolated and alone as she goes through this hard time.
3. Self-care: You may notice you are feeling frustrated or overwhelmed at first. Habit stack practicing self-care strategies when these feelings arise so you can consistently offer a coregulation space and trauma-informed care.

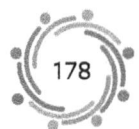

4. Clarify the barrier/need: Hani doesn't have any family or friends here. Any mother with 3 older kids and a new baby finds it challenging to maintain routines. When you are alone and living in a motel, it magnifies the stress of this scenario. For this family, they are also new to the country, so they have likely lost all the geographic and cultural resources that helped them maintain previous routines. Video chats can be a meaningful way to maintain connections if this approach is feasible.[1]

5. Cocreate a plan: Ask if Hani would like referrals to your clinic's community health workers, public health nurses, or other family outreach or support services. If video chats are desirable, identify options for free internet access (eg, a public library).

6. Follow up: Make sure you arrange follow-up to find out if these referrals "worked" and if Mom was able to connect with the intended services and those connections helped address the unmet need. Have a system for outreach that takes into account how maintaining cell service when facing SDOH is dependent on multiple variables. Just being able to take a call to set up an intake appointment can be challenging if a family communicates primarily through WhatsApp or does not have cellular service. One alternative system is to have a support person make calls to connect the family with intended services or resources before the family leaves your office.

Routines

1. Family strength(s): Mom's ability to regulate her own emotions under stress.

2. Identify a barrier: The family members have been unable to maintain routines given family disruption and they may be unable to follow your standard recommendations around maintaining routines.

3. Self-care: If you notice you are feeling like this is too much, habit stack practicing some form of self-care. When you regulate your own nervous system, you can more consistently model offering a coregulation space.

4. Clarify the barrier/need: Ask what routines they had as a family that they really enjoyed before they arrived here. What makes it hard to keep those going?

5. Cocreate a plan: Are there any ways they can re-create familiar routines here? If nothing seems possible, you can pivot to a standard, like having dinner as a family. Eating as a family at the table can be literally impossible if you are sheltered in a motel or facility without tables. You can ask what their space is like where they are living and where and how they eat. Maybe a solution is having a floor picnic together at the end of the day or a breakfast together on an outdoor picnic table. Traditional food security questions can be followed with something like *Do you have anything your children will actually eat?* This can help illuminate if the only thing they are getting from WIC or the food

bank that the older kids will consume is juice or rice.

6. Follow up: Ensure that you have a system for the nurse or community health worker to call to see how things are going and ask if the family needs any more support.

Spending Time With Older Children

1. Family strength(s): Mom has been managing the older children's needs through the birth of her baby and everyone is safe and growing well.

2. Identify a barrier: For Hani, it feels like she's spending all her time with her children. The idea of having individual one-on-one time with her older children may feel logistically impossible.

3. Self-care: You are in the midst of a busy workday, and perhaps this is the last patient before lunch and you are hungry. Take time to get a snack before you go into the room, and practice self-care as needed when you feel overwhelmed during the visit.

4. Clarify the barrier/need: Even though they are all feeling the stress as a family, they may not be used to talking about their feelings and exploring the emotional component of their shared experiences. Shifting the focus away from physical one-on-one time to emotional one-on-one time may be more feasible.

5. Cocreate a plan: The VIVA (Validate, Inform, Validate, Ask) approach helps you share relevant positive childhood experiences (PCEs), such as the protective power of just talking about feelings and feeling supported by each other as a family when going through hard times. This might sound something like *It is really hard to be in such a different setting without the supports and resources you are familiar with.* (Validate) *We know that talking about your feelings as a family helps everyone feel supported as you go through this and can help decrease the impact of any adversity on the children's long-term health.* (Inform) *This is something that most parents don't realize is such a powerful protective factor.* (Validate) *Are you interested in exploring this idea more and together coming up with a few strategies to support talking more about feelings as a family?* (Ask)

In a clinical scenario when the family speaks English or Spanish, you can use the 4 building blocks of HOPE (Healthy Outcomes from Positive Experiences) worksheets to further celebrate the family's strengths and identify areas where the family wants to try creating new dynamics or habits. When you're working with an interpreter and have limited time, identifying one thing in each building block that they want to restore or enhance helps cocreate a plan.

6. Follow up: Have the nurse or community health worker call to see how things are going and ask if the family needs any more support.

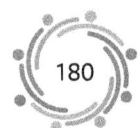

Maternal Health

Mohamed's mom has been through so much recently, while being pregnant. She doesn't have support, and at this point, it seems the baby's father is still en route to the country. We often notice potentially stressful parental scenarios like this and feel like we need to defer addressing them to adult clinicians since we are pediatricians. But we're not swerving out of our lane as pediatricians when we invite a deeper conversation around parental wellness and the family's health. Caring for the relational health of the parent-child dyad is a fundamental part of anticipatory guidance. Ask things like *Many new parents feel more stress than they expected after a baby is born. How are things going for you? Often we have an idea of what things will be like after a baby is born, but then once it happens, everything is totally different and can feel overwhelming. How has it felt for you since your baby was born?* Sharing a simple problem-solving approach with Mohamed's mom can help her respond to challenges in a less stressful manner. This can include sharing the concept of PDSA cycles for problem-solving, SUNBEAM (See, Unhook, Nurture, Breathe, Emotionally Aware, Mindful, Meditation) for when she is feeling overwhelmed, and the "back the bus up" approach when things have gone sideways.

Literacy and Access to Information

1. Family strength(s): The family has been able to navigate the health care system through the birth of the new baby in a foreign country and with a language barrier.
2. Identify a barrier: Mohamed's mom doesn't speak or read English, which can present an obstacle to integrating anticipatory guidance since many of us use print handouts and send them home because of time constraints in the office.
3. Self-care: It's normal to feel pressed for time when working in the context of a language barrier. Use self-validation and practice self-care as needed so your stress doesn't become its own barrier for the family to attain what they need.
4. Clarify the barrier/need: The Bright Futures parent handouts are currently only available to print in English and Spanish for children older than 2 years. For children 2 years and younger, they are also available in Arabic, Bengali, Chinese, French, Haitian Creole, Hmong, Korean, Polish, Portuguese, Russian, Somali, and Vietnamese. Be mindful that even if you are able to print these in your patient's primary language, not all parents are comfortable reading a handout even if it is in their most comfortable speaking language.
5. Cocreate a plan: Google Translate or another similar mobile app can be a resource for families, although it is not 100% accurate and it should never replace an actual interpreter. But this type of tool can allow parents to

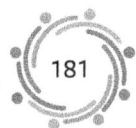

take a picture of something in English and the app will attempt to translate the document into their preferred language. Again, this is not ideal but may allow families to access more information from English sources when resources are not available in their language.

When available in the family's language, video links may be helpful to provide. This type of resource can be particularly helpful for stepwise instructions or visual aids for occasionally perplexing tasks such as installing a car seat. Be aware of any subconscious assumptions you make about which types of anticipatory guidance a family may not "need" at a certain visit. For example, if families don't have a car, it doesn't mean they don't need car seat guidance. Families may depend on a taxi, Uber, or Lyft ride to get to appointments and still need this essential advice.

Sharing/modeling graphic representations, diagrams, and strategies on paper in the office can help augment access to more complex concepts when combined with an interpreter. You can also direct parents to the SPARKS video series (www. sparksvideoseries.com, available in Spanish and English), which is designed to help families access relational health strategies for each health supervision visit.

6. Follow up: Make sure you have a system for the nurse or community health worker to call a week or so after the appointment to see how things are going and ask if the family needs any more support.

Case 2: Lyla's 15-Month Visit

Lyla comes in to her 15-month health supervision visit with her grandmother, Bella, and 3-year-old sister, Lucy. Bella declines filling out any of the screening forms, saying she is just here for vaccines. She is new to your practice, and your medical assistant shares that Bella argued with the front desk staff about what time the appointment was and they felt she was being rude. After you introduce yourself and welcome the family to the practice, you ask Grandma how things are going. She says, "It's really been just too much." She became the kids' legal guardian after Mom experienced a recurrence of substance use but now lost her car because she couldn't make the payments anymore. "I really care about these kids, but I'm just too old for this and they are too expensive." Bella shares that they were late because they had to walk from the shelter where they've been staying since they got evicted for not paying rent on time. You validate how challenging things are for the family at the moment ("It's OK to not be OK") and ask if Bella would like to start with her questions and concerns. She says she is worried that Lyla isn't talking at all yet. She thinks Lucy talked more by this age but notes that the kids were still with their mom then so she doesn't really know.

You observe that Bella is holding on to Lyla tightly during the whole visit and won't let her explore. Lyla is getting upset and starts to hit her grandma, who tells

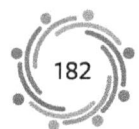

her to quit it and behave. She also sternly directs Lucy to sit still in the chair beside her, and when Lucy tries to get up, Bella grabs her arm and yanks her back into the chair. You say it's OK for Lucy to get up and look out the window, and Grandma says no, because Lucy was not behaving before they left the shelter and was being "a drama queen, like usual," so she has to sit there; she is in a time-out.

You do your exam and notice that, aside from mild speech delays, Lyla's development appears largely age appropriate. Lyla reaches out to you and wants to be held. While you are doing your exam, Bella starts arguing with Lucy about why she isn't letting her get up. As you are reviewing the sleep hygiene guidelines, Grandma says she uses the iPad to get the kids to fall asleep at night because it is so loud at the shelter. You validate her experience and then give them the 15-month Bright Futures handout and ask if they need any help with food resources or diapers. Bella says yes to both. You offer to do a Child Development Services referral and an audiology referral to ensure that there is not a hearing issue contributing to the speech delay. Bella says yes to the referrals, and you also provide the number to call to arrange a ride. See if your state participates in the national Help Me Grow initiative (https://helpmegrownational.org), which facilitates follow-through on early childhood referrals and usually involves a separate referral but can help ensure that families are actually connected with the services they need.

Regular Family Mealtimes

1. Family strength(s): Despite limited resources, Grandma has managed to support Lyla's growth and development and genuinely cares about both children.
2. Identify a barrier: This family is facing multiple SDOH and barriers to maintaining routines such as eating as a family.
3. Self-care: Honor how your first response may be to avoid responding to the SDOH because it feels like opening Pandora's box. When you notice this feeling, habit stack a form of self-care to support regulating your own nervous system and keeping your prefrontal cortex "online," which allows for collaboration.
4. Clarify the barrier/need: They are in a shelter where Grandma has no control over where or when they eat or what food looks like. Similarly to Mohamed's family, they may not have an actual table where they can eat and they may not have access to toddler-friendly foods. Many times, families in these challenging transitional times have no bandwidth to worry about details when it comes to sitting at a table or getting balanced nutrition.
5. Cocreate a plan: Bella shares that Lyla is currently living on mostly juice from WIC and refuses to eat anything the shelter serves. You show Bella the website to apply for SNAP and provide her a list of local resources for food

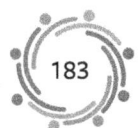

banks. You use the VIVA approach to discuss Lyla's and Lucy's nutritional needs and then cocreate a plan with the intent to incorporate alternatives to living on juice and ideas for having routines other than sitting at a table for meals.

6. Follow up: If you have a social worker or community health worker, have them call to see how things are going in 1 to 2 weeks and inquire if the family needs any more support.

Avoiding Arguments

1. Family strength(s): Bella clearly loves her granddaughters and has developed a bond with them. She is seeking care appropriately and advocating for the kids.

2. Identify a barrier: Lyla's grandma likely has her own adverse childhood experiences (ACEs) and is interpreting both girls' behaviors as a threat, which unintentionally leads to a harsher parenting approach.[2]

3. Self-care: When a caregiver is responding harshly to a child's behaviors in the exam room, it can feel stressful, and depending on your own nervous system state, you may realize that you have ended up in your own fight, flight, or freeze response. Habit stacking self-care into the visit as you notice this response supports a coregulation space.

4. Clarify the barrier/need: If Bella didn't experience people asking her to talk about her feelings when she was little, it is unlikely she will naturally prioritize this with her granddaughters. Encourage her to talk about feelings with Lyla, even at an age that may seem oddly early to many adults, especially from this generation. At this point, Lyla and her grandma are in one of those negative reinforcement cycles. Lyla's night-waking pattern will likely continue until she feels more safe and secure in her relationship without the attention she has begun to rely on during those nocturnal interactions. Even if they are entirely negative, at least they are predictable.

5. Cocreate a plan: Encouraging Bella to try toes-to-nose with Lyla at bedtime will help them get out of this negative cycle and bring a new, relational health–promoting routine into their daily schedule. Remember that just saying something like *Try to avoid arguing with your child* to a caregiver who hasn't ever experienced anything else may just mean they angrily send their child away to a time-out instead of continuing to argue with them. If Grandma is struggling with the 3-year-old having public meltdowns and that is why she is being so strict with her, you can offer the Anatomy of a Meltdown approach from Chapter 6, Using Relationship-Based and Trauma-Informed Anticipatory Guidance (see the Anatomy of a Meltdown section) and the "Back the Bus Up: A Parenting

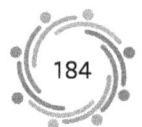

Problem-Solving Approach" handout from Appendix R. Recommending the SPARKS video series here may help foster relational health as well.

6. Follow up: Have the nurse or community health worker call to see how things are going and ask if the family needs any more support.

Child-Directed Speech, Bonding, and Playing

Making choices that foster relational health and connection with a toddler requires that a parent or caregiver think clearly about age-appropriate options.

1. Family strength(s): Bella has been able to keep Lyla and Lucy in safe housing despite the turmoil.
2. Identify the barrier: Bella is experiencing toxic levels of stress and is interpreting her granddaughter as a source of that stress. This makes it seem like play and connection are luxuries they can't afford at the moment and everything is about enforcing rules.
3. Self-care: This patient is the last one in your day. Perhaps you're trying to get to your child's soccer game and feeling frustrated and rushed. Habit stack 5 Big Deep Breaths when you notice the rushed feeling to help you regulate your own stress level and give yourself permission to prioritize. Choose one specific skill or strategy to share.
4. Clarify the barrier/need: We have to help Grandma see that she needs to put on her proverbial oxygen mask first so she can help Lyla and Lucy. And in doing this, we are promoting that affiliate response so she can see that Lyla is actually not the source of danger here; she is her loved one.
5. Cocreate a plan: We are modeling this ourselves and can share NICER (Notice, Identify, Connect/coregulate, Explore, Review/repair) parenting and SUNBEAM with Bella, reviewing how important it is for her to offer a coregulation space for the girls to develop self-regulation skills. If you have time for only one strategy, try SUNBEAM. When her sympathetic nervous system feels calmer (after breathing, meditation, or mindfulness), Bella can better understand the unmet need or unmanageable emotion behind Lyla's and Lucy's behaviors. You can also use VIVA to explain how unwanted behaviors often become the means for connection and suggest they try a playful framework for chores to foster connection instead. Send them home with the Five-Minute Connection strategies from Attachment, Regulation, and Competency (ARC; https://arcframework.org/wp-content/uploads/2020/03/Five-minute-connection-activities-updated.pdf).
6. Follow up: Try to have a nurse or community health worker call to see how things are going after a few weeks and ask if the family needs any more support.

Avoiding Harsh Discipline and Promoting Caregiver Self-Care

Sharing SUNBEAM with stressed caregivers not only helps them understand how to take a moment to take care of themselves, so they can avoid harmful harsh discipline tactics, but also illuminates how they are modeling responses to unpleasant, stressful situations for their children.

1. Family strength(s): Bella is invested in her grandchildren and wants them to do well in life. She is open to help and ideas to begin using more positive parenting skills.
2. Identify the barrier: For Lyla's grandma to shift from responding harshly to Lyla's and Lucy's behaviors to cultivating options for gentler discipline and distraction, she has to feel safe.
3. Self-care: Feeling overwhelmed in this setting is normal. Habit stack grounding yourself in your body when you notice the part of you that's saying you can't handle all of this. Practice self-care as needed so you can regulate your own nervous system.
4. Clarify the barrier/need: Continue with open-ended questions and active listening. Explain the "fire-truck brain" analogy to Bella and how, when her grandma is stressed, Lyla is tuning into this and sensing it.
5. Cocreate a plan: Use the VIVA approach to explore how it is normal for Bella to be stressed in this situation, and cocreate a path to more options for caregiving responses that promote relational health and decrease the chance of harsh discipline. For Bella to be able to praise Lyla and Lucy for anything other than being obedient, she has to first feel safe and have her basic needs met. Asking only about what brings her joy when it comes to Lyla or caregiving may just bring up shame if she is not enjoying it at all. Validate how hard it is to raise children, inform how common it is for caregivers to experience burnout, validate how easy it is to react more harshly than you intend when the kids are acting out and you are stressed, and ask if she wants to try "backing the bus up" to understand what is behind Lyla's unwanted behaviors. VIVA helps you avoid pathologizing typical responses to high levels of stress while supporting caregiver habit-stacking strategies that promote relational health.

Bella is clearly used to feeling as though she is in an unsafe environment, so unpacking this a little bit with her may be helpful. Once her stress is validated and she's able to use SUNBEAM, she can start discerning the settings where she can let her child explore versus the ones where she needs to be vigilant and hold her child close.
6. Follow up: Send a message to your nurse or a community health worker to call in a few weeks to see how things are going and ask if the family needs any more support.

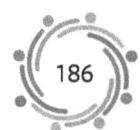

Media Use and Support Systems

Keeping in mind this book's earlier discussions about not over-pathologizing media use, you can cocreate a PDSA cycle with Grandma if she is interested in decreasing their dependence on the iPad at bedtime. For example, if Lyla is currently watching a favorite show at bedtime, they could transition earlier to watching ocean waves on YouTube and then slowly decrease the brightness of the screen and shift, eventually, to just a sleep white noise machine or app. These strategies combined with toes-to-nose can alleviate many bedtime screen battles.

1. Family strength(s): The family has strategies they are using to mitigate stress and has tried ideas to foster better sleep.
2. Identify the barrier: Bella shares that she has lost her support system and feels isolated at the moment. This makes her feel more stressed and like she never gets a break from her grandchildren. The iPad feels like a welcome relief at bedtime.
3. Self-care: When you notice that all you want to do is share your "limit screen time" blanket advice, habit stack a self-care strategy and lean in with curiosity.
4. Clarify the barrier/need: Bella may appreciate support exploring how and where she could connect with other caregivers who may have similar lived experience because it can help decrease her sense of isolation.
5. Cocreate a plan: Share with Bella your local resources for child care subsidies. Being able to obtain stable child care for her 3-year-old might increase her bandwidth for one-on-one time with Lyla. This is a wonderful opportunity to use Amy King's Circle of Support tool,[3] which includes drawing concentric circles on the exam table paper and identifying whom she might be able to call on for support and help with the kids.
6. Follow up: Tell Bella that you are looking forward to seeing how everything is going at the 18-month health supervision visit but she can call sooner if the family needs any more support.

Case 3: Rodrigo's 2½-Year Visit

Rodrigo is here for his 2½-year health supervision visit with his dad, Javier. At the top of Dad's list of concerns is that Rodrigo gets out of bed every night and comes into his parents' bedroom. Dad wants to know how to get him to stay in his own room. Both Mom and Dad work full-time but take opposite shifts so one of them is always able to be with the kids since they can't afford child care. Also, Rodrigo doesn't want to eat meals; he likes just Goldfish crackers and juice. You have had concerns about indoor smoke exposure in the past.

Reducing Smoke Exposure

1. Family strength(s): Javier is engaged in the care of his son and comes to the appointment with a list of questions about how to help him raise a healthy child.

2. Identify the barrier: The family lives in Maine: it's winter and below zero outside. You have talked with Javier before, encouraging him to smoke outside. When you bring this topic up today, he says everything is fine. He appears frustrated and says he knows about your ideas, but it's his house and he chooses to smoke in it.

3. Self-care: You may notice a wave of anger or frustration since you have been working on this for a long time. Notice the feeling, habit stack a self-care strategy, and then lean back in with curiosity and open-ended questions.

4. Clarify the barrier/need: Use VIVA to respond to Javier's frustration, validating that it's frustrating to hear the doctor keep asking the same questions; informing him that it's a good idea to avoid smoking in any room where the kids sleep, play, or watch TV; validating that figuring things out like this often takes different ideas; and then asking if he would like to explore some other options with you.

5. Cocreate a plan: Dad says yes and, now that you mention it, he is constantly having to yell at Rodrigo for unplugging the TV. Javier says he puts him in a time-out "like you told us to do at the last visit" but can't get Rodrigo to stay in his room for 3 minutes. Dad physically restrains him in his recliner. You respond again with VIVA: *Wow. That must be frustrating.* (Validate) *We know that for some kids, time-outs don't work and can actually trigger new behaviors.* (Inform) *Any parent would try things that come to mind to try to manage such disruptive behaviors.* (Validate) *Would you like to review a few different strategies?* (Ask)

Dad says he would like ideas and he's at the end of his rope. You offer Javier NICER parenting and discuss the "back the bus up" strategy for responding to these behaviors. You also share how behaviors can be Rodrigo's attempt to connect with Dad, and one-on-one time may decrease these behaviors. You explore ideas for outdoor play together and cocreate a plan for Javier to kick a ball with him before dinner. You share how this type of interaction will support Rodrigo's development and celebrate how Dad will be supporting him with emotion coaching with this new response to his behavior, which supports his long-term mental and physical health.

6. Follow up: At the end of the visit, you give Javier the Bright Futures handout in Spanish (you checked, and that is Dad's preferred reading language even though he is fluent in English) and ask Dad to schedule Rodrigo's 3-year checkup on the way out.

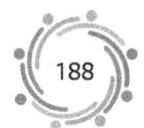

You ask if there is anything else you could help them with today. Dad shrugs and says, "Only if you have a cure for the terrible twos! He's just always trying to ruin the day. I told him no bedtime stories when he talks back to me." By saying this to you at the end of the visit, Dad is expressing that after all the guidance you've given, he may still not think it will work for his situation and/or might have realized you could be a good resource for parenting tips. This is one of those classic "doorknob" moments. Even though you are worried about getting behind, you feel confident you can help with a quick PDSA cycle for them to try and plan on a follow-up. You take a deep breath and ask him to tell you more about what the hardest part has been with Rodrigo's behavior, other than the TV. This helps you clarify what he really is asking for help with so you can cocreate a path forward. Don't worry, the strategies here will help you both address his concerns and stay on schedule.

Behavioral Concerns

Javier says, "Well, I didn't want to bring it up because it's not really about his health. But he is starting to act violently, and I am worried he is bipolar. You know it runs in our family." The other day, Rodrigo pushed his sister over right when she had just learned to walk. Dad looks at you and says he doesn't know what to do. He doesn't want him to think he can get away with things like that. Javier goes on to say he took away all of Rodrigo's toys; he says this was Mom's idea. She follows a parenting coach on TikTok, and this person recommends using this strategy and then making the child earn the toys back one by one.

1. Family strength(s): Javier and Rodrigo's mom are actively looking for ways to help them raise a child who understands boundaries and is well-behaved.
2. Identify the barrier: The current strategies they are using for behavior management are not anchored in connection or coregulation.
3. Self-care: Do you notice a wave of frustration hearing that the advice you gave was not implemented, but the TikTok parenting coach's advice was implemented? It's totally normal to feel frustrated! Habit stack a self-care strategy as soon as you notice the frustrated feeling. Acknowledge it and then lean in with open-ended questions and learn more. This helps you build the trust that is essential for engagement.
4. Clarify the barrier/need: Use VIVA to validate how challenging these behaviors are, inform Javier that this strategy may not be aligned with Rodrigo's developmental stage, validate how normal it is for parents to worry when their child shows aggressive behaviors, and ask if it's been working. Dad says no, things have just gotten worse and he thinks maybe the TikTok person is wrong. Javier says they are worried that no preschool will take him because his behavior is so bad. You respond by validating this concern, informing him that big emotional states and unmet needs can lead to behaviors, validating

how hard it is to understand what led to the aggression, and then asking if they would like to try a different approach.

5. Cocreate a plan: You review how to use the "back the bus up" approach in conjunction with NICER parenting. You explain fire-truck brain and have Javier make a list of 10 things he and Rodrigo can do for self-care to help the fire truck go back into its garage.

6. Follow up: When you ask if he wants to follow up in a few weeks to see how things are going, Dad says he can't come in again, but he thinks it would help for Mom to hear what you're saying and they will schedule a follow-up. This is also an opportunity to offer 4 formal Resilience University (RU) sessions with the family to help them understand how they can respond to Rodrigo's behaviors in a way that promotes relational health and emotional growth.

Bedtime Routine

1. Family strength(s): Dad is trying to find useful ways of working with his son's behaviors.

2. Identify the barrier: At the moment, the family is unable to practice a bedtime routine that supports relational health and sleep hygiene.

3. Self-care: Often our blanket advice feels easy and reassuring because we know what to say and trying a different approach can feel overwhelming. Habit stack one self-care strategy before you further clarify what the barrier or unmet need looks like. Give yourself permission to address the next barrier at a different appointment.

4. Clarify the barrier/need: You explain that at this developmental stage, Rodrigo's parents will likely need to wait until he is older to extinguish co-sleeping if he is used to it. His need for connection and safety can feel stressful and overwhelming to the family, leading them to try things that are not ideal.

5. Cocreate a plan: The family can try a "bedtime pass" (explained in Chapter 5, A Structured Approach to Resilience Coaching, in the outline of RU session 2) and work on sleep hygiene. Ask Dad what his bedtime routine was like when he was little, then you can ask Mom the same question when she comes in at the follow-up visit. What do the parents each want for Rodrigo? By the end of the day, each parent may be so tired and stressed that reading feels like a chore and they would rather not do it. Stay curious and see if there is a different time of day reading might work better, and suggest they try a mutually soothing bedtime routine such as 5-4-3-2-1, singing, or toes-to-nose. Send the chosen handout home with them, and suggest they try integrating 5-4-3-2-1 and/or toes-to-nose into the bedtime routine. Share how they can use habit stacking to develop a new routine.

6. Follow up: Make a note in the record to follow up on how this is going at the next visit, or you can schedule a follow-up sleep visit.

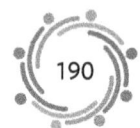

Support System and Engagement

Use a strengths-based approach and VIVA when exploring this family's support system and framing connections in the community to support Rodrigo's PCEs.

1. Family strength(s): Celebrate how well Rodrigo is growing and developing and how you have seen them do hard things as a family, like when the little sister was born early and had to spend weeks in the neonatal intensive care unit.
2. Identify the barrier: Rodrigo's parents are both stressed and working hard with little downtime to connect with him one on one. They are feeling isolated and without support in the community. You can ask *Tell me about your support system* or *Where do you feel like you can go for support within the community?*
3. Self-care: It is understandably easier to hand a family a piece of paper with scripted advice, so it may at first feel cumbersome and like "too much" to offer tailored advice. Notice this feeling and breathe in through your nose and out through your mouth a few times as you listen to the family respond to your open-ended questions. Sometimes I think of it with an internal family systems lens: *Part of me feels overwhelmed. That part can rest. And the part of me that wants to promote equitable access to resilience can take over.*
4. Clarify the barrier/need: Use VIVA to clarify needs, validate their experience, and invite them to work with you on addressing this barrier. Validate for Javier how it is normal to feel exhausted and tired of parenting, especially now that they have 2 kids; inform him about the importance of having non-parent adults involved in the kids' lives and how important it is for parents to have a support system; and validate how both the parents are working hard, yet there are still financial constraints. Ask if they would like ideas about how to find a way to get Rodrigo enrolled in child care.
5. Cocreate a plan: Dad is eager for any advice you can provide on getting Rodrigo into child care, because the family can't afford it. Share your state's subsidized child care resources (www.ccrcca.org/parents/funded-child-care-options or https://childcare.gov), and make sure they can access the internet to explore these options. If they don't, you can have a community health worker or case manager (if they have one) help them explore these options.
6. Follow up: Make a note to follow up on this when you see the family back about the behavioral issues.

When Mom comes in with Rodrigo at the next visit, you can explore her self-care strategies and resources for support. You can ask what she does to "fill her bucket" when she feels frustrated or exhausted. Who can she count on for support? How does she communicate with them? Perhaps it is harder know because Grandma used to help a lot but has moved out of state; encouraging them to do video chats

can help maintain the support system. You can also ask what activities they all enjoy, which are fun as a family, and if there are currently barriers to doing them. You can give them the building blocks worksheets (in Spanish) to take home and plan to follow up at the next visit to review the sleep and behavior concerns.

Enforcing Limits/Time-Outs

Use VIVA to explore how the family can enforce limits and discipline in a way that promotes family health in the context of behavior problems.

1. Validate: Validate how hard parenting moments feel when a young child is being aggressive with pets or siblings or friends.
2. Inform: Share with the parents how they can use emotion coaching and the "back the bus up" approach to help them remain curious about what is leading to each behavior.
3. Validate: Honor how hard it is when they start to feel angry or afraid because of their child's behaviors.
4. Ask: Inquire if they want to try an alternative to time-outs. If the family says yes, you can share SUNBEAM and fire-truck brain along with NICER parenting. These concepts help everyone understand what is happening with their brains and nervous systems when the aggressive behaviors happen. Cocreate a PDSA cycle for the unmet needs or big emotions that led to Rodrigo pushing his sister over. Review the NICER parenting steps with Dad at the first visit and Mom at the follow-up. Arrange to see Rodrigo back again in 2 weeks with a new cocreated PDSA cycle if things are still not going well when Mom comes in with him. Emphasize how you are right there with them, supporting them through this; just like when they had to go through the hospital stay with their daughter, you are there to help and want them to tell you how things are going. You'll help them in whatever way they need.

Screen Time

You know from caring for this family that both parents experienced adversity as children, and your trauma-informed understanding is that they are using screens to help mitigate their own stress.

1. Family strength(s): The parents are clearly trying to help their son grow up healthy and attain what he needs.
2. Identify the barrier: From talking with the family, your assessment is that they are currently experiencing overwhelming stress.
3. Self-care: Again, notice when you feel overwhelmed yourself, and model practicing self-care often so you can consistently offer a coregulation space.

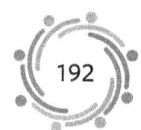

4. Clarify the barrier/need: Framing the TV use as an accessible coping mechanism for stress reduction helps us understand why TVs can be left on perpetually in some of our patients' households. Learning healthy coping skills and having a strategy to integrate them can support less reliance on screens.

5. Cocreate a plan: Lean in with curiosity (if it isn't already clear) and invite the parents to think about why, when, and how they are using the TV. Does it help them feel less stressed? You can again use VIVA here: validate how TV is a commonly used coping strategy; inform them that other strategies may provide longer-term benefit for them and their kids; validate that you've talked about a lot today, and if this is not something they want to address today, you totally understand; and ask what they think. If they are interested in integrating other coping skills into the day, you can explore if other stress-reducing tactics could be useful and how they could use habit stacking to create new, media-free stress-relieving routines (use the stress-buster wheel, writing the ideas in each quadrant, or a stress reduction plan for the family).

6. Follow up: Make a note to follow up on this when you next see the family.

Reading, Simple Requests, and Choices

Invite the parents to share what their own experiences were around reading books or reading in general when they were little. Did they like it, or did it feel like a chore or a punishment?

1. Family strength(s): Rodrigo's parents are engaged and interested in learning ways to foster resilience.

2. Identify the barrier: Dad shares that he was ridiculed for not being able to read well in his early educational years and it's never been easy for him. He prefers to let Mom do the reading. When you talk with Mom at the next visit, she says she can't read to Rodrigo because he will never let her leave once she starts.

3. Self-care: Honoring that this may initially feel like a lot, you may catch yourself wanting to just respond with generic advice. You use your trauma-informed awareness, however, to help you avoid this by pausing for a few deep breaths as you ask more about what happens when she tries to read to him.

4. Clarify the barrier/need: You can use VIVA here to validate how frustrating this situation must be, to inform her that Rodrigo may be needing extra reassurance because of his baby sister, to validate how challenging it can be to juggle the needs of 2 kids, and to ask if she wants to explore options for doing time-ins and connecting one on one with Rodrigo.

5. Cocreate a plan: If Mom accepts the invitation to work together, you can explore if it helps for her to make a specific request for Rodrigo to choose one special book for her to read after she puts the baby sister to bed. Or perhaps planning

a game or activity for them when his sister is napping would help, just like they are planning for Dad to kick the ball around with him before dinner. These strategies may need to be habit stacked into the parents' days to make sure they remember to try them and increase the chance that they are consistent.

6. Follow up: When you see Rodrigo back in the office after this second PDSA cycle with Mom, you observe her speaking negatively about him. She says he is always whining and "acting like a baby" to try to get his way. You can use VIVA to reframe what is happening here and help her unpack this idea that he is somehow intentionally trying to manipulate her. This involves normalizing how whining is really just an emotionally driven form of communication: it can sometimes feel ineffective and frustrating to parents, but really, Rodrigo is just trying to express a need. You can also normalize how common it is for parents to miss the mark when we're trying to figure out what our child needs, emphasizing that this is actually the case most of the time for most parents under typical stress. Then you can share the importance of relational health rupture repairs and how simple these can be. If you feel like Mom and Dad need more ideas for connecting and repair, start with the ARC list of Five-Minute Connection activities or suggest the SPARKS video series.

Case 4: Ngoc's 7-Year Visit

You have cared for Ngoc's family for years, but they have missed most of their health supervision visits. When Ngoc is sick, her mom (May) tends to take her to the emergency department. You haven't done a health supervision visit since Ngoc was 4 years old when Mom needed a form filled out to enroll her in a new preschool. At that point, you noted she had been suspended from the closest preschool and kicked out of 3 in-home child care settings prior. May had called asking for help when Ngoc was sent home nearly all the time from kindergarten for "bad" behavior; you had requested they come in for an office visit, but they did not keep that appointment.

Ngoc is here now for her 7-year checkup. You use a Vietnamese phone interpreter to translate. May tells you that school is going poorly again this year. Ngoc is hitting other children and, last week, punched the ed tech teacher who was trying to help her during math class. May met with the principal, and her understanding was that Ngoc has to be put on medication or she won't be allowed to keep coming to school. Mom is angry with the school and feels like they aren't teaching her daughter anything; they just keep sending her home. Mom grew up in foster care and feels like Ngoc is ungrateful for everything she has. May says she gives Ngoc "everything she wants," and "she doesn't even appreciate it." Ngoc looks off into the distance with her arms tightly crossed on her chest. She occasionally looks at her mom with an angry expression.

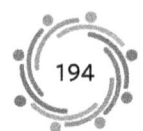

When you ask about media use, May says the TV is on all the time, because she can't stand silence. She proudly shares how she saved up and got a second TV for her daughter's room to help her sleep. She doesn't understand why even with playing Ngoc's favorite movie at bedtime, Ngoc still ends up in Mom's bed every night. Mom tried locking Ngoc's door so she couldn't get out at night, but then she screamed so loud, the neighbors reported her; the landlord says that if that happens again, they will get kicked out. May is very frustrated and says you need to put Ngoc on medication so she doesn't get kicked out of school and make them lose their housing. Ngoc says she doesn't care, that she wants to get kicked out of school because it is stupid and she hates the school and everyone in it.

Problem-Solving Strategy

You can start with modeling how to approach layered problems like this so the family can learn to do it themselves.

1. Family strength(s): Ngoc clearly loves her daughter and wants her to get an education. Start with something like *You both have been through a lot since I saw you last time. It sounds like sometimes things have gotten really hard and stressful. I am so glad you came in for this visit.*
2. Identify the barrier: This is 2-fold: the family's stress and your feeling of overwhelm. This is a lot, and with the interpreter, the visit may feel like it is moving slowly. Instead of narrowing your scope, expand it.
3. Self-care: Do 5 Big Deep Breaths while you are listening to the family share their concerns. Honor that this is stressful and overwhelming, and share the It's OK to Not Be OK approach. You may feel frustrated that this family has missed so many opportunities for care, or it may cross your mind that you can't offer everything so you will just stick to the medical basics. Notice if you are feeling that addressing anything more is out of your scope and brings up big unpleasant feelings. If you feel overwhelmed as you're reviewing the phone notes in the record or shared data repository before you go into the room, try walking meditation as you go from your office to the room. If you are already in the room and all this information feels overwhelming in the moment during the clinical encounter, take a minute to breathe.
4. Clarify the barrier/need: As you talk with the family, it becomes clear that the stress of her daughter's behavior is feeling overwhelming and making it difficult for May to see what is within her power to change to help support Ngoc. Ngoc is feeling stuck.
5. Cocreate a plan: Include May and Ngoc in choosing some self-care strategies; ask them what might work. You could do 5 Big Deep Breaths with them, or if you have supplies for a glitter jar, you can start there. Next, review firetruck brain and backing the bus up and ask if they would like to explore how

everyone can respond differently to these stressful moments and maybe even make school feel less stressful for Ngoc.

6. Follow up: Schedule a follow-up appointment in 2 to 4 weeks to see how things are going, and you can offer formal RU sessions at that point if the family would like to work with you more.

Responding to Harsh Parenting

Start by celebrating strengths before you cocreate a path.

1. Family strength(s): Embrace that May is parenting in the best way she knows how, which may reflect some of the harsh parenting styles her biological and/ or foster parents used. Point out how you have seen them do hard things in the past, like when Ngoc broke her leg on the playground and had to have surgery.

2. Identify the barrier: May's neurohormonal stress response is currently framing her daughter as the source of danger. Neither parent nor child is able to put the affiliate response to use in this scenario.

3. Self-care: When parents come into the office with these urgent needs and high stress levels, we can feel stressed and pressured to prescribe when there is no clear diagnosis. Notice this feeling and habit stack a healthy coping skill so you can continue to offer a coregulation space. Remind yourself that engagement moves at the speed of trust.

4. Clarify the barrier/need: After you use VIVA to set the stage and ask for permission, sharing NICER parenting and SUNBEAM can help May understand that in the moment, her most important job is not actually to make Ngoc do or not do something but instead to notice if she herself is triggered and needs to put on her own oxygen mask first, before she parents.

5. Cocreate a plan: Review with May that part of her role in supporting Ngoc's emotional development is to just hold space for Ngoc's big emotions. You can share the Leveling Up Your Container of Love approach with her. This might feel stressful for May, who is already worried about whether her daughter's behaviors may jeopardize their housing. But as May and Ngoc become more aware of which feeling states tend to derail the day and end up with yelling, they can proactively integrate appropriate, accessible strategies for practicing self-care and mitigating stress. Landlords may be legally allowed to evict a family for noise violations, even if the noise is developmentally appropriate. You can still advocate and write a letter for the landlord that says when children express emotions loudly at this age, that is developmentally appropriate and not a reason to take away their housing. If they need legal help, you can give them the site where they can search for free legal aid (www.americanbar.org/groups/legal_services/flh-home).

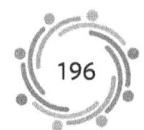
Ngoc and her mom are in a dysfunctional pattern of mutual dysregulation; that pattern is how they are connecting, which is part of the reason it is continuing. Even though they probably both want something different (Ask Ngoc if she wants to get into trouble less!), they feel stuck and don't know how to shift things. You can use VIVA to frame a PDSA cycle around activities they can do to connect (share the Five-Minute ARC resource). Cocreate a next step that supports relational health and promotes PCEs and protective factors.

6. Follow up: Ensure that they feel confident trying the tools you provided, and schedule a follow-up (telehealth or in person) in a few weeks.

"Spend Time With Your Child": Relational Health as a Long-Distance Event

1. Family strength(s): Ngoc's mom doesn't want to re-create her own childhood and is trying everything she can to help her daughter succeed.

2. Identify the barrier: Despite doing everything as best she can, Ngoc is re-creating some of the scenarios she probably promised herself she wouldn't do and having trouble integrating positive parenting.

3. Self-care: You have a busy morning and are seeing this family in between acute care visits. You have a child with low oxygen saturations getting a nebulizer treatment in one room and a teen in suicidal crisis waiting for intervention in the other. You notice your mind jumping around and realize you are not 100% in this room with this family. Practice a short body scan (toes-to-nose) to ground yourself and arrive fully in the room.

4. Clarify the barrier/need: Parents may specifically want to re-create some of their favorite childhood memories. Yet when toxic levels of stress arise, things inevitably go sideways. May wants to do things differently, but she needs a strategy for change and stress-mitigating techniques.

5. Cocreate a plan: Support May's intentions as you cocreate a parenting plan that integrates relational health and PCE-promoting strategies with her deepest wishes for Ngoc. Ask May if it would be helpful to write it down, and give her a pen and paper (unless you can write in Vietnamese). Start by asking May for 3 things she most certainly wants Ngoc to experience as a child. Invite her to explore any core values around raising kids that she feels align with her truest intentions for raising kids. Without a language barrier, you can scribe for them, writing these on a plain piece of paper they can take home and put on the fridge or in some central location. Include Ngoc in this process by asking her what she enjoys doing with her mom.

May will also need strategies for how to get back on track when things drift; it's important to normalize this process. You ask for 3 things May definitely does

not want Ngoc to grow up with. May immediately shares that she doesn't want Ngoc to grow up with yelling, but she finds herself yelling all the time. Reassure her that this is not the end of the world and they can use these moments of disconnect to repair and strengthen their relationship. Normalize how common it is for relationship ruptures to go unrepaired, and cocreate ideas for relational health repairs. The first step for May to engage in the repair process is to regulate her own nervous system and then reconnect with Ngoc. Offer strategies such as Authentic Apologies as well as activities for connection or playful chores.

6. Follow up: Make a note to ask how this is going when you do the telehealth or in-person follow-up.

Talking About Feelings

Ngoc and May appear to have had a breakdown in their communication, and now the focus is entirely on Ngoc's behaviors. Use VIVA to validate how hard the behaviors are, and inform May that this type of behavior can be a normal way of maintaining connection for children. If May and Ngoc can develop new strategies to talk about feelings and Ngoc's worries, they may be able to reconnect without behaviors taking center stage. One approach could be to put a family feelings chart in a central location in the house.

With NICER parenting, May can lean in with curiosity and may learn that worries are leading to some of the behaviors that are upsetting her. Model asking Ngoc how she was feeling and what happened before she hit the support person at school. You can use the "Back the Bus Up: A Parenting Problem-Solving Approach" handout to facilitate this discussion.

You ask Ngoc how she was feeling when she punched the ed tech teacher; she just shrugs and looks away.

1. Family strength(s): Ngoc shares that even though she hates school, she loves gym class and her PE teacher. Ngoc also shares that she is tired of always getting into trouble.

2. Identify the barrier: Honor that Ngoc is probably not used to talking about how she feels and May was not raised with an "emotion coaching" approach, so this is a new concept.

3. Self-care: You can invite May and Ngoc to do glitter jar meditation with you and share with May that she can use this same strategy at home to more consistently offer a coregulation space for her daughter.

4. Clarify the barrier/need: Even though Ngoc is not used to talking about feelings, she is used to people talking at her about how she behaves. You can start with asking her if she wants to brainstorm some ideas for getting into

trouble less. Behavior discussions are familiar to her, so starting with behaviors and using backing the bus up and emotion coaching can help May and Ngoc see how the two are connected.

5. Cocreate a plan: Share the emotion coaching approach and the "Resilience University Emotion Coaching" handout with May. Encourage Ngoc to share what she needs to make school feel more comfortable. Ask about her friends and peer interactions. You may want to encourage them to ask for a learning evaluation through the school if specific subjects are particularly frustrating for Ngoc. Invite Ngoc to make her list of "10 Things I Can Do When I Feel Yucky," and cocreate a PDSA cycle (or two!) that sounds realistic to both of them.

6. Follow up: Make a note to see if they need ideas for additional PDSA cycles at the follow-up appointment.

Chores, Rules, and Consequences

When families are stuck in frustrating cycles of yelling and disobedience, enforcing the rules can become a surrogate for connection. When chores aren't completed, consequences can escalate, leading to harsh discipline. None of this supports relational health or PCEs. As pediatricians, we can provide support so families can find the exit ramp from these frustrating loops and repair the relational health ruptures that lead to these cycles. Supporting May in genuinely shifting her dynamic to one that is more likely to promote PCEs and protective factors fortunately just requires that you use the same strategies you've learned from this book. SUNBEAM is helpful for supporting "asynchronous discipline," where we are giving the parent permission to wait until their own nervous system is regulated and their prefrontal cortex ("that good-thinking part of your brain") is back online. That way, they can parent the way they truly intended instead of feeling like the child's behaviors are always tanking their intentions and derailing the day.

Case 5: Dakota's 14-Year Visit

Dakota has been your patient since she was born. Her parents got divorced a year ago, which was hard on her mom, and she hasn't seen or heard from her dad since. Dad struggled with substance use, and there was a lot of yelling and fighting in the home before the divorce. Dakota has always been a very quiet person with borderline scores on the PHQ-9 Modified for Adolescents. You have tried to get her into counseling for years, but she declines. Her mother, Aponi, was unable to pay rent after losing her job when she showed up to work intoxicated. They lost their apartment, and while Mom is in a substance use treatment facility, Dakota is temporarily sheltered in one of Aponi's friend's houses. The

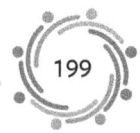

friend's name is Talulah. Dakota now has to watch Talulah's kids after school. Talulah and Dakota are here for Dakota's checkup, and Talulah shares how Dakota has "turned into a total stranger" recently and says, "Maybe you can figure out what's wrong with her. She never used to act like this. I don't know if it's because her mom is in rehab or if she's bipolar."

You talk with them together at the beginning of the visit, and you validate that it sounds like things have gotten really challenging and ask if there are any other concerns. Dakota says, "No one even cares about me. They don't even care that I hate sharing a room with 2 kids I barely know!" Talulah seems visibly upset, raises her voice, and yells, "You know, none of this is my fault. I'm helping you. Will you quit blaming me? We're all doing the best we can. You need to quit freaking out about everything and learn how to deal!" Talulah asks to talk with you privately in the hallway. You've normalized talking with the caregivers and teens separately for years, so you agree and reassure Dakota you'll be right back to talk with her alone. You ask her to complete the recommended, validated screening questionnaires (eg, PHQ-9 Modified for Adolescents, CRAFFT [Car, Relax, Alone, Forget, Family/Friends, Trouble], Guidelines for Adolescent Preventive Services) while you talk with Talulah.

Talulah shares she's worried that Dakota has started smoking weed because she smells like it when she comes back from her friend's house. She also says she thinks Dakota may have had sex because there was a boy who was always coming around, but then he suddenly stopped coming around. Since then, Dakota seems to be crying more. Talulah took away her phone and grounded her for smelling like weed and turning off her Life360 so Talulah couldn't tell where she was. But she says "it didn't work" and Dakota just yells at her, saying she hates her, and has recently been refusing to talk with her at all. Talulah says she told her she was grounded until she "starts to behave." But it has now been 2 weeks and things are just getting worse. She thinks she saw something like lines on Dakota's arms, but Dakota is always wearing long sleeves. Talulah asks how she can make her stop cutting and get out of her room and do her chores.

Responding to Overwhelming Stress

Use VIVA to validate Talulah's concerns and prioritize next steps. Emphasize connection and that you understand a lot is going on and you'll want to work with them closely until they get set up with all the resources and supports they need. Validate how hard this situation is for Talulah, inform her that cutting is often a way for kids to transform unbearable emotional pain into something more tolerable, validate how scary it can be as a guardian to realize this is happening, and ask if she wants to come up with ideas together for next steps.

Use VIVA with similar language to validate how it's normal for Talulah to be worried about Dakota using substances, to inform her that this is often a

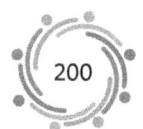

less-than-ideal coping mechanism for teens, to validate how any caregiver would try things that may have worked in the past or with other kids to try to get her to stop, and then to ask if she would like some other strategies since it seems like this time, grounding Dakota doesn't sound like it is having the effect Talulah wanted. The American Academy of Pediatrics provides support for how we can talk with caregivers and parents about marijuana use,[4] and you can share relevant pieces of information with Talulah. She appreciates the resources and would like a counseling referral for Dakota to someone who also does family therapy. You have Talulah wait in the waiting room as you continue the visit with Dakota.

When you talk with Dakota by herself, you validate how it sounds like things have been hard. She nods. You ask if you can review the questionnaires she filled out. As she hands them to you, you ask about what has been going well or anything she's proud of that she wants to share with you. She says, "Nothing." You note that on her questionnaires she disclosed cannabis use to self-medicate and being sexually active. She says she can't tell Talulah because "she will freak out." She shares that Talulah screams at her in the car all the time, calling her "worthless," and that Talulah says she's ruining her life and she's going to end up a mess like her mom. Dakota rolls her eyes and says she is sick of it and thinking about running away. You ask if she thinks Talulah has any idea about how hard this situation is for her. Dakota shrugs and says she isn't talking with Talulah and is just staying in her room when she's not babysitting to avoid getting yelled at. You validate how challenging this must be and ask if it is OK with Dakota if you bring Talulah back in at the end of the visit to explore some different ideas.

Dakota looks alarmed and physically shrinks away from you when you say that Talulah noticed her arms and was worried she was cutting. You are careful to frame your response nonjudgmentally by saying she's not in trouble, and you know that sometimes, when kids are in a lot of emotional pain or distress, it is easier to turn that pain into something physical so they can tolerate it better. You remind her it's OK to have unpleasant feelings—they are all OK—but "maybe now is the time to have a little more help because it sounds like things have gotten a lot harder for everyone." Dakota likes the idea of a counselor. When you share that the referral process sometimes takes a few months and offer to share other coping skills in the meantime, she says great, because she used to do guided meditation on YouTube to fall asleep, but since Talulah took away her phone, she can't fall asleep. You teach her toes-to-nose and relaxation breathing.

Encouraging Responsibility and Preventing Substance Use

As kids develop more independence and want to try to make their own decisions, they may need support in developing a decision-making process, especially when they have grown up with varying levels of toxic stress that required most of their mental bandwidth.

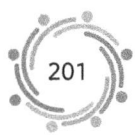
1. Family strength(s): Dakota is trying to take care of herself in the best way she can figure out while she is going through this stressful time.
2. Identify the barrier: When children grow up in a setting where adults are modeling substance use to manage stress, this may seem like a reasonable option, and the availability of substances for youth is alarming.
3. Self-care: Suppose you have a 14-year-old teen as well and you just discovered that they were experimenting with weed. Talking about this with Dakota and Talulah brings up your own big feeling of fear. Notice this; don't judge yourself, and do relaxation breathing.
4. Clarify the barrier/need: Dakota has grown up watching her parents both use substances to manage stress, but this behavior has not been talked about, other than Talulah making comments about how Dakota will turn out like her mom.
5. Cocreate a plan: Shifting this dynamic to one that is more supportive of PCEs includes talking with Dakota about how she takes care of herself when she has unpleasant emotions. Share the concept of emotional awareness and a stress reduction plan. The building blocks worksheets could also help Dakota and Talulah explore other resources or supports.
6. Follow up: Plan to follow up on how things are going with Dakota when they come back in to see you in 2 weeks. You can ask if they need any supports or resources to integrate what they wrote on the stress reduction plan or building blocks worksheets.

Promoting Positive Childhood Experiences

1. Family strength(s): When you ask what things Dakota and Aponi enjoyed doing together in the past, Dakota's face lights up and she says that she and Mom used to love going to community ceremonies together, but they haven't done that since she was little.
2. Identify the barrier: When you ask Talulah if she could take Dakota and the kids to one of these ceremonies again, you discover that Talulah has anxiety around social situations, and that is why they don't go to these ceremonies.
3. Self-care: Notice how you are feeling and habit stack self-care strategies during the visit as needed to support coregulation and this nonjudgmental, collaborative problem-solving space.
4. Clarify the barrier/need: Talulah welcomes the idea of working on her anxiety, but she doesn't have any accessible strategies. She has tried breathing but often panics and can't catch her breath.
5. Cocreate a plan: Support Talulah with habit-stacking ideas for using other mindfulness, body-based healthy coping skills to manage anxiety and stress (eg, toes-to-nose, sensory grounding, or walking meditation), and encourage

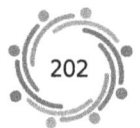

her to reach out to her own doctor if she feels like she needs more support. Review the PCEs and how enjoying participating in community traditions can help support children through adversity. Ask if, in the meantime, maybe another friend or family member could take Dakota to these gatherings.

6. Follow up: Make a note to ask Talulah if they have identified any community events she thinks they might be able to participate in and if they need anything else to make this happen (ie, resources for transportation).

Shifting From Transactional to Relational Responses to Behaviors

When parents have used punishment for years to compel their child to behave, it can often lead to children avoiding or fighting with their parents when they are around Dakota's age, the early teen years.

1. Family strength(s): Talulah is one of the nonparent adults who genuinely cares about Dakota. Dakota and Talulah have had a good relationship in the past.

2. Identify the barrier: Used to their parents essentially bartering their love (connection) for behavior, youth may dig their heels in even more to make it clear they will no longer do what is required to "earn" the caregiver's love (connection). At the moment, Dakota and Talulah have had a series of unrepaired relational health ruptures and they are not communicating well.

3. Self-care: Perhaps you are going through something similar with your teen and notice that parts of this conversation are triggering big feelings in you. Breathe in through your nose and exhale slowly as you listen.

4. Clarify the barrier/need: Talulah is genuinely worried about the trajectory Dakota is on and unleashing a "shock and awe" campaign to try to get her behaviors back on track. If we simply recommend that a dysregulated caregiver spend more time with a dysregulated teen, we are setting everyone up for more adversarial interactions. Use VIVA to validate how disconnected they feel and explore options for repairing the rupture(s) in their relationship. This does not have to be a long conversation. You can validate that things are hard and it may feel stressful and exhausting to be constantly having trouble communicating.

5. Cocreate a plan: Cocreating a path forward for this family, where Dakota actually wants to spend time with Talulah, is unlikely to happen quickly; but you can help them build a bridge. In addition to doing a referral for counseling, offer tools to improve their ability to connect emotionally and communicate effectively (ie, SUNBEAM, NICER parenting) while they are waiting for the first appointment. Emphasize that each person is responsible for soothing their own nervous system, and when someone is having a big emotion, it's

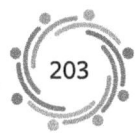

their job not to hurt anyone else, anything else, or themselves while that big feeling is there.

6. Follow up: Plan on close follow-up: have them return in about 2 weeks to see how things are going, and offer to stay closely in touch until Dakota starts her individual counseling.

Coregulation for Teens

We encourage caregivers to be there for teens and support them as they figure out ways to deal with stress.

1. Family strength(s): Talulah genuinely cares about Dakota. Explore with Dakota what she loves and what her interests are.

2. Identify the barrier: Talulah is resorting to harsh discipline because she is afraid that Dakota's behaviors are "out of control." When caregivers and children are simultaneously stressed, trying to be there can just result in yelling and door slamming. Talulah is trying to keep Dakota safe and is trying to be present for her in a way that feels firm but loving. Dakota is behaving in a way that makes Talulah feel like she has to be even stricter.

3. Self-care: Maybe you yelled at your teen and imposed a shock and awe campaign just last night and this is hitting close to home. Remember to put on your own oxygen mask first so you can regulate the room.

4. Clarify the barrier/need: Talulah needs tools and strategies to hold space for a stressed teen when it feels like they are suddenly morphing into a mysterious porcupine. Without being prepared for this, it can feel impossible, especially when the teen takes an adversarial stance. When both teen and caregiver are dysregulated and stuck in a sympathetic response to each other (fight, flight, or freeze), it can even result in the adults kicking the teen out of the house or the teen running away. Dakota is at risk of running away. More than half of youth who run away identify family dynamics, including conflict with caregivers, as a reason they ran away.[5,6]

5. Cocreate a plan: Help Talulah and Dakota understand their current dynamic, how they can put the affiliate response to use and stop seeing each other as a source of danger, and how this supports building relational health and repairing ruptures. Fortunately for us, the same tools support this essential shift. You can draw a "back the bus up" diagram on the exam room table paper and use it to explore what is happening when Talulah and Dakota end up in a yelling match and how they can restore communication. Sharing emotion coaching, NICER parenting, and SUNBEAM with Talulah can help her shift into a less adversarial caregiving stance and be more able to put the affiliate

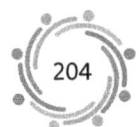

response to use. Once they are communicating better, Talulah can focus more on supporting Dakota's emotional health and long-term goals instead of punishing her.

6. Follow up: Plan to follow up with them either in person or by phone in 2 to 4 weeks, and check in on how this is going and if they are feeling like they can communicate more effectively.

Decision-Making Process

As noted earlier, when a family is experiencing high levels of stress for long periods, it decreases the family's bandwidth for decision-making in general, and all the attention goes to the most essential needs (ie, food, shelter, safety).

1. Family strength(s): Dakota is trying to practice self-care strategies. She is aware she is anxious. Talulah is paying attention to Dakota's behaviors and is concerned about risk.

2. Identify the barrier: At the moment, smoking weed is the only coping skill that helps Dakota feel calm.

3. Self-care: Notice if you feel overwhelmed and keep thinking about your own family's experience. Integrate self-care into how you respond. You may want to model 5 Big Deep Breaths and invite the family to join you.

4. Clarify the barrier/need: Explore if Dakota has tried anything else for her anxiety and what has happened with the things she tried.

5. Cocreate a plan: Offer alternative ways for her to take care of herself when she feels anxious while she waits for the counseling appointment. She may not feel like there is anything else that could help her at first. Practice a few ideas, like toes-to-nose and relaxation breathing, in the office and see if she finds them helpful. These can be listed on her stress reduction plan so they are easier for her to remember. Judicious use of medication may be helpful if her Generalized Anxiety Disorder 7-item scale or Screen for Child Anxiety Related Emotional Disorders form is consistent with a diagnosis of anxiety while working toward comanagement with a mental health professional.

6. Follow up: If you do start medication, you will follow up in 2 to 4 weeks, and this coincides with when you would want to ask how practicing the healthier coping skills is going.

Responding to Harsh Parenting

Talulah is terrified about Dakota's behaviors. She shares with you that she is overwhelmed and is just trying to make sure Dakota isn't ruined for life. She doesn't like it when she yells at Dakota or calls her names, but the stress from everything that is happening feels like too much. You can validate how the stress can cloud

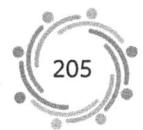

her ability to make clear decisions and feel like she is able to solve problems as they arise. Framing Talulah's responses as some version of "fight," "flight," or "freeze" can help you cocreate a new path. You can reflect back that it sounds like she is so stressed that her nervous system is constantly in danger mode.

You can use the fire-truck brain analogy with teen-friendly language to explain to both Dakota and Talulah the effect the stress may be having on their relationship and ability to communicate. Talulah is caregiving in fight mode: the stress means she isn't able to unlock her prefrontal cortex's full potential, and it feels overwhelmingly like Dakota's behavior is a source of danger. At times, caregivers may be in flight mode, or they step away and distance themselves from their child. Stressed caregivers can also enter into freeze mode, when they essentially shut down in response to situations that feel intolerable and are unable to support or connect with their child. All these modes are typical, neurobiochemical stress responses. And all parents can befriend their nervous systems, put the affiliate response to use, and work through this stress. As Talulah learns to use SUNBEAM, she can notice when she is in this stressed, sympathetic mode and use strategies to shift to a parasympathetic mode before they try to solve issues or make important decisions about Dakota.

Activities and Responsibilities

Dakota is somewhat involuntarily working as a live-in babysitter, which is what has made this housing situation work, at least in the short term. As you explore things with them, stay curious and try to avoid judgments. We have to consider the financial and social implications of any recommendations with regard to activities or sports, especially when a family is experiencing homelessness, toxic stress, or other SDOH. But it also sounds like this is a source of frustration for Dakota: she feels like she didn't sign up for it and doesn't enjoy it. Finding an activity that is fun and that Dakota likes may sound great in theory but feel completely out of reach. It may also be financially impossible. Help the family reframe what fun, helpful activities are, even if it includes making chores more playful and fun. Model telling Dakota how much she is helping by watching Talulah's kids. Ask Dakota what she thinks the worst part of this new situation is. What is one thing she thinks she could do differently to make it feel a little less stressful (eg, stress reduction plan)? What is one thing Talulah could do to support her in her interests? Have they had conversations about what Dakota would like to be doing after school instead of watching these kids? Do they want help connecting with resources to find another housing situation for Dakota? Sharing the Authentic Apologies tool may facilitate a repair of the underlying relational health rupture here, especially if Talulah is feeling guilty about the dynamic but doesn't know what to say.

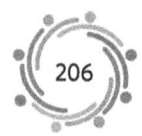

Strategies for Reconnecting

For Talulah, praising Dakota probably feels out of reach at the moment. She is angry with her, and Dakota is angry with Talulah. If she could show sincere appreciation for Dakota in a way that shows she is actually right there with her in this difficult journey, it could facilitate a repair in their relationship rupture. You can share with Talulah that even in the best of times, parents accurately attune to their child's needs about only one-third of the time. In situations like these, that might be even lower because of the toxic levels of day-to-day stress. You can reframe Dakota's behaviors in a way that will help Talulah see past the behaviors and understand how Dakota is struggling. Highlight that Dakota is having a hard time and this is an opportunity for Talulah to model healthy coping skills and a healthy response to stress.

Sometimes you find that caregivers and parents may not currently be able to integrate many or any healthy coping skills. If you feel like Talulah is too over-whelmed to be able to digest SUNBEAM and NICER parenting, consider sharing just the 6 Steps to Connect and then offering to briefly check in with her when you see Dakota back in 2 weeks. Modeling language for Talulah to praise Dakota could sound something like *Wow, it sounds like you and Dakota have been having a hard time connecting lately. Is there something she's been doing that you appreciate?* Encourage Talulah to not frame the praise with things that could make it sound like it's really all about her own needs, because Dakota will catch on to that quickly. Instead, encourage her to frame the praise with regard to Dakota's hard work and effort.

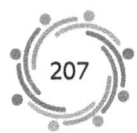
References

1. Gaudreau C, King YA, Dore RA, et al. Preschoolers benefit equally from video chat, pseudo-contingent video, and live book reading: implications for storytime during the coronavirus pandemic and beyond. *Front Psychol*. 2020;11:2158 PMID: 33013552 doi: 10.3389/fpsyg.2020.02158
2. Hanetz-Gamliel K, Dollberg DG. Links between mothers' ACEs, their psychopathology and parenting, and their children's behavior problems—a mediation model. *Front Psychiatry*. 2022;13:1064915 PMID: 36620690 doi: 10.3389/fpsyt.2022.1064915
3. King A. Designing and using efficacious interventions to support early relational health and heal trauma. In: Gillespie RJ, King A. *The Trauma-Informed Pediatric Practice: A Resilience-Based Roadmap to Foster Early Relational Health*. American Academy of Pediatrics; 2024 doi: 10.1542/9781610027410
4. Ryan SA, Ammerman SD, Gonzalez PK, Patrick SW, Quigley J, Walker LR; American Academy of Pediatrics Committee on Substance Use and Prevention. Counseling parents and teens about marijuana use in the era of legalization of marijuana. *Pediatrics*. 2017;139(3):e20164069 PMID: 28242859 doi: 10.1542/peds.2016-4069
5. Fact sheet. National Runaway Safeline. Accessed November 13, 2024. https://www.nationalrunawaysafeline.org/wp-content/uploads/2021/02/NRS-Fact-Sheet-2021.pdf
6. Noh D, Kim E. Experiences of family conflict in shelter-residing runaway youth: a phenomenological study. *J Fam Issues*. 2021;42(10):2335–2352 doi: 10.1177/0192513X20979624

Chapter 8

Universal Integration in Practice

I remember when my teachers said in medical school that by the time I finished my training, a large percentage of what I had learned would already be obsolete. This is true not only in regard to treating complex medical diseases but also from a biopsychosocial perspective. One of the things that probably has always been the same but is only just becoming part of our overt conversations is how every symptom a patient and their family brings to us is part of a bigger web of relationships, stressors, resource networks, and histories. How do trauma and overwhelming stress play a role in disease process or relational health rupture, and how does resilience illuminate a path back to health?

When we embrace trauma-informed care as a universal precaution offered across the population, it can be seen as a primary, secondary, and/or tertiary response.[1,2] From this perspective, the tools and strategies you learn from this book can be applied in any clinical encounter. At the core of this type of trauma-informed care is an assumption that trauma affects everyone's life at some point. Instead of only using trauma-informed care after asking if a family has experienced trauma, we apply it universally.

Use a trauma-informed response the next time a worried parent asks if their child is OK, even if you end up using that billing code "complaint unfounded." We have to validate their worry to build trust and engage families in care. Often we want to quickly reassure them that everything is OK, perhaps even before we are really sure that everything is actually OK, to help soothe palpable parental fear. Of course we want to reassure the parents. That is a normal human response and often part of our clinical practice. We can help parents accept the idea that everything is actually "OK" even when things are "not OK." We can normalize fluctuations in the 4 building blocks of HOPE (Healthy Outcomes from Positive Experiences) just like we do in different organ systems as a part of any human's life trajectory. Integrating emerging knowledge from developmental neuroscience and epigenetics research into the visit means we can not only

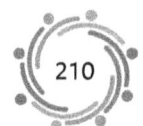

treat the ear infection but also address the parents' fears about why their child is constantly getting ear infections: *Is it because I am working full-time and sending him to child care? Am I hurting him by not being home? Is it because Dad smokes in the house? Is it because I can't stop giving him a bottle at bedtime even though I know you said I should have stopped doing that months ago?* Remain curious about the meta-message behind the ear infection and how can you address that in a simultaneous, seamless, and trauma-informed manner.

Honoring the parents' fears and concerns does not have to take all day. Don't worry: with these stepwise skills and strategies, I find that we often stay more on time with our days than we may have in the past while being able to feel like we didn't ignore those elephants in the room. We can order the lab workup for immunodeficiency and treat the 10th ear infection without falling behind because the skills we're developing for talking about hard things become as well honed and natural as the skills we have in deciding which antibiotic is best for that bulging, erythematous pus drum. We can get to the heart of the parents' concerns, have fewer questions that leave us feeling helpless, and proactively uncover what the family may not have historically felt comfortable bringing up. This decreases what leads to "doorknob moments," those far-reaching concerns or questions that the family brings up just as we are about to leave the encounter.

Parents are asking us for this kind of help and guidance. When we view their worries and concerns through the lens of resilience, the real ask looks a little different. Parents may be asking for your advice about whether they should stop working and take their child out of child care: *Would that help my child with the recurrent ear infections be healthier?* Of course, that question is not really one for you to answer. What is the parent really saying? *I'm worried. Is my baby going to be OK? Are the choices I am making hurting him? How do I know what is the right thing for his health? How can I help him grow up to be healthy and happy and not have to struggle with the same things that have plagued me my whole life?*

General Parenting Guidance

The surgeon general's 2024 advisory about parental stress highlighted how 48% of parents feel that most days their stress is overwhelming,[3] compared with 26% of nonparent adults. Barriers to implementing parenting recommendations have been studied[4,5] and the role of parental stress highlighted as an area that needs to be addressed for any parenting intervention to be effective. Part of the benefit of the tools and strategies discussed in this book is that they use mnemonics and other easy-to-remember frameworks both for us as stressed clinicians and for stressed parents. Mnemonics help us remember things when we may be temporarily in fight-or-flight mode and trying to function mostly from our "fire-truck brain." In medical school, we often used them to retrieve complex information

under the pressure of taking tests; in residency, they helped us remember differential diagnoses; and we still use them universally for emergency responses. In the middle of a stressful parenting encounter, caregivers can walk themselves through the steps of SUNBEAM (See, Unhook, Nurture, Breathe, Emotionally Aware, Mindful, Meditation) and NICER (Notice, Identify, Connect/coregulate, Explore, Review/repair) parenting. In the middle of a stressful patient care moment, you can still access VIVA (Validate, Inform, Validate, Ask).

We can use the strategies and tools in this book to teach caregivers about noticing their own feelings as part of our routine parenting guidance. Being able to access tools and skills in the moment can transform problematic or stuck parenting patterns. You can first validate the parents' feeling in the moment and then show them how validation supports emotional processing. In this process, you are modeling for a caregiver how they can do this for themselves as well as the children they care for.

For example, the first step is trying to label the feeling or feelings. What unpleasant emotion or unmet need is coming up for you, the caregivers, or the kids? Is it fear or frustration? Exhaustion? Hunger? Aloneness? Whatever it is, you can practice yourself and coach families in identifying feelings. Remember, it is OK to start with just "unpleasant," "hard," or "yucky." The next step is to identify a healthy coping skill or a way to address barriers to meeting any unmet need (eg, getting food when hungry, resting when tired, getting a coat or blanket when cold). Some parents may have readily accessible healthy coping skills and strategies for overcoming barriers, whereas others may not be as familiar with these concepts and may welcome the new tools and skills. As parents internalize this simple rhythm of noticing, identifying, and connecting with their own feelings or with someone else having an unmet need or big emotion, fewer needs go unmet and parents naturally adopt an emotion coaching response, which we've discussed throughout the book.

Taking the time to reflect and honor the parent's or caregiver's own emotions allows them to understand how they landed where they are in their parenting. Otherwise, they end up doing what I affectionately call "accidental parenting," where they are not at all aware of how they got to where they are, and if they wanted to change something, they couldn't. Think of *The Wizard of Oz*, when Oz is taking off in the hot-air balloon and Dorothy calls out to him, asking him to wait and come back, and he says, "I can't! I don't know how to work this thing!" Emphasizing how you have seen the family do hard things is the strengths-based foundation of this problem-solving approach, looking at the timeline of behaviors and connecting them with experiences and emotions. The adults raising the children can understand how feelings and resilience intertwine through the framework of relational health and emotional growth and then proactively make intentional decisions about how they want to relate to their kids in difficult moments.

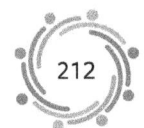

This approach can also be helpful when the question itself arises from something that does not have a traditional Western clinical basis for concern. This may include things like vaccine hesitancy, nonclinical food sensitivities or avoidance, or school choices. If you approach these with a dismissive strategy, you will lose many parents' trust. I have always taken the stance that if it is important to the parents, it needs to be equally important to me so I can understand how this concern is affecting their parenting and their child's access to health and wellness.

On one level, we are clinical experts, with years of training and experience offering scientifically proven strategies for healing while embracing the delicate art of practicing medicine. On another level, I can lightheartedly see myself as a kind of "fancy waitress." Physicians are experts who know the "menu" of Western medicine inside and outside, forward and backward. While it is our job to explain to our patients and their parents all the different options for care so we can proceed with shared decision-making, at the end of the day, the parents are the ones who choose the care model they think is best for their children. My lived experience helps me validate how scary it is to have a sick child and how hard it is to think clearly when you are frightened beyond belief. A parent who is afraid is trying to use just their fire-truck brain to figure out what treatment plan they should pick from the options we offer. This can result in the familiar sympathetic nervous system response patterns: "fight" (arguing), "flight" (declining care), or "freeze" (being unable to decide). Normalize how no one talks about how important it is to have accessible strategies and skills to shift out of that sympathetic nervous system mode, so we can unlock our prefrontal cortices again and consider all the options and variables. As pediatricians, we can coach caregivers in this process so they can make good decisions for their children. By modeling a path for parents to understand their own nervous system, we can work with them so their fire-truck brain doesn't get in the way and freeze or hijack their decision-making.

We can also honor an almost constant, often unspoken parenting feeling: fatigue. Especially if a parent has a child with a chronic or serious health condition, decision fatigue[6] can be overwhelming and itself a source of toxic stress. In the past decade, researchers have explored what happens with our brains when we are asked to make decision after decision. This process is exhausting to the brain, and we have only so much energy for it during the day. When we reach our limit, we become irritable and make more split-second decisions. Parents experience decision fatigue all the time, and it rarely gets validated. Talking openly about how decision fatigue plays a role even in more mundane settings, like the spontaneous candy purchase at the checkout or the parent's response to a meltdown at the shoe store on back-to-school shopping day, can help parents and patients understand

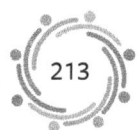

that all these experiences are normal. Just like a muscle that is exhausted after being used for hours, the brain needs regular rests from making decisions.

We can also validate how often parents feel overwhelmingly stressed and how changing that feels impossible. Mitigating the impact of parental and caregiver stress on children involves another version of "backing the bus up," where we support parents in unpacking the myriad of feelings and unmet needs that have led to their own feelings of unmanageable stress. In doing this, we help them see how they can connect to resources and integrate healthy coping skills to decrease the allostatic load. Regardless of whether stressed parents are also feeling either fatigued and worried or frustrated and hungry, there are almost always multiple feelings involved with any sort of prolonged stressor, including those that involve a medical or mental health journey. When we understand this tendency and help our staff understand it as well, we may see how a stressed parent who arrives appearing angry about a small scheduling change is also frustrated and hungry and experiencing decision fatigue, so the whole idea of another decision at that point may just feel like too much. Through a resilience-informed lens, we understand and normalize how the family is experiencing our office and the day-to-day frustrations of obtaining medical care. Staff can be trained in the same tools we are sharing with families so they can respond in a meaningful way, further mitigating stress.

Examples of Clinical Scenarios

Working with families who are currently experiencing stress or trauma may feel challenging. You may feel frustrated, as though nothing, including the trauma-informed strategies from this book, could "work" in these situations. But with a little self-care, and a trauma-informed stepwise approach, we can usually support integrating at least one strategy with any family. Even in situations where you uncover an acutely neglectful or abusive dynamic and need to make a report to social services, you can still use these tools for your own self-care and for your staff as you discuss with the family your obligation to report and go through that process.

Often parents with children who have complex health care needs have already tried a handful of approaches, and if they are coming to you, most likely these have not worked or haven't been helpful enough. Many of the initial approaches are behavior based and advise parents to withhold attention, privileges, or access to toys or coveted things to try to bring about behavior change. But many children who are neurodivergent or have special health care needs struggle even more than children without those to effectively express their emotional needs. This can result in more behavior concerns and affect caregiver well-being.[7,8] We can help relieve stress from this struggle.

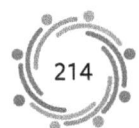

When a Child Is Neurodivergent

Children on the autism spectrum flourish with support in understanding interpersonal interactions. All parents intermittently struggle to understand what their children need, and with neurodivergent children, overstimulation or sensory overload may more frequently trigger an unmanageable behavioral state. The traditional applied behavioral analysis (ABA) approach has garnered criticism for discouraging behaviors without acknowledging their emotional component.[9] We can support strategies for emotional awareness and self-care to help parents manage their own unpleasant feelings as well as their child's big emotions while the child works on ABA therapies. Studies have shown that how parents respond to their children's big emotions can help autistic children with emotional regulation and social adjustment.[10]

More research is needed to understand the role parents can play in helping neurodivergent children learn emotional regulation, but studies indicate that a combination of prompting the child to discuss their emotions and passively following the child's lead when they talk about their feelings may be effective for school-aged children with ASD.[11] A pilot study showed that physical exertion was helpful with emotional regulation and behaviors such as meltdowns, self-injuries, or aggression in children with ASD,[12] indicating that high-energy coping strategies may be a good approach for the "10 Things I Can Do When I Feel Yucky" list in this subset of children.

Children with ASD may need to use strategies other than a mindfulness approach to their emotions because of their literal and concrete thought processes. Cognitive reappraisal, or using the mind to reframe an unpleasant experience, can also be a helpful tool to add, specifically for children with ASD, and increase emotional regulation.[9] When supporting families, encourage parents to still try to be mindful that they don't label emotions as "bad" or "good" and try to avoid blaming the emotion on a specific external factor. Even though it may seem like an older child's anger is related to riding in the car next to a little sibling, we can point out that when the older child's nervous system is calm and regulated, they can tolerate sitting there without hitting or yelling at their little sibling. It is only when they are dysregulated and don't feel good at baseline that these tasks are experienced as impossible—for both the child and the caregivers! As parents gain confidence in using these skills, they can model self-care, talk about the temporary nature of emotions, and work with their children on emotional regulation.

Intellectual or Physical Disabilities

Children who have physical or intellectual disabilities are often very aware that things are harder for them than for their peers. Many parents raise their children with the mindset that they can do anything they want to if they just set their

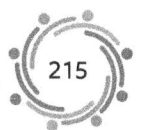

mind to it. These families often struggle with meltdowns when things are difficult or the child gets exhausted trying to accomplish something. Both parents and children in these families can benefit from the Resilience University tools and strategies, so they can try out different approaches and integrate time for self-care. Just giving the family language to acknowledge experiences and validate feelings can help the child process how skill acquisition and their learning journey may be different for them.

The role that unmanageable emotions play in difficult behaviors has been studied with children who have intellectual disabilities. Research shows that how parents respond to their child's emotions can help children who have intellectual disabilities learn to regulate their emotions.[13]

Suicidality

Elevated adverse childhood experience scores are associated with an increased likelihood that an individual will attempt suicide.[14] Given that suicide is the second leading cause of death in adolescents aged 14 to 18 years and that suicidality has increased from 2009 to 2019,[9] pediatricians are much more likely to encounter this regularly. We need meaningful responses both for when we need to escalate care and for when we can safely send the child and family home with an outpatient plan. For the children who have a plan or intent to harm themselves, we are providing a bridge while they wait for a higher level of care. For the children who do not have a plan or suicidal intent, we are also providing a bridge to services (eg, counseling, medication, support services), which may not start to help as quickly as we hope. In that space, between when a child presents with suicidal thoughts and when the family gets established with needed support and services, our support is crucial to the child's well-being.

When a child expresses that they wish they were dead or that life is too hard, it feels terrifying for parents. All too often, the core of what the child is trying to express gets lost in their parents' fear. A loving, terrified parent may start yelling or taking away privileges or time with friends in an effort to change this behavior because this is a reflexive parenting response. These parenting responses are understandable and come from Skinner's[10] operant conditioning studies, which are the cornerstone of behavior-based parenting approaches. But a child expressing suicidality needs emotional connection, coregulation, and validation of how hard things are for them, not behavioral modification techniques.

More often than not, children who attempt suicide are not trying to end their lives; they are crying out for help.[11] Only 20% of children and adolescents who attempt or die by suicide have a psychiatric history, and more than half of pediatric suicides are preceded by a specific precipitating event, most commonly conflict with a romantic partner.[12] We know that almost 20% of teens

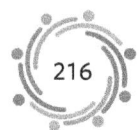
have seriously considered suicide,[9] which means this phenomenon is happening within almost every adolescent friend group.

Some parents want to pull us out into the hallway, away from their child, to talk about suicidal ideation. But when a child has suicidal thoughts, talking about it openly and validating the feelings can help shift a stressful dynamic. Other parents are not aware their children have been thinking about suicide when we discover this on the PHQ-9 Modified for Adolescents. I always ask the child first if it is OK if I talk about the answers on the questionnaire with their parents or guardians. Depending on age, I prefer to do this when I am with the child alone, but I have developed a way of asking even if a parent is still in the room. I'll say to the child, *Is it OK with you if we talk about your answers on this questionnaire with [caregiver] here, or do you want them to step out for a minute while we talk?* Sometimes, speaking with the parent alone, without their child, can further pathologize whatever is happening. I intentionally try to normalize that a mental health issue is the same to me as a case of cellulitis or diabetes. And I wouldn't want a child to think they can somehow get better on their own without help or that they should be hiding how they are feeling from their parents. By explaining suicidality this way, we can often work past the stigma and families' cultural and functional ideas around mental health.

We commonly refer patients with suicidal ideation to a counselor who will start some form of evidence-based therapy, such as cognitive behavioral therapy or dialectical behavioral therapy. Often we also start a prescription, such as a selective serotonin reuptake inhibitor. Both these interventions take time to start helping. Children and families can use the healthy coping skills, emotional regulation tools, and problem-solving strategies you teach them when thoughts arise that life is too hard and they feel like they don't want to be here anymore. Emotion coaching and the trauma-informed parenting approach of SUNBEAM allow parents to lean in with curiosity, notice their own natural fear in response to what their child is experiencing, and, rather than reflexively resort to fear-based punishment to try to stay in control, stay connected. Families can become more comfortable talking about feelings as they go through this difficult experience, by using emotional awareness and healthy coping skills, and foster connection. Talking about unpleasant feelings and using the same stepwise problem-solving strategy (Plan-Do-Study-Act, or PDSA, cycles) for addressing barriers to integrating healthy coping skills and necessary resources in the context of suicidality can help make the stress feel more tolerable.

Self-Harm

Children who experience suicidal ideation are 7 times more likely to also experience non-suicidal self-injury (NSSI).[15] With both increasingly presenting to primary care clinicians, having language to work with families is helpful. Finding out that a child is engaging in self-harm (eg, cutting, burning, hitting themselves)

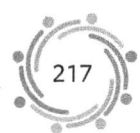

can be overwhelming and terrifying for parents. Caregivers often have a sympathetic nervous system overload and understandably act from that space of fear, sincerely trying to protect the child from self-harm by punishing them for doing it. Emotion coaching and SUNBEAM give parents language and strategies to help them respond to self-harm behaviors, shifting the parents' focus away from the viscerally alarming behavior and toward the underlying issue. When parents can see that their child is struggling (not just doing something that alarms them), they are often able to put the affiliate response to use within the space of sympathetic overload and shift from trying to control to trying to connect with their child.

When you are seeing children with NSSI, first, make sure the child is safe and there are no urgent safety concerns you need to address. Second, screen for suicidal ideation, depression, and anxiety. Self-harm is not always a direct precursor to suicide, but we would never want to miss a cry for help. Then you can help the family process and understand what is happening with the child (eg, by using the analogy that emotions are like ocean waves: they come and go with their own rhythm, and it's our job to learn to care for ourselves while the big emotion is there so we don't hurt ourselves, anyone else, or anything else).

Encourage families not to punish the child for self-harm. Ensure they get the counseling and tailored support the child needs as soon as possible. For many communities, however, rapid access to counseling and teen support services is not available. Sharing breathing exercises, meditation skills, and mindfulness practices can give the child ways to care for themselves while they await the referral(s). Emotion coaching and trauma-informed parenting strategies give the family a way to understand and respond to what is happening. Plan-Do-Study-Act cycles can help the family problem-solve areas that may be contributing to the child's emotional distress and help repair any relational health ruptures to provide more connection and emotional support.

We know that for the child, self-harm is not an intentional act to defy parents' rules. Some research, however, indicates that NSSI is more common when children report experiencing their parents as invalidating, controlling, punitive, and non-supportive.[16] Cutting, or any self-harm act, is a less-than-ideal coping skill that the child has figured out helps them tolerate otherwise unbearable emotions and feelings. Like with any unhealthy coping skill, punishing them for using it without supporting them with new, functional healthy coping skills doesn't set them up for success. Once parents understand that the behavior is coming from a deeper, more complex emotional state, they can respond in a more compassionate way. Encourage parents not to shame or belittle this behavior as well as not to focus too much on it, to the point where the child feels that the self-harm is the most effective way to get parents to notice their emotional needs. Reconnecting with adults for support is very important; that process can

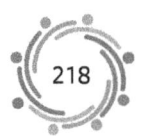

begin in your exam room when you become a trusted adult who understands what is happening and can guide the worried parents down a path to reconnect with their struggling child. If talking about feelings is not part of the family culture, using a family feelings chart can help destigmatize the feelings underlying concerning behaviors. Supporting parents with the "NICER Parenting" and "SUNBEAM: A Parent's Antidote to Meltdowns" handouts can serve as a blueprint for a different response.

Patient-centered PDSA cycles can help the child come up with a set of different coping strategies that don't cause harm to their body or anything else. Cocreate a plan integrating healthy coping skills with a list, as long as possible, of things the child can try when they feel like self-harming. We can work with the parents to support the child in using habit stacking to try one of the healthy skills instead of NSSI when unpleasant thoughts or emotions arise. Explaining the time-versus-emotion curve to the parent and child can help as well, since allowing thoughts to amplify feelings over time can increase the intensity of the urge to self-harm and make the other coping skills feel less effective.

Sometimes, replacing the act of cutting with something noninjurious that still has a sensory skin component can act as a bridge while the child builds healthier responses to overwhelming emotions. Techniques with direct use of the skin may be helpful early in the process, such as rubbing the skin, taking a shower, using an ice cube on the skin, or snapping a rubber band on the wrist. Different strategies will be more or less effective depending on the child and the situation. These can help lead the way to the generalized coping skills we've discussed throughout the book: mindfulness, meditation, breathing exercises, exercise, art or writing, calling a friend, or singing/music, to name a few.

Another helpful step is for parents to remove the items the child is using for NSSI. This cannot be the only response and has to be done in a nonpunitive way. Because of the natural fear response many parents have, they may appreciate coaching on how to communicate with their children about this and help initiate the conversation in the office: *When someone is healing from self-harm, it is an important part of the process to keep their space safe. Can you share what you are using to self-harm now?* Once the child has disclosed the current self-harm devices, you can turn to the parents and say, *Do you think you can help your child by keeping those somewhere else for now so she can have a safe space to heal?* Use the conversation in the exam room to normalize the child's use of a common but unhealthy coping strategy, and help the parents see how they can support choosing healthier options. Caution the parents not to expect this shift to happen overnight and to avoid shame or blame for using less-than-ideal strategies. When parents can remain connected without letting their fear or frustration come between them and their child, they can be more effective in responding to their child's underlying

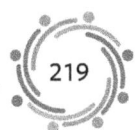
needs. With SUNBEAM and PDSA cycles on emotion coaching, we can support parents in consistently regulating their own nervous systems to allow them to respond in a more validating, supportive, nonpunitive, noncontrolling manner.

Substance Use

Like with self-harm, many tweens and teens are using vaping (nicotine and/ or cannabis) to help with anxiety and other unpleasant feelings. Remember that for teens, saying *Don't do XYZ* may actually make them want to do it more. Reactance[13] makes teens want to do whatever is off-limits to regain a freedom they feel is threatened, while amplification[17] guarantees that the off-limits thing (ie, drugs) will get more bandwidth in their minds. With 30% of high school students currently reporting daily e-cigarette use,[18] just making these things illegal for kids and telling them not to do it is ineffective.

While the data may be hard for us to digest as clinicians, the actual experience is impossibly stressful for the parents. As caring adults in the tweens' and teens' lives, we need to care for our own fear and frustration, regulate our nervous systems, and create a space where youth can feel safe, heard, and held as they work through their relationship with these readily available substances. As we do this, we can model language and self-care strategies for parents that they can use to repair relational health ruptures and better understand their child's experience and needs.

We can support parents to respond in a meaningful way when they discover their child is using substances. The traditional, punitive parenting response would be to take away the phone, ground the child, and confiscate any drugs and paraphernalia found in the child's possession. If the child is routinely turning to nicotine, cannabis, or another substance for self-medicating, this approach may backfire. Without guidance on how to approach this situation differently, many parents go with the "shock and awe" parenting approach we discussed in Chapter 7, Examples of Tailored Anticipatory Guidance: Vignettes, consisting of yelling, berating comments, and removal of the child's connection with friends as punishment. A frightened parent with their child's best interests at heart may react with harsh verbal discipline, saying things like *How could you be so stupid!* Or, *Haven't we raised you to know better? What on earth is wrong with you?* Or, *What are you thinking? You are choosing to be a drug addict after all I've done for you?* Isolating a child or teen after this type of encounter could be triggering and leaves them vulnerable and alone.

Recent data from Maine show that an average of 76% of high school students felt that a kid who used cannabis would be caught by the police and knew that their parents would disapprove, yet more than 25% of high school seniors also reported using cannabis within the past month and 43% of seniors had tried it.[19]

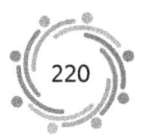

Our threat of punishment and our disapproval alone are not enough to protect children from the harms of substance use.

If, instead, we approach youth substance use with a nonjudgmental, curious attitude and use a similar framework to the ones we are using elsewhere in this book, we will increase trust and understanding. When we assume drug use is secondary to an underlying emotion or feeling state, we can be curious about what is going on. Approaching substance use scenarios by using a similar technique to what we laid out for self-harm can help parents respond in a way that fosters relational health and resilience.

One way to start is simply to frame substance use as an unhealthy coping skill and work to extinguish it while integrating new, healthier coping skills. Explaining positive childhood experiences (PCEs) to parents can help them understand why isolating children is counterproductive. If you notice parents are stuck in a harsh discipline pattern, try using the VIVA approach to inform them about the long-term harm associated with calling a child names or screaming at them.[20] It can help to normalize this pattern by sharing that some historical studies have shown that 90% of US parents report using harsh discipline.[21]

An example of VIVA might go as follows: *It's completely normal to feel angry when you find out your child is smoking weed.* (Validate) *We know that when your child is struggling, they really need connection and support.* (Inform) *Most parents get angry with their kids in this scenario and often feel terrified too.* (Validate) *Would you be interested in ideas to help stay connected through this? I'm honored to be here for you, just like when he was hospitalized for asthma.* (Ask). Assuming the family says yes, you can follow with another VIVA: *It's normal to feel reluctant to talk about this since it has already brought up some really big feelings.* (Validate) *Research has shown that feeling like you can talk about your feelings with your family and like you have been supported by friends are 2 of the protective factors that can offset the long-term impact of any adversity.* (Inform) *All families struggle with talking about feelings from time to time, and it can be a normal parenting strategy to "ground" a kid when they break the rules.* (Validate) *Do you want to explore a different strategy?* (Ask)

With unhealed trauma and ongoing stressors, teens may be more at risk for self-medicating. For a caregiver to view friends who rely on vaping simply as a "bad" friend choice may miss the point and remove the teen's access to that crucial, supportive connection with peers. Just like with any other unwanted behavior, we may end up where we want to go sooner if we start with radical acceptance of what is happening and then look underneath the surface, lean in, and be curious about why it is happening. Blaming friend groups is problematic as well since often it is shared unpleasant or traumatic experiences that will bring a set of teens together for support.

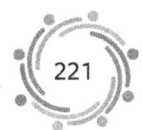

Of course, medical interventions and additional referrals may also be warranted. If a teen is addicted to nicotine, they may need medication for nicotine use disorder or some alternative approach to be able to stop vaping. If the resources are available in your community and the family is accepting of the referral, you can also include teen substance use counselors or support groups. Because this topic brings up so many feelings for both parents and teens, it can be difficult to get traction with outside referrals and is one area where leveraging the trust that the family members have in you, as their primary care clinician, can help support the family system as they experience this stressor.

Depression and Anxiety

In addition to your routine screening questionnaires and referrals, you can integrate emotion coaching, PDSA cycles, healthy coping skills, and trauma-informed parenting practices to help patients and parents manage symptoms while waiting for a prescription to work and/or for referrals. Many times, caregivers have a hard time understanding the severity of their child's depression or anxiety. Depending on the age and family milieu, many children work hard to hide their symptoms from their parents, especially if the family is undergoing major life stressors. By the time they bring the concern to you, the family health may have already been affected, and responding with a resilience-informed approach can help restore relational health and promote other protective factors.

In Western culture, it's common for parents and patients to come to you with the hope that a prescription will fix everything. Yet helping them understand that prescriptions are only part of the treatment for mental health issues can help launch a discussion about healthy coping skills and connecting to additional resources and supports. For so many families, feeling sad or angry or worried has historically been framed as "bad" or unwanted. Start by explaining that feeling sad or worried or angry is unpleasant but also a normal part of being human. We get to the point of prescribing medication when these feelings are interfering with what the person wants or needs to do in their life. I point out that it's normal to feel worried about going to school, but if the worried feelings are keeping the child from going to school, then we need to rethink what is going on and find a way to keep the feelings from derailing the day. For anxiety and depression, I say that prescriptions are sort of like a bridge. The child is at point A, and we need to get them to point B. For children not experiencing anxiety or depression, there is a straight path along even ground from point A to point B. For a child who is struggling with anxiety or depression, it may feel like the Grand Canyon lies between these points. It may seem that the only way across is to shimmy down one side and climb up the other, but medication offers the

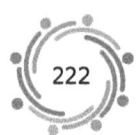

possibility of building a bridge. I always emphasize that medication is offered *in addition to*, not instead of, working with the feelings and learning healthy coping skills. We have to do both simultaneously. Since the medication may take a few weeks to start helping, the first step is healthy coping skills.

If a family is willing to accept a referral to counseling, I place that and share the anticipated wait time until the counselor will be able to see the family. This often involves validating the family's frustration in how long it will take to get in since in our area, there are often long wait lists. Next, I offer to help them come up with some strategies and tools that might help make things feel a little less hard while they are waiting for the counseling. Emphasize how this is not all about the child; it is important for the parent or caregiver to have skills, tools, and strategies as well. This is also an important place to frame your suggestion through a strengths-based lens (eg, *Remember when you all realized that Josie had diabetes? That felt so overwhelming at first, didn't it? And look at you all now: you could manage her insulin in your sleep. I've seen your family do hard things and I am here to support you, no matter what*).

If younger kids want to come up with strategies, I have them make a list with either my help or the parent's of 10 things they can do when they feel "yucky" (eg, "box" or "square" breathing, glitter jar meditation, sensory grounding with 5-4-3-2-1, drawing, singing). For older kids, I help them fill out a stress reduction plan or put the list into their phone and I help them come up with realistic, accessible ideas for self-care (eg, singing, listening to music, doodling, 5 Big Deep Breaths, toes-to-nose, journaling). I make sure the parents understand that self-care may need to take priority over other activities at the moment and that anything needed for self-care should never be taken away as part of discipline. If missed school and catching up on work are contributing to the stress level and disrupting relational health, frame this as a solvable problem. You can recommend they check with the school about a Section 504 plan and support the family in asking for any other necessary accommodations to allow the child to continue to get their education.

When youth are struggling with their mental health, they may engage in NSSI or substance use or express suicidal thoughts. Integrate the approaches from those sections of this chapter into your work with families as needed.

Oppositional Behaviors, Aggression, and Impulsivity

Aggression, trouble focusing, and impulsivity can all be signs of trauma. Sometimes they are associated with a larger diagnosis, but often they manifest before the diagnosis is made. They may be isolated symptoms causing impairment at school and difficulties at home and with friends. Teasing out "pure" attention-deficit/hyperactivity disorder (ADHD) from trauma-related symptoms can be impossible even with psychiatric evaluations and neuropsychological testing.

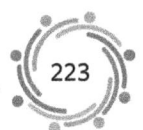
For example, bring to mind a time when you were seeing a patient for behavioral problems and the parent was convinced they had ADHD except the symptoms were present only at home. Perhaps you felt pressured by the parent to put their child on medication, but you were clinically certain it was more of a relational issue. Hyperactivity and impulsivity can be symptoms from trauma and overwhelming stress. You can use VIVA in this scenario to validate the parent's frustration, inform them that this isn't consistent with ADHD, validate how that information may feel terrifying, and then ask if they want to explore other strategies that may help improve the behaviors and relationships at home. If the family is interested, you can share NICER parenting and emotion coaching while you're making a glitter jar with the child. You can see the family back and cocreate PDSA cycles to integrate these new skills into the household dynamic. In a setting where the child is having behavioral issues at school as well, encourage the family to share useful tools and strategies with the school so they can incorporate them into any behavior management plan, Section 504 plan, or individualized education program.

When mutual dysregulation happens, we can offer a bird's-eye view of what is happening so parents can respond differently to a child who is not following directions. Framing oppositional behaviors and defiance as a symptom of a ruptured child-parent bond helps you direct the family toward interpersonal strategies, healthy coping skills, and resources to help repair this. You can coach caregivers so they can begin to see how stalemate standoffs between them and the child may not actually be the child's fault. Often families are stuck in a cycle and just need an external nudge to stop revolving in the same orbit around the same problem. When parents bring a problematic behavioral situation to us, we're able to help them find a different path around the same obstacle just like we would work with them on weird-colored baby poop. Sharing strategies like NICER parenting, SUNBEAM, emotion coaching, the time-versus-emotion curve, and healthy coping skills allows parents to turn what is now a source of conflict into an opportunity for connection and PCEs.

Mindfulness, meditation, and breathing exercises can help parents manage their own frustration and implement change when their child's neuropsychological evaluation results are inconclusive. Many parents have been waiting for months to get the results of a neuropsychological evaluation, sure it will make things easier, only to receive complex information about family systems and behavioral modification strategies that might feel out of reach, especially for families with multiple social drivers of health (SDOH) and toxic levels of stress. Similarly, a diagnosis without any role for medication can feel overwhelming for families. They may feel like they have already tried everything and that without medication, nothing can improve. Yet you can authentically reassure them: you are with them in this journey with tools and strategies for the behaviors. Then, together,

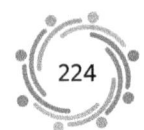

cocreate a plan that works. Encourage parents to try looking at things through a resilience-informed lens, highlighting the power of caring for yourself when unpleasant feelings and experiences arise. We can also encourage parents to parent asynchronously (unless the situation is a true emergency) if they are overwhelmed, by using SUNBEAM and NICER parenting. Parents can shift their focus from extinguishing unwanted behaviors to using emotion coaching and validating experiences.

When impulsive, aggressive, or oppositional behaviors result in a physical injury, patients often land in the emergency department. When you see them in follow-up, you can use the VIVA approach for parents, integrating how "It's OK to not be OK." If the family consents to working on new strategies with you, you can suggest the parents try the "back the bus up" approach along with the time-versus-emotion curve. Perhaps in that process, you learn that the child punched the wall only after a parent took away their phone and called them stupid. Here you can offer VIVA again, normalizing how occasional harsh discipline happens and supporting restoration of a coregulation space in those moments. If the family would like to try something new, you could cocreate a path with PDSA cycles around identifying feelings earlier and choosing healthy self-care approaches for the child and for the parent, trying SUNBEAM and emotion coaching instead of the harsh discipline. By doing this in the clinical setting, we are normalizing how "Big behaviors happen when you have big emotions" and "Your job is to take care of yourself while the big emotion is there and not hurt anything or anyone else, including yourself." Families where anger is often expressed as aggression may find the Authentic Apologies tool useful as a step toward relational health rupture repair.

When a Child Is in Foster Care

When a child enters the foster care system, the changes in living situation, relationships, and routines can decrease the chance that they will maintain existing PCEs. Ensure foster parents are aware of the PCEs and able to connect with resources for support as they try to implement trauma-informed parenting, which may look very different from how they have parented their own children.

Validate how different and challenging things may feel for the child and foster family. Normalize that behaviors may arise simply from previous patterns or in response to new situations, and encourage everyone to remember that behaviors are a sign of underlying feelings, unmet needs, or unmanageable emotions. These feelings are important and require a response, either meeting the need or practicing some form of self-care or healthy coping strategy. What form this takes may differ depending on the behaviors, family structure, age of the child, and other factors. To help with difficult transitions, foster parents can use breathing exercises, singing, or meditation or mindfulness tools. One example

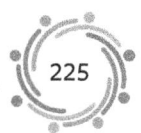
would be to start singing the ABCs with the child and then say *We need to be in the car by the time we get to Z* to make it a fun, connected game as well as a healthy coping skill. Caregivers can implement NICER parenting as an alternative to time-outs since those can be experienced as traumatic for children with a history of abuse or neglect. We can provide a valuable safety net for information for foster parents, who may not have been told that discipline strategies that worked for their biological children may be harmful to a foster child. We can cocreate problem-solving cycles with the foster family as well, to help the child adjust to new routines and environments and the foster family's culture (see Chapter 4, Process for Stepwise Change). If you are seeing the child when they are entering care, the new caregivers are still getting to know this child, so it may take a few visits to figure out what helps lower stress and foster connection in different situations. Reassure the foster parents that you are right there with them, just like you would be for an asthma exacerbation. Normalize how the foster child has been through a lot of change and that this can feel hard, but there are some things that can help make it feel less hard over time. You can draw the HOPE building blocks of environment and engagement on the exam table paper and see if you can identify safe areas of continuity for the child within each block. You can share with the new caregivers how it is protective over the long term to maintain connections with 1 or 2 safe nonparent adults (eg, previous teacher, minister, or coach) and facilitate a sense of mattering and belonging (eg, cultural traditions, community groups, after-school activities).

When a Family Member Is Sick

If a parent or sibling has an illness, acute or chronic, it can disrupt the family's normal routines and structure. If there is a sense of fear for the family member's life or well-being, this can be experienced in a traumatic way for children. The same approach we've discussed throughout this chapter works here too: validate the emotions and experience, inform caregivers that less-than-ideal behaviors may arise, validate how challenging these may be, and ask if they are interested in identifying useful coping skills and resources. Community-based or online peer support groups for parents are wonderful resources and can provide them with a space to connect with others and express frustration or exhaustion, so it doesn't end up getting blamed on their children. If a child is sick, the siblings may not be getting as much attention from the parents as they are used to; on top of this, they are likely afraid for the well-being of their sibling. This underlying fear and change in routine can lead to unwanted behaviors. With the parents already stressed and afraid, parental responses to the other siblings may be reactive and less intentional than what the parents would do if they were in a different setting.

Toes-to-nose can be modified and used when a child is "whining" and the parent or caregiver is busy tending to the child's sibling with chronic health care needs.

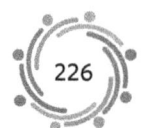

Share with the parent that they can ask the "whining" child to check in with their body bit by bit, starting with their toes and going up to their head. The parent can have the child tell their body that everything is OK, promise to come check on them in a minute, and ask for a report on how things are. Box breathing is also a wonderful tool to help siblings take care of themselves when they have to wait or are not feeling like anyone is paying attention to them. You can encourage the family to start a family feelings chart to help them talk about what everyone is experiencing. Preparing parents with emotion coaching skills, validation language, and SUNBEAM can help them model a healthy way to respond to unpleasant feelings so everyone can support each other through the hard times.

Pain Management for Psychosomatic Symptoms

So many children are used to getting a hug, a kiss, and a bandage for little bumps and bruises that they can sometimes *somaticize* emotional pain. This refers to when the child doesn't have a physical injury or abnormality causing pain; rather, the pain is emerging in response to unmanageable emotional pain. Stomachaches are a common scenario where this arises. We had traditionally thought of symptoms as being "all in your head" versus "real," but now that we understand the mind-body connection better, we can see this thinking is not helpful in responding to a child's very real distress.

Teaching parents that they can guide their child through toes-to-nose to check in with their whole body when something is hurting can help balance the mind's attention so they don't fixate on the one thing that is hurting. This also provides the parent with a way to connect with their child, and honor that their child needs attention, without focusing on the complaint itself. Parents often become frustrated when they believe the child is "exaggerating" or attention seeking, and then the opportunity for meaningful connection and for validation of the child's distress is lost.

If you are seeing a patient back after a referral to a subspecialist (eg, gastroenterologist for abdominal pain, neurologist for tics/involuntary movements) and there seems to be no organic cause for the pain, these strategies are helpful. Parents can be extremely frustrated in this situation, exhausted and just hoping for the symptoms to resolve. Specialists will often say that the symptoms are related to stress, worry, or the child's mood but then not give the family tools and strategies to address it. Offering a follow-up appointment to see how things are going and what may be getting in the way of using the new tools can help normalize how hard it can be to change the family dynamic. As always, we can tailor which tools and strategies we discuss to what seems to be the most relevant for the family, the child's symptoms, and the triggering factors.

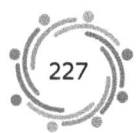

Offsetting Clinician Stress

Once you're familiar with these strategies and approaches, it makes sense to revisit the old saying *Physician, heal thyself.* We don't realize how much we put our own feelings and emotions aside to become doctors. We dismiss our own needs for rest, food, and time with family to get through the training process. Then, once we are out in the "real" world, for a while we are so grateful to no longer be an intern or pediatric intensive care unit resident; we feel a sense of luxury in being able to lie down in our own bed at night and to not be in the call room. We appreciate being able to eat when we are hungry and not having to pretend we are fine until an operating room case is finished.

But to bring our whole self to work, we have to be able to feel like everyone at home is OK. This can be hard if we have family members with acute or chronic illnesses or if we are going through high levels of stress ourselves. Remember, stress can become toxic when you're experiencing it for a prolonged period without adequate supports and resources. If you are struggling and trying to put on a brave front at work and at home, you may end up isolating yourself and magnifying the impact of the stress.

If you have been compartmentalizing your stress, it can help to turn your doctoring toward yourself. Visualize your calm self welcoming your stressed self into your office, and care for yourself in the way you care for others. Sometimes, if you are a parent, you can imagine parenting yourself in the way you would parent your child if they were experiencing the same thing. Often this type of practice helps us have compassion for ourselves, which for whatever reason seems to be one of the hardest things to do.

We spend so much time in the clinic seeing patients that it is important to have a strategy for integrating self-care into our workday. Keeping a glitter jar on your desk or at the nurse's station can be a good visual reminder to stop and take a minute for meditation throughout the day. Another strategy is to use walking meditation as you go between exam rooms. This allows you to center and clear your mind for the next patient. You breathe in as you walk, counting a few steps, and then breathe out to the same number of steps. Mindfulness exercises can be incorporated into the workday. For example, if your feet are hurting, you can use toes-to-nose to draw your attention away from the pain in your feet and notice that the rest of your body is actually OK. Breathing exercises are simple and universally available, even when you are in a stressful meeting or patient interaction. Remember, you have to take care of yourself before you can take care of anyone else.

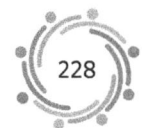

Resilience applies to the office as well, not just to you as an individual. You can share these strategies with your entire staff so they can start to see how undesirable behaviors at work and outside the office are related to big emotions or unmanageable feelings. Administrative skills can be transformed with this approach as well. If you are in a leadership role and you focus on how people are feeling, not just how they are behaving, you can become a more trauma-informed office and reinvent your practice, becoming nimbler when responding to changes and adapting to your community's changing needs. Try this approach for patients who are chronically late, a medical assistant who is distracted, or an administrator who is dismissive. If you can maintain a mindset of calm understanding, you can look past how other people are behaving and find a meaningful way to respond.

Integrating Resilience University for Practice Enhancement and Self-Care: An Example

You have been covering the nursery and were up all night with a sick newborn. You are seeing patients in the clinic. A mom calls, distraught, having found out that her 13-year-old was cutting and had a vaping device inside the pocket of her hoodie at school. You agree to add on one more patient at the end of the day.

Clinician Self-Care

Take a minute to take care of yourself (eg, walking meditation, 5 Big Deep Breaths) and address any of your unmet needs (eg, snack, bathroom break, quick video chat with own your toddler).

Patient Care

Mom says she told her daughter she would kick her out of the house if she found another one of those vaping devices and asks you what she needs to do to make her stop cutting.

Findings from the SDOH screening are negative. The PHQ-9 Modified for Adolescents is not diagnostic for depression; she shows mild anxiety on the Generalized Anxiety Disorder 7-item scale.

What You Might Have Done Before Resilience University

Place a referral for counseling to someone who is familiar with teen substance use. Provide a handout on the dangers of vaping. Ask how much nicotine she is using, and offer medication for nicotine use disorder through a patch if needed.

What You Can Offer After Resilience University

In addition to the above, use VIVA to share how both these things (cutting and vaping) can be less-than-ideal strategies for coping with difficult emotional or physical states. If the parent and/or teen is interested in responding differently, cocreate a plan using the following healthy coping skills:

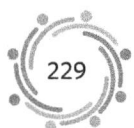

For the Teen

Discuss the mild anxiety; explore if this is related. Identify what other feelings might precede vaping or cutting, and make a list of things she can do when she feels like that. Offer meditation, mindfulness, and breathing exercises if she is not sure what to try. Reassure her that changing habits takes time. Cocreate a PDSA cycle that she thinks she can do, and plan to follow up in 2 weeks.

For the Parent

Share SUNBEAM with Mom, and discuss how important connection is, especially during these hard times, framed in the context of PCEs. Use VIVA to cocreate a plan for Mom to take care of herself (if she doesn't have ideas about healthy coping skills, you can offer meditation, mindfulness, or breathing exercises) when she feels worried or angry about something her daughter is doing. Share the validation sandwich tool with Mom (see Figure 4-2), and encourage her to use the "back the bus up" strategy to support her daughter as she works to make changes. Follow up in 2 weeks.

References

1. Ashworth H, Lewis-O'Connor A, Grossman S, Brown T, Elisseou S, Stoklosa H. Trauma-informed care (TIC) best practices for improving patient care in the emergency department. *Int J Emerg Med.* 2023;16(1):38 PMID: 37208640 doi: 10.1186/s12245-023-00509-w

2. Forkey H, Szilagyi M, Kelly ET, et al; American Academy of Pediatrics Council on Foster Care, Adoption, and Kinship Care; Council on Community Pediatrics; Council on Child Abuse and Neglect; and Committee on Psychosocial Aspects of Child and Family Health. Trauma-informed care. *Pediatrics.* 2021;148(2):e2021052580 PMID: 34312292 doi: 10.1542/peds.2021-052580

3. Office of the Surgeon General. *Parents Under Pressure: The U.S. Surgeon General's Advisory on the Mental Health & Well-Being of Parents.* US Dept of Health and Human Services; 2024. Accessed December 18, 2024. https://www.ncbi.nlm.nih.gov/books/NBK606667

4. Weisenmuller C, Hilton D. Barriers to access, implementation, and utilization of parenting interventions: considerations for research and clinical applications. *Am Psychol.* 2021;76(1):104–115 PMID: 32134281 doi: 10.1037/amp0000613

5. Rostad WL, Moreland AD, Valle LA, Chaffin MJ. Barriers to participation in parenting programs: the relationship between parenting stress, perceived barriers, and program completion. *J Child Fam Stud.* 2018;27(4):1264–1274 PMID: 29456438 doi: 10.1007/s10826-017-0963-6

6. Pignatiello GA, Martin RJ, Hickman RL Jr. Decision fatigue: a conceptual analysis. J *Health Psychol.* 2020;25(1):123–135 PMID: 29569950 doi: 10.1177/1359105318763510

7. Heslon K, Hanson JH, Ogourtsova T. Mental health in children with disabilities and their families: red flags, services' impact, facilitators, barriers, and proposed solutions. *Front Rehabil Sci.* 2024;5:1347412 PMID: 38410177 doi: 10.3389/fresc.2024.1347412

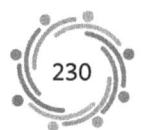
8. Smith AM, Grzywacz JG. Health and well-being in midlife parents of children with special health needs. *Fam Syst Health.* 2014;32(3):303–312 PMID: 24749680 doi: 10.1037/fsh0000049

9. Ivey-Stephenson AZ, Demissie Z, Crosby AE, et al. Suicidal ideation and behaviors among high school students—Youth Risk Behavior Survey, United States, 2019. *MMWR Suppl.* 2020;69(1):47–55 PMID: 32817610 doi: 10.15585/mmwr.su6901a6

10. Winokur S. Skinner's theory of behavior: an examination of B. F. Skinner's *Contingencies of Reinforcement: A Theoretical Analysis. J Exp Anal Behav.* 1971;15(2):253–259 doi: 10.1901/jeab.1971.15-253

11. Theodorou CM, Yamashiro KJ, Stokes SC, Salcedo ES, Hirose S, Beres AL. Pediatric suicide by violent means: a cry for help and a call for action. *Inj Epidemiol.* 2022;9(1):13 PMID: 35395936 doi: 10.1186/s40621-022-00378-6

12. Molina DK, Farley NJA. A 25-year review of pediatric suicides: distinguishing features and risk factors. *Am J Forensic Med Pathol.* 2019;40(3):220–226 PMID: 30994496 doi: 10.1097/PAF.0000000000000485

13. Steindl C, Jonas E, Sittenthaler S, Traut-Mattausch E, Greenberg J. Understanding psychological reactance: new developments and findings. *Z Psychol.* 2015;223(4):205–214 PMID: 27453805 doi: 10.1027/2151-2604/a000222

14. Dube SR, Anda RF, Felitti VJ, Chapman DP, Williamson DF, Giles WH. Childhood abuse, household dysfunction, and the risk of attempted suicide throughout the life span: findings from the Adverse Childhood Experiences Study. *JAMA.* 2001;286(24):3089–3096 PMID: 11754674 doi: 10.1001/jama.286.24.3089

15. Burke TA, Bettis AH, Walsh RFL, et al. Nonsuicidal self-injury in preadolescents. *Pediatrics.* 2023;152(6):e2023063918 PMID: 37916265 doi: 10.1542/peds.2023-063918

16. Fong ZH, Loh WNC, Fong YJ, Neo HLM, Chee TT. Parenting behaviors, parenting styles, and non-suicidal self-injury in young people: a systematic review. *Clin Child Psychol Psychiatry.* 2022;27(1):61–81 PMID: 34866412 doi: 10.1177/13591045211055071

17. David S, Congleton C. Emotional agility. Harvard Business Review. November 2013. Accessed November 13, 2024. https://hbr.org/2013/11/emotional-agility

18. Cooper M, Park-Lee E, Ren C, Cornelius M, Jamal A, Cullen KA. *Notes from the Field:* e-cigarette use among middle and high school students—United States, 2022. *MMWR Morb Mortal Wkly Rep.* 2022;71(40):1283–1285 PMID: 36201370 doi: 10.15585/mmwr.mm7140a3

19. *2023 Maine Integrated Youth Health Survey High School Report.* Maine Dept of Health and Human Services, Maine Dept of Education; 2023:508, 523. Accessed November 13, 2024. https://www.maine.gov/miyhs/sites/default/files/2023_Reports/Detailed_Reports/HS/MIYHS2023_Detailed_Reports_HS_State/Maine%20High%20School%20Detailed%20Tables.pdf

20. Bender HL, Allen JP, McElhaney KB, et al. Use of harsh physical discipline and developmental outcomes in adolescence. *Dev Psychopathol.* 2007;19(1):227–242 PMID: 17241492 doi: 10.1017/S0954579407070125

21. McKee L, Roland E, Coffelt N, et al. Harsh discipline and child problem behaviors: the roles of positive parenting and gender. *J Fam Violence.* 2007;22(4):187–196 doi: 10.1007/s10896-007-9070-6

Conclusion

More than 15 years ago, when my son was born, we thought he was going to be a healthy baby. So much so that even though I was in my late thirties and had given birth to my other 2 children within arm's reach of a neonatologist, my obstetrician convinced me that it was perfectly safe for me to have my third child at the convenient community hospital. Everything seemed to go smoothly. After he was born, I could feel his heart beat as he laid on my chest, sleeping comfortably after nursing. I marveled at how amazing it was to hold your very own baby, how I'd forgotten this feeling from my daughters who were a few years older.

The following morning, the pediatrician listened to him and told me he had a large hole in his heart. Stunned, I realized I had been feeling the thrill from his prenatally undiagnosed almost-tetralogy-of-Fallot heart condition. They sent me home to "watch for heart failure" as we waited for surgery. The days, weeks, and months that followed were a perfect example of toxic stress. I never knew if his tachypnea was the start of heart failure or was normal periodic breathing. I was always terrified, and although I was using what coping skills and resources I had, they were not adequate for the situation. My terror taught me something invaluable about being the parent of a child who needs medical care.

I'd always validated for parents that it is terrifying to rely on a system you are not familiar with to protect your child. Offering education, coping skills, and social support to parents of children who have been hospitalized improves outcomes for both parent and child.[1] But even though I was familiar with the system and support services as a pediatrician, the entirety of medicine felt unfamiliar to me as a parent. I knew where I was supposed to enter the hospital as a doctor but not as a mom. I was used to receiving other people's children into care, not to vulnerably presenting my own precious baby to be poked and prodded and found to be defective and broken. Of course, no one actually said that aloud. But I felt like they said it with their eyes, their body language, and their hurried looks and sad eyes. When my obstetrician offered for me to meet with the counselor at a postpartum visit in their office, I felt confused and insulted, not supported. *Of course I am anxious. It's normal to feel anxious. Anyone would feel anxious when their newborn baby has a life-threatening heart condition. Why are you now telling me that something is wrong with me too?*

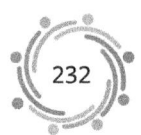

In that process, I learned how essential it is to frame what we are offering to families who are under stress within a strengths-based approach and to validate and normalize difficult feelings as we care for a child's physical and emotional needs. I also learned that when families are asking if something is wrong with their baby, you are seeing only the tip of the iceberg. Even if the family is not consciously aware of it, there is a vast sea of unexpressed feelings underneath that single moment in the office. This sea can lead to dysregulation and tip over the proverbial boat or, when acknowledged and cared for, can help everyone get safely through their journey.

Physicians are being asked to do more and more documentation and screening in less and less time. We often feel potentially toxic stress during our workdays, unable to practice healthy coping skills to respond to the demands of the modern health care and insurance systems. We often do not have adequate resources for our patients within our communities, leaving us feeling helpless. Almost half of pediatricians reported experiencing burnout in 2022—often related, at least in part, to these issues.[2] The art of medicine can feel like a fairy tale, describing a time long ago that seems incompatible with current care models. And yet, when we incorporate stepwise approaches to respond to stress in our day-to-day practice, we can reimagine what the art of medicine looks like within this new world we are living in and cocreate tailored paths forward with our patients and their caregivers and families.

Whether it is a new diagnosis of a boxer's fracture from punching the wall or it is the 6 frustratingly unsuccessful medication follow-up appointments, incorporating a resilience-informed approach enables you to respond with a depth and breadth that rejuvenates the art of medicine. Each time you do a screening or referral, order a test, or adjust a medication dose, you can simultaneously connect and concisely respond to the unspoken asks before the family brings them up when your hand is on the doorknob and you are ready to leave. Honoring the other factors that led your patient or their parents or caregivers to ask for your help restores connection within our modern, often harsh and pressured medical system. Relational health and resilience-building strategies have a role in almost every appointment, even a seemingly straightforward ear infection visit. We can embrace opportunities to lower the stress levels of the parents and patients by validating experiences, normalizing the journey, and reinforcing healthy coping strategies and resources when things are hard.

I hope you feel inspired to start using these tools and strategies to respond to that sea of feelings and unmet needs that are intricately connected to your patient's chief concern(s) and that it revitalizes your practice as it did mine.

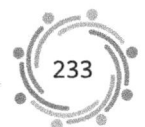

References

1. Doupnik SK, Hill D, Palakshappa D, et al. Parent coping support interventions during acute pediatric hospitalizations: a meta-analysis. *Pediatrics*. 2017;140(3):e20164171 PMID: 28818837 doi: 10.1542/peds.2016-4171

2. Nigri L, Carrasco-Sanz A, Pop TL, et al. Burnout in primary care pediatrics and the additional burden from the COVID-19 pandemic. *J Pediatr*. 2023;260:113447 PMID: 37120131 doi: 10.1016/j.jpeds.2023.113447

Handouts and Tools

Electronic Resources Available

Electronic resources, including printable color versions of the handouts in this Appendix, are available online for purchasers of this book.

Print book users: Please see the inside front cover for instructions and a unique code to grant you access.

eBook users: Please visit www.aap.org/coachingfamilies for access.

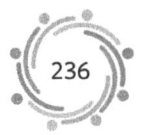
Appendix A

Using 5 Big Deep Breaths to Calm the Nervous System

5 Big Deep Breaths

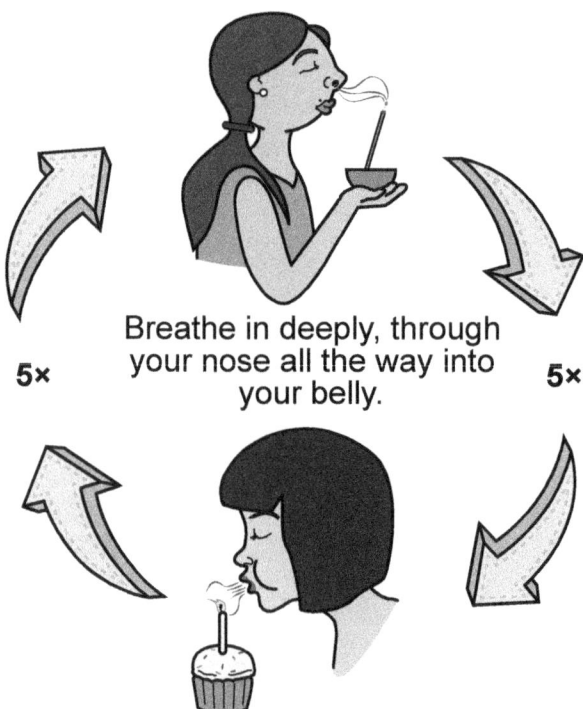

5×   Breathe in deeply, through your nose all the way into your belly.   5×

Blow out through your mouth like you're blowing out a candle. Try to exhale for longer than you inhale.

Repeat at least 5 times!

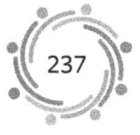
Appendix B

Box Breathing

Breathe OUT to the count of 4

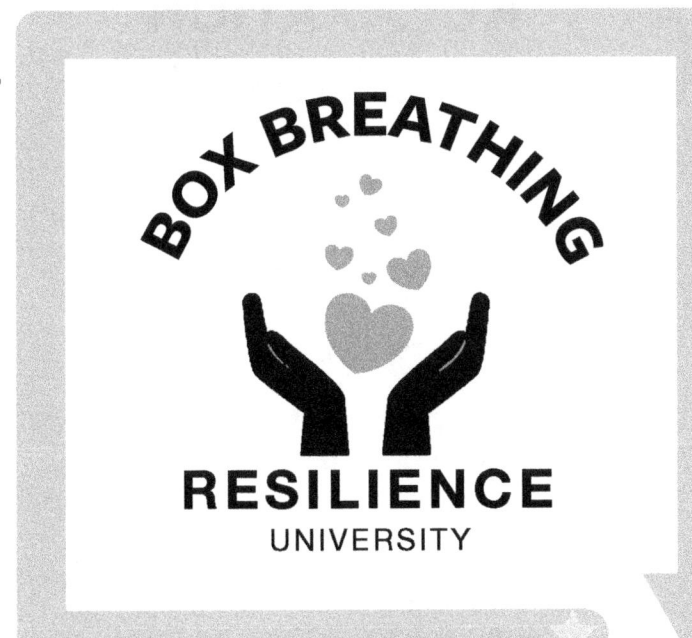

HOLD to the count of 4

WAIT to the count of 4

Breathe IN to the count of 4

Repeat at least 4 times.

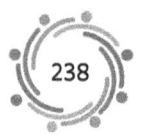

Appendix C

Relaxation Breathing

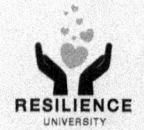

RESILIENCE
UNIVERSITY

RELAXATION BREATHING

Breathe in, saying:
"I am OK."

Hold your breath, saying:
"This feeling will come and go."

Breathe out, saying:
"I am loved and I can do this."

Single copies of this quick reference sheet may be made for noncommercial, educational purposes.

Appendix D

Use Your Breath

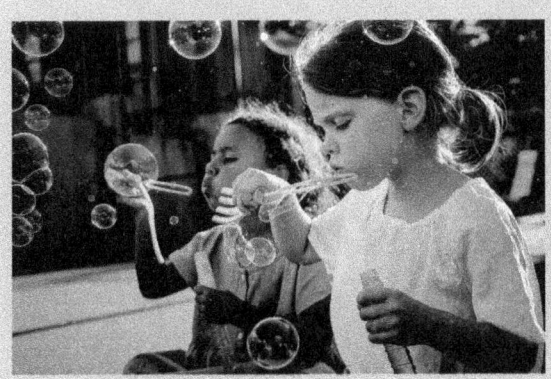

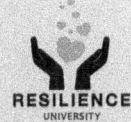

USE YOUR BREATH

Simple things we already do as parents, such as singing songs and blowing bubbles, can lower stress and help children regulate their emotions.

The trick is integrating these nervous system–soothing solutions into the day BEFORE things disintegrate and then it is too hard to get kids to use these self-care strategies.

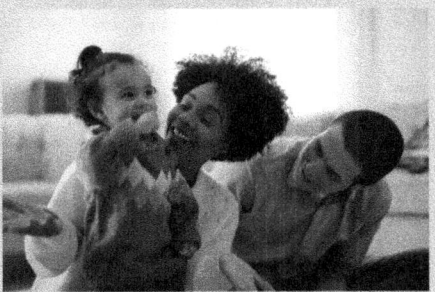

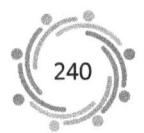

Appendix E

Glitter Jar Meditation

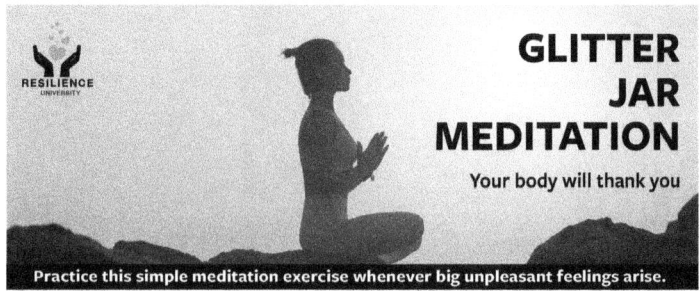

GLITTER JAR MEDITATION

Your body will thank you

Practice this simple meditation exercise whenever big unpleasant feelings arise.

1 **MAKE A GLITTER JAR**
1 plastic Voss still water bottle + 2 glitter glue tubes + 1 packet of glitter. Mix together and shake!

2 **WATCH THE GLITTER SETTLE**
Shake the glitter jar and sit (or stand) with the jar in front of you.
Allow your eyes to rest on the glitter as it settles.

3 **BREATHE**
Watch the glitter settle, breathing in through your nose, like you are smelling something good, all the way into your belly. Then breathe out through your mouth like you are blowing out a birthday candle.

4 **REPEAT**
Still feeling yucky?
Shake the glitter jar and repeat.

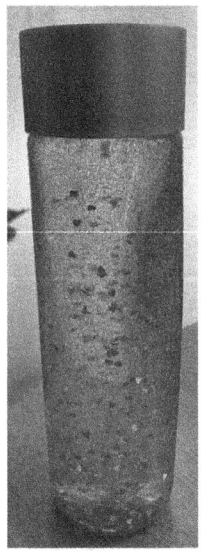

CAREGIVERS, MODEL THIS FOR YOUR KIDS!

Next time you notice you are feeling irritated, angry, annoyed, or anxious, pause to meditate.

Just like you teach them to get food when they are hungry, modeling this will teach them to meditate when they don't feel good.

Single copies of this quick reference sheet may be made for noncommercial, educational purposes.

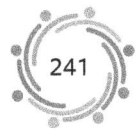

Appendix F

Emotional Awareness

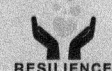

Emotions are like ocean waves.

Some are big.
Some are small.
None of them last forever.
Your job is to take care of
yourself while they are there so
they don't wash you out to sea!

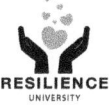

10 THINGS I CAN DO
TO TAKE CARE OF MYSELF

1. _____

2. _____

3. _____

4. _____

5. _____

6. _____

7. _____

8. _____

9. _____

10. _____

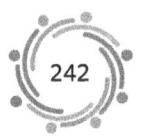

Appendix G

Loving-Kindness Meditation for Parents and Caregivers

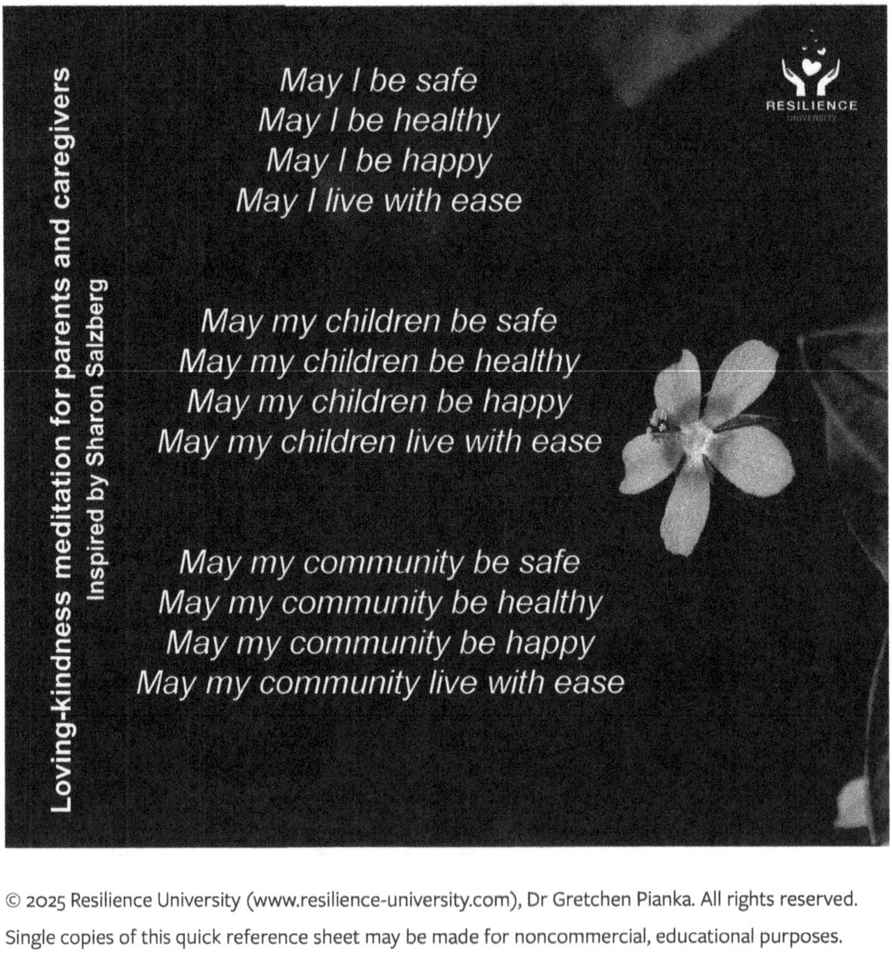

Loving-kindness meditation for parents and caregivers
Inspired by Sharon Salzberg

RESILIENCE
UNIVERSITY

May I be safe
May I be healthy
May I be happy
May I live with ease

May my children be safe
May my children be healthy
May my children be happy
May my children live with ease

May my community be safe
May my community be healthy
May my community be happy
May my community live with ease

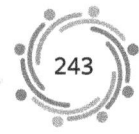
Appendix H

Loving-Kindness Meditation for Older Children and Teens

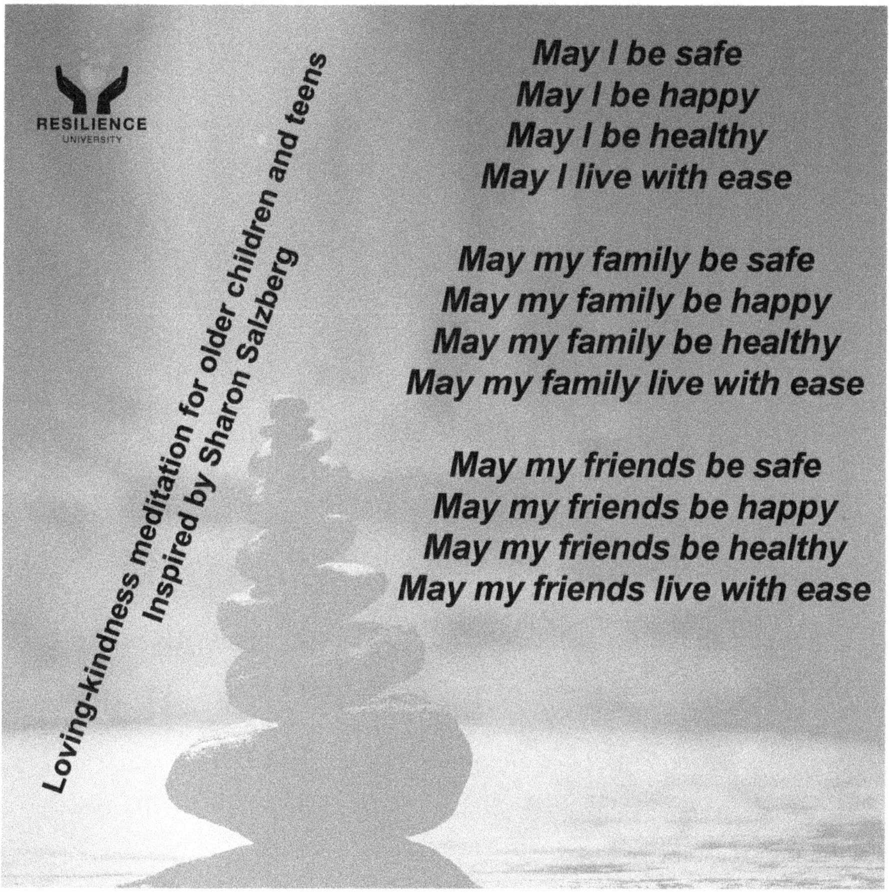

RESILIENCE
UNIVERSITY

Loving-kindness meditation for older children and teens
Inspired by Sharon Salzberg

May I be safe
May I be happy
May I be healthy
May I live with ease

May my family be safe
May my family be happy
May my family be healthy
May my family live with ease

May my friends be safe
May my friends be happy
May my friends be healthy
May my friends live with ease

Appendix I

Walking Meditation

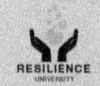

Walking Meditation

As you are walking toward the room where
you hear screaming,
BEFORE you talk with your children,

breathe in 2, 3, 4...
breathe out 2, 3, 4...

repeat until you arrive at the chaos!

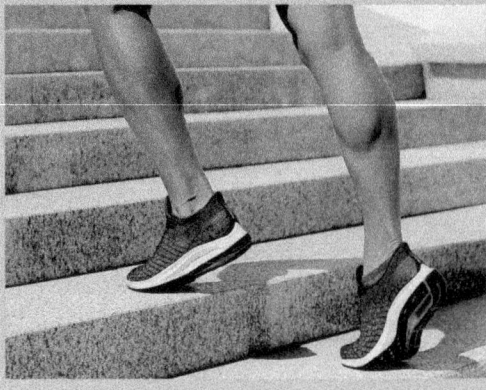

Appendix J

Mindfulness Using 5-4-3-2-1

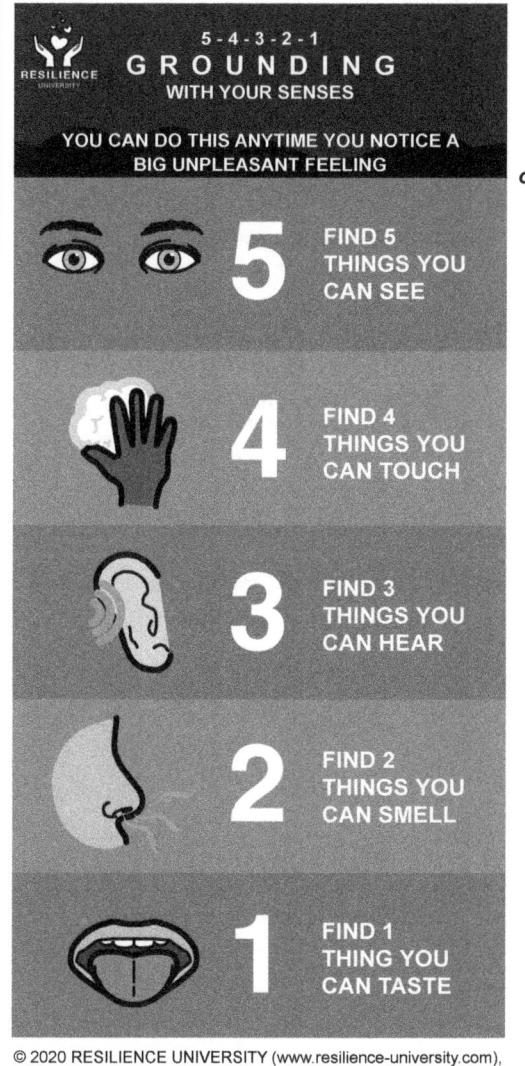

Tips:

Remember, traumatic memories are stored in our senses, so when our "fire-truck brain" is activated, sometimes the only thing that can help calm it is soothing sensory input.

You can simplify this on the go using these other options.

Find me 5 things that are blue.

What are 4 things you can touch?

Can you tell me 3 things you can hear?

Imagine your 2 favorite smells.

Describe 1 of your favorite foods to me.

Let's find the alphabet together on the signs here.

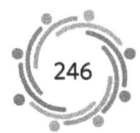
Appendix K

Mindfulness Using Toes-to-Nose

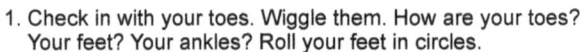

1. Check in with your toes. Wiggle them. How are your toes? Your feet? Your ankles? Roll your feet in circles.

2. Check in with your legs. Bend your knees. How are your legs? How are your hips? Your stomach? Are you hungry?

3. Check in with your heart. Put your hand on your chest; see if you can feel your heart beating.

4. Check in with your lungs. Take a few big deep breaths.

FEELING NERVOUS? WORRIED? BORED?

RESILIENCE
UNIVERSITY

5. Check in with your hands, wrists, and elbows. Roll your shoulders and neck. Are you tight?

6. How is your jaw? Eyes? Head? Nose?

TRY TOES-TO-NOSE!

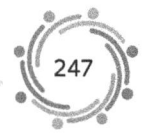

Appendix L

Applied Mindfulness: The Fire-Truck Brain Analogy

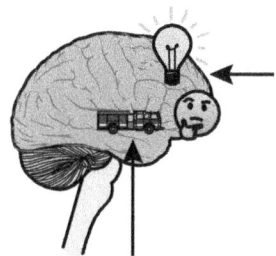

The Prefrontal Cortex
This is that good-thinking, problem-solving part of the brain that can do math, answer questions, read books, and figure things out.

Fire-Truck Brain
Our "fire-truck brain" stays in a "garage" in the center of our brain, ready to help in an emergency. It shows up sirens blaring, hoses ready, lights flashing, and ready to put out the fire. But it can't do math, read a book, or problem-solve.

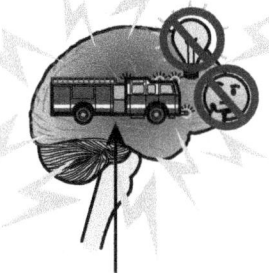

Stress Response
When a big emotion takes over, our good-thinking part of our brain goes "offline" and we are being driven by our fire-truck brain! When we feel calmer, our good-thinking brain comes back "online" and the fire truck goes back into its garage.

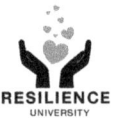

RESILIENCE
UNIVERSITY

Inspired by Dan Siegel's "flipping your lid," *Mindsight,* Bantam, 2010.

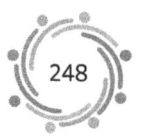

Appendix M

Building Block Worksheets Using the HOPE (Healthy Outcomes from Positive Experiences) Framework

Building Blocks for Health

These 4 building blocks are important factors in growing up healthy. Share what's working and your provider will brainstorm with you for solutions to anything that's not working.

Engagement

What is one thing you like to do as a family outside the home?
Where do you feel most connected to others?

Environment

Describe a place you love to go or play. Where is your safe space?

Relational Health

What do you like to do at home with your family?
Who is someone outside your family that really cares about you?

Emotional Growth

What feelings do you talk about at home? With whom do you talk about feelings? How can you take care of yourself when you have big feelings?

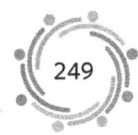

Build a "tower" with your blocks!

Emotional growth: What feelings do you talk about at home? With whom do you talk about feelings? How can you take care of yourself when you have big feelings?

Environment: Describe places you love to go or play. Describe your safe space(s). What is your favorite place in your house?

Relational health: What do you like to do at home with your family? Who outside your family cares about you?

Engagement: What do you like to do as a family outside the house? Where do you feel connected to others? Describe a favorite outing.

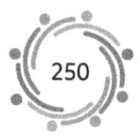

Appendix N

Conversation Topics to Support the HOPE (Healthy Outcomes from Positive Experiences) Building Blocks

Strengths-Based Building Block Conversations

Engagement

- Suggest after-school programs.
- Explore summer camps and community programs.
- Identify a local YMCA: Can the family connect to this resource? Are there scholarships? Are there transportation barriers to address?
- Offer parenting resources (eg, positive parenting resources, community groups).
- Identify youth programs, outreach, and school and community groups.
- Offer a list of local places of worship or spiritual centers and resources.
- Identify parent support groups, online or in person.

Relational Health

- How are things at home? What is hard for the parents?
- Are the parents able to play with their kids? Read with them?
- What is the parent proud of?
- How high is the stress level at home?
- Are there specific things or times of day that are hardest?
- Name the nonparent adults who can help; identify barriers to asking them for help.
- Identify community resources that can reduce barriers and decrease isolation.
- Provide a list of community groups and supports.
- Provide books and library resources.

Environment

- Provide a list of local housing resources.
- Provide a list of food banks.
- Provide a list of transportation options.
- Review gun safety.
- Review medication safety.
- Brainstorm about safe play areas.
- Brainstorm about options for trips and outings.
- Offer a list of community resources for outdoor activities.
- Offer trail/park maps and resources (eg, state park passes).

Emotional Growth

- Ask the parents if they feel like they know how to help their child when their child is angry, frustrated, worried, or scared.
- Ask the parents how they take care of themselves when they are stressed, sad, angry, or frustrated.
- Make a family feelings chart and encourage them to ask, "How do I know I am feeling this way?" and "How can I take care of myself while this feeling is here?"
- Teach at least one breathing exercise (glitter jar, box breathing, or 5 Big Deep Breaths).
- Teach one strategy for anger (eg, playing "angry" ball with a Nerf ball, going outside to run around).
- Teach one mindfulness strategy, such as toes-to-nose or 5-4-3-2-1 (ie, using all 5 senses).

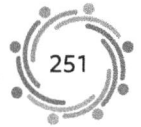

Appendix O

Stress Reduction Plan for Teens

Stress Reduction Plan

Name:

Date:

| Friends/Family | Sleep | Nutrition |

| Mental Health | Mindfulness | Nature |

| Movement |

Inspired by the California surgeon general's Roadmap for Resilience stress-buster chart. www.acesaware.org/managestress

Appendix P

9-5-2-1-0 Checklist

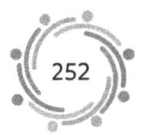

9-5-2-1-0	Monday	Tuesday	Wednesday	Thursday	Friday	Saturday	Sunday	✓ = I totally did it. ☆ = I tried to do it. ✗ = I didn't try this one.
7–9 hours of sleep								
5 or more servings of fruits or veggies								
2 hours or less of screen time (doesn't include homework!)								
1 hour or more of physical exercise or active play								
No sugary sweetened drinks								

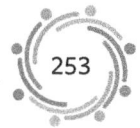
Appendix Q

Plan-Do-Study-Act Approach in Resilience University

PDSA CYCLE: WHAT ISSUE ARE WE TRYING TO ADDRESS?

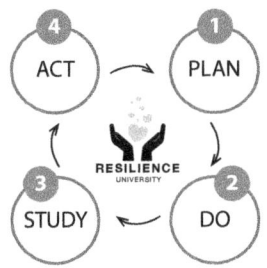

Identify a shared goal: _____

1 Plan: A change or test aimed at supporting resilience. Cocreate a plan:

_____

_____

2 Do: Carry out change (on a small scale).
Do the plan for _____ (amount of time; eg, 2 weeks).

3 Study the results: Did it help? What went wrong?
Discuss how things went in person, then follow up by phone or through a patient portal:

_____

_____

_____

4 Act: Adopt the new strategy or abandon it and run another cycle.
Discuss if this "worked" or if a new plan is needed:

_____

_____

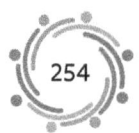

Appendix R

Blank "Back the Bus Up" Timeline

Back the Bus Up

A Parenting Problem-Solving Approach

RESILIENCE
UNIVERSITY

Precipitating
behavior or
event:

My child/I was feeling? _____

Next time, I can try this to take care of that feeling: _____   Unmet need,
emotion, or
other stressor:
_____

Unmet need,
emotion, or
other stressor:

My child/I was feeling? _____

Next time, I can try this to take care of that feeling: _____
_____

Unmet need,
emotion, or
other stressor:

My child/I was feeling? _____

Next time, I can try this to take care of that feeling: _____
_____

Unmet need,
emotion, or
other stressor:

My child/I was feeling? _____

Next time, I can try this to take care of that feeling: _____
_____

My child/I was feeling? _____

Next time, I can try this to take care of that feeling: _____
_____

Original unmet
need,
emotion, or
other stressor:

My child/I was feeling? _____

Next time, I can try this to take care of that feeling: _____
_____

Appendix S

Feelings Sticker Chart

When I feel bored, I can... 😊	I did it!			
Draw or write in my journal				
Use 5-4-3-2-1				
Listen to music				
Go for a walk or play with the dog				

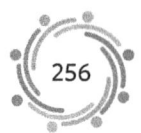
Appendix T

Family Feelings Chart

Family Feelings Chart

Angry Mad Frustrated Annoyed Irritated	
Sad Lonely Left out	
Hungry Famished Starving	
Confused Worried Scared Overwhelmed	
Cold Freezing	
Tired Sleepy Exhausted	
Happy Joyful Loved	
Overwhelmed Stressed Freaking out	

Add a sticker, a check mark, or a comment when you notice you are feeling a certain way. Have each person in the family use a different sticker or color. See if you can start talking with each other about your feelings.

Appendix U

"10 Things I Can Do When I Feel Yucky" List

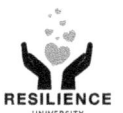

**10 THINGS I CAN DO
WHEN I FEEL YUCKY!**

1. _____
2. _____
3. _____
4. _____
5. _____
6. _____
7. _____
8. _____
9. _____
10. _____

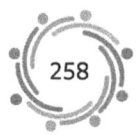

Appendix V

Validate, Validate, Validate

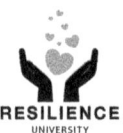

Validate, Validate, Validate

One of the most powerful tools we have as parents is to validate our child's emotions. You don't have to agree with what your child is saying to validate what they are feeling. Even if what they are saying or how they are behaving is not what you would like to hear or see, remember: validate first. Once they have returned to a calm baseline, you can problem-solve.

The following 3-sentence framework can help your child feel heard, understood, and as though you care about their feelings; remember to use this language:

- "I get…"
- "I totally understand…"
- "Anyone would feel…"

Example: Johnny comes home from school and throws his backpack onto the floor. You ask how his day was. He yells that he hates you and hates the school and hates his teachers and he never wants to go to school again! Then he stomps up to his room.

You can validate the feeling (even though you are not agreeing with everything he just said or giving him a free pass for his behavior) by saying

- "I get that you are angry."
- "I totally understand being frustrated with your teachers and the school."
- "Anyone who had a frustrating day like that would feel like they don't want to go back to school."

and

- "When you say you hate me, I feel sad, and I'm wondering how you are feeling. Is now a good time to talk about how you feel, or do you need some time to take care of yourself first?"

Then, pivot back to the list of "10 Things I Can Do When I Feel Yucky." Once the big feeling has come and gone, you can start problem-solving about what happened to make Johnny feel that way.

Appendix W

NICER Parenting

NICER PARENTING

Big behaviors are a bid for connection.
We can help our kids one messy moment at a time.

IN THE MOMENT WHEN YOUR CHILD IS MISBEHAVING:

1. Notice

Notice that your child is having a big emotion. This often coincides with unwanted behavior. Don't focus too much on the behavior. Behaviors will improve as you help your child with their big unpleasant emotions.

2. Identify

Help your child identify how they are feeling. Don't worry too much about details. Start with basics (eg, sad, angry, afraid) or just generally "yucky."

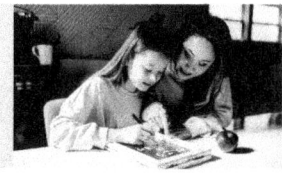

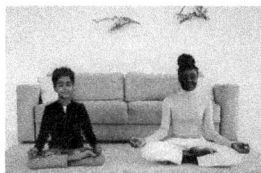

3. Connect/Coregulate

Big feelings can be scary. Let them know you feel the same way sometimes. Talk about how you care for yourself when you have this feeling (eg, go for a walk, listen to music, draw, write, meditate, do breathing exercises).

LATER, AFTER THE FEELING HAS COME AND GONE:

4. Explore

Develop 10 self-care strategies your child can do next time a big unpleasant feeling arises. Make a self-care nook in their room.

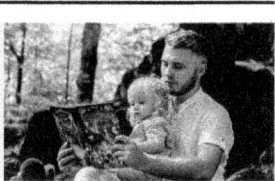

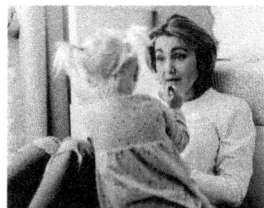

5. Review/Repair

Talk with your child about the feeling. What did they do while it was there? Is there a need for a relationship repair? It is their job not to hurt themselves, anyone, or anything while the yucky feeling is there. If consequences are necessary, make sure they are natural, and don't take away anything your child needs for self-care.

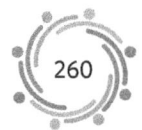

Appendix X

SUNBEAM: A Stress-Lowering, Trauma-Informed Parenting Practice

SUNBEAM

RESILIENCE
UNIVERSITY

A PARENT'S ANTIDOTE TO MELTDOWNS

 1. SEE: Is your child misbehaving? Did their unwanted behavior trigger an unpleasant feeling in you?

2. UNHOOK: By now, you have a habitual way of responding to this unpleasant feeling. Notice the feeling, but don't take the bait!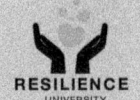

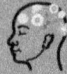 **3. NURTURE:** Pause to take care of yourself before you respond to your child, by using one or more of the same skills they are learning.

• BREATHE: Breathe in deeply through your nose all the way to your belly and blow out through your mouth. Box breathing and 4-7-8 breathing are alternatives. If you can't incorporate breathing, try mindfulness.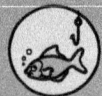

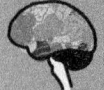 **• EMOTIONALLY AWARE:** Remember, each feeling is like an ocean wave. It may feel big or small, but it won't last forever. Take care of yourself. This is temporary!

• MINDFUL: Check in with your body, starting with your toes; use 5-4-3-2-1; or just find 5 things that are blue. Trauma is stored in our senses, so mindfulness can be powerful if you have a trauma history.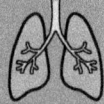

 • MEDITATION: Sit, allowing your eyes to rest on the glitter as it settles while you breathe deeply.

Single copies of this quick reference sheet may be made for noncommercial, educational purposes.

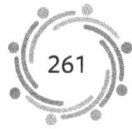

Appendix Y

Emotion Coaching for Parents and Caregivers

RESILIENCE UNIVERSITY EMOTION COACHING

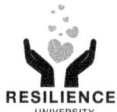

RESILIENCE
UNIVERSITY

Applying the Concept of Emotion Coaching in Resilience University

Many people have studied emotion coaching to help parents work with their children on emotional growth, so we know it has a protective effect. Sometimes it takes time to learn how to do it and it's not intuitive if no one coached us as kids on how to do it. But it's just like learning a new sport!

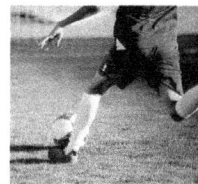

I use an analogy of learning how to play soccer. Let's say you wanted your child to be a professional soccer player. You wouldn't expect them to just go out and be that player out of the blue, right? You would start with kicking the ball around in the backyard. Occasionally, the ball might end up in the neighbor's living room. Oops! You don't give up. Maybe you pivot and practice at the soccer field or have your child kick in the opposite direction. You want them to learn this, so you keep helping them. You will inevitably learn along the way too.

Think of yourself as your child's coach for learning about and understanding their emotions. It is OK if you are learning along with them! Remember, sometimes you will have to do breathing exercises to hold space for your child's unpleasant emotions. Take care of yourself so you can help them understand their emotions.

Basic Concepts

1. How to identify your emotions and take care of yourself while they are there is not something kids learn how to do without help.
2. When you lean in, listen, and validate their feelings, you help your children learn how to do this.
3. Learn how to help your children identify their emotions and take care of themselves. There are no bad or trivial emotions, so try not to ignore or dismiss the unpleasant ones. Separate unwanted behavior from the emotions that led to it, and don't punish your child for having emotions.
4. As parents, we did not always get this help because our parents didn't get it from their parents, their parents didn't get it from their parents, and so on. Start now and change the family culture.
5. You can help your child learn something new, just like you can help them learn soccer even if there hasn't ever been someone in your family who has played soccer before, by taking an interest in learning about emotions as well, working on them with your child, and not giving up when something goes wrong!
6. Just like learning to play soccer, occasionally, things may go sideways and you may wish you'd done something differently. Don't give up entirely! These are opportunities for do-overs. Talk about what happened, pivot your approach, and then try again.

If you are interested in learning about the Gottman "emotion coaching" approach, check out the blog: www.gottman.com/blog/an-introduction-to-emotion-coaching.

Derived from Lunkenheimer ES, Shields AM, Cortina KS. Parental emotion coaching and dismissing in family interaction. *Soc Dev.* 2007;16(2):232–248.

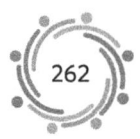

Appendix Z

Resilience University Enrollment Form

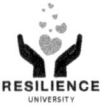

To be filled out by a parent or guardian (One form may be used for multiple children.)

Date: _____

Name of Person Filling Out This Form:_____

Current Address:_____

Contact Methods:
Phone—please provide preferred number: _____

Email—please provide preferred email: _____

Child/Children Enrolling:

Name:_____ DOB:_____ Relationship: _____

Name:_____ DOB:_____ Relationship: _____

Name:_____ DOB:_____ Relationship: _____

Name:_____ DOB:_____ Relationship: _____

Do you have any concerns about your child's mood, development, or behavior? If so, please explain: _____
_____
_____
_____
_____

Anything else you want to make sure your clinician is aware of: _____
_____
_____
_____
_____
_____

Appendix AA

Resilience University Certificate of Completion

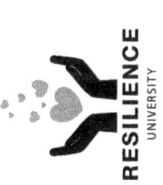

RESILIENCE
UNIVERSITY

CERTIFICATE OF COMPLETION

This certifies that on this ___ day in the month of ___ in the year ___

has satisfactorily completed
Resilience University
and now has
emotional agility superpowers!

_____
CLINICIAN'S SIGNATURE

_____
PATIENT'S SIGNATURE

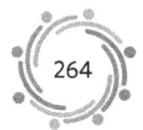

Appendix BB

Other Feeling Chart Templates

When I feel sad, I can... 🙁	My Self-Care Superpowers I did it!			
Cuddle my pets or my stuffies				
Hug Mom or Dad				
Glitter jar				
Listen to music				

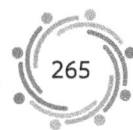

When I feel worried, I can... 😟	My Self-Care Superpowers I did it!
Meditate with my glitter jar	
Use 5-4-3-2-1	
Sing	
Do box breathing	

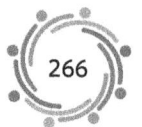

When I feel overwhelmed, I can... 😣	My Self-Care Superpowers I did it!			
Meditate with my glitter jar				
Use 5-4-3-2-1				
Take a break and listen to music				
Go for a walk or play with the dog				

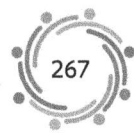

When I feel bored, I can...	My Self-Care Superpowers I did it!			
Draw or write in my journal				
Use 5-4-3-2-1				
Listen to music				
Go for a walk or play with the dog				

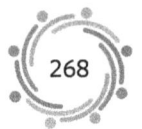

When I feel _____, I can...	I did it!	

My Self-Care Superpowers

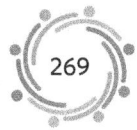

Appendix CC

Self-Care Nook

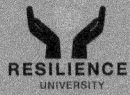

SELF-CARE NOOK

A COZY SPOT WHERE EVERYONE CAN PAUSE TO TAKE CARE OF BIG FEELINGS

RESILIENCE
UNIVERSITY

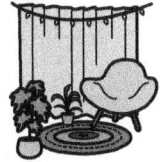

CHOOSE YOUR LOCATION
Inside or outside

You can set this nook up in a bedroom, the basement, the backyard, or even a closet. Hang up an old shower curtain or regular curtain and some holiday lights or fairy lights.

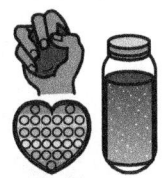

GLITTER JAR
Be creative

Your family's glitter jar lives here, on the floor or a little footstool, small table, box, or windowsill. It should be easy to see it when you or your child is sitting.

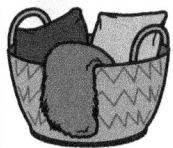

COMFY SEAT
Cushions and more cushions

Add a few squishy pillows and a favorite soft blanket. Your child can also bring a few favorite stuffed animals for cuddling.

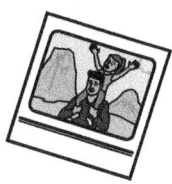

FAVORITE PHOTO
Any photo that helps the family member using the nook feel loved

Try a photo of you or your child as a baby or toddler. If you don't have something to put it on, you can simply stick it to the wall with tape.

JOURNAL OR PAD OF PAPER
For drawing or writing or just doodling

Include a pad of paper, a journal, or scraps of paper to write or draw on. For the family member using the nook, draw how you are feeling or write about your feelings and thoughts.

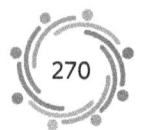

Appendix DD

Printable Glitter Jar Labels

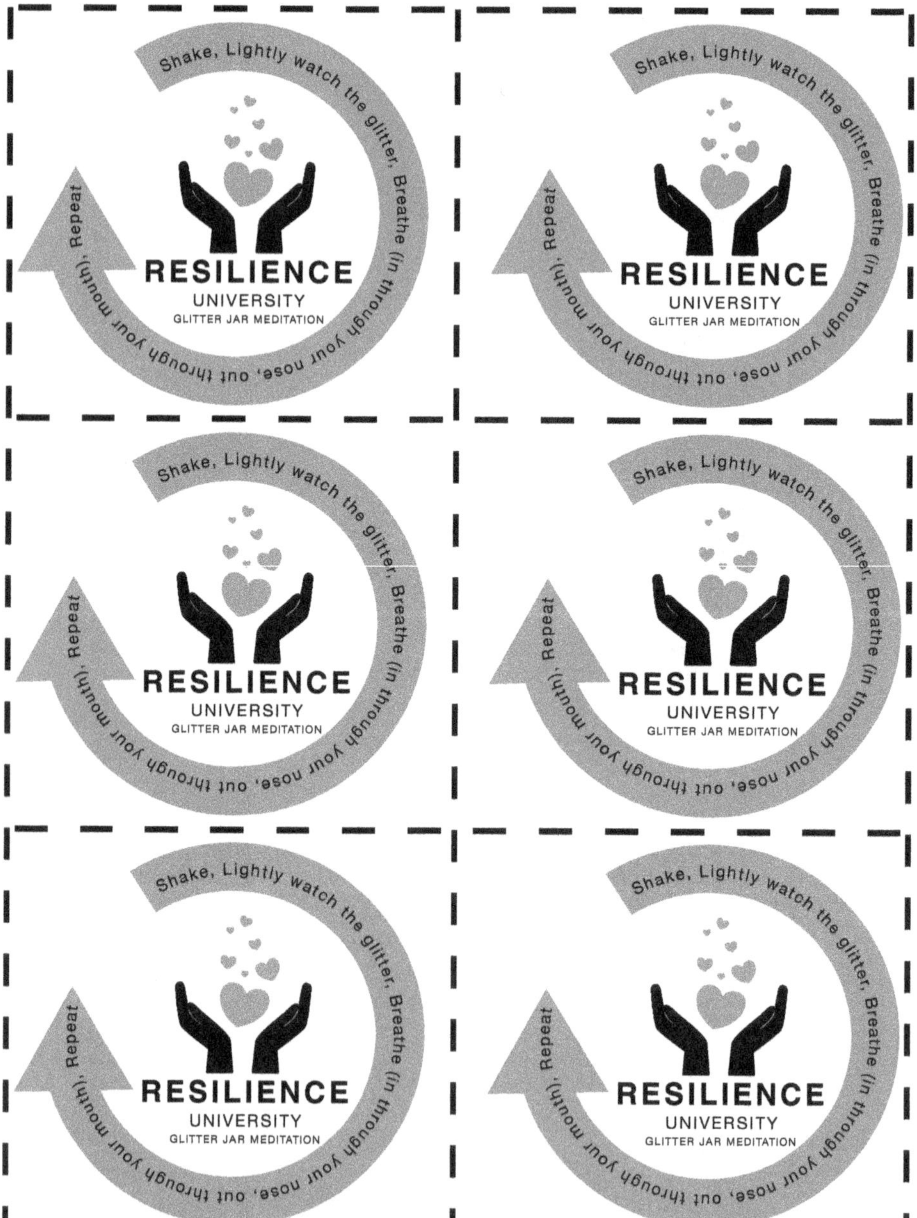

Appendix EE

6 Steps to Connect

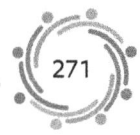

6 STEPS TO CONNECT
when both you and your child are stressed

a collaboration between
the Maine AAP & Resilience University

1

SEE:
WHAT YOUR CHILD IS DOING HAS TRIGGERED YOU.

2

UNHOOK:
DON'T TAKE IT PERSONALLY!

IF YOU HAVE A HABITUAL WAY OF RESPONDING WHEN YOUR CHILD DOES THIS, TRY NOT TO DO IT.

3

NURTURE:
PAUSE TO TAKE CARE OF YOURSELF.

REGULATE YOUR NERVOUS SYSTEM FIRST, BEFORE YOU RESPOND TO YOUR CHILD'S BEHAVIOR.

4

NOTICE:
THERE IS SOMETHING ELSE BEHIND YOUR CHILD'S BEHAVIORS.

5

IDENTIFY:
TRY TO IDENTIFY WHAT IS DRIVING THE BEHAVIOR(S). IS YOUR CHILD HUNGRY? SAD? FRUSTRATED?

IT'S OK TO START WITH "THIS IS YUCKY/ HARD."

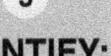

it's OK to feel
your feelings

6

CONNECT:
COREGULATE. OFFER A COPING SKILL THAT HAS HELPED YOUR CHILD & DO IT WITH THEM.

Index

Page numbers followed by *f* indicate a figure; by *t*, a table; and by *b*, a box.

A

AAP. *See* American Academy of Pediatrics (AAP)

Acceptance and commitment therapy, 23

Active listening, 153, 154*f*

Activities and responsibilities, anticipatory guidance on, 205

Adverse childhood experiences (ACEs), 6, 8, 13, 121
  screening for, 40
  toxic stress and, 12

Adversity, 5, 39. *See also* Resilience
  positive childhood experiences for offsetting, 6, 23
  resilience interventions for offsetting, 14–15

Affirmations, 58, 70–71

Agency, 33

Aggression, 222–224

American Academy of Pediatrics (AAP), 13, 14, 40, 73, 149, 170

Anticipatory guidance, 36, 40
  activities and responsibilities, 205
  addressing food and housing insecurity, 176–179
  avoiding arguments, 183–184
  avoiding harsh discipline and promoting caregiver self-care, 185
  bedtime routine, 189
  behavioral concerns, 188–189
  case 1: Mohamed's newborn visit, 175–181, 177*f*
  case 2: Lyla's 15-month visit, 181–186

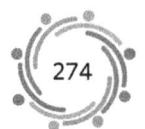
Anticipatory guidance (*continued*)

    case 3: Rodrigo's 2½-year visit, 186–193

    case 4: Ngoc's 7-year visit, 193–198

    case 5: Dakota's 14-year visit, 198–206

    child-directed speech, bonding, and playing, 184

    chores, rules, and consequences, 198

    coregulation for teens, 203–204

    decision-making process, 204

    encouraging responsibility and preventing substance use, 200–201

    enforcing limits/time-outs, 191

    maternal health and, 179–181

    media use and support systems, 186

    problem-solving strategy, 194–195

    promoting positive childhood experiences, 201–202

    reading, simple requests, and choices, 192–193

    reducing smoke exposure, 187–188

    regular family mealtimes, 182–183

    relational health as long-distance event, 196–197

    relationship-based, trauma-informed. *See* Relationship-based, trauma-informed anticipatory guidance

    responding to harsh parenting, 195–196, 204–205

    responding to overwhelming stress, 199–200

    screen time, 191–192

    shifting from transactional to relational responses to behaviors, 202–203

    strategies for reconnecting, 206

    support system and engagement, 190–191

    talking about feelings, 197–198

    tools for. *See* Tools, anticipatory guidance

Apologies, Authentic, 169–170

Applied behavioral analysis (ABA) approach, 214

Applied mindfulness, 76–77

Apps, meditation, 86

Arguments, avoiding of, 183–184

Attention-deficit/hyperactivity disorder (ADHD), 39, 49, 96, 99, 166–167, 222–223

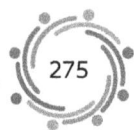

Autism spectrum disorder (ASD), 214

Autonomy, 39

B

"Backing the bus up" approach, 102, 103*f*, 138, 139*f*, 152, 213

Barriers, identification of, 154–157, 157*t*

Bedtime routine, 189

Behavioral concerns

    anticipatory guidance on, 188–189

    oppositional behaviors, aggression, and impulsivity, 222–224

    positive parenting for shifting, 109–110*b*, 109–111

Behavioral health guidance, 34–38

    shifting from transactional to relational responses to behaviors, 202–203

Blanket advice, 164

Body scan, 74–76, 132

"Box" breathing, 63–64, 64*f*, 132

Breathing exercises, 60*t*, 62–66

    "box" breathing, 63–64, 64*f*, 132

    5 Big Deep Breaths, 37, 62–63, 176

    other ways to use breath, 65–66

    relaxation, 64–65

Bright Futures, 36, 149

Brown, Charlotte Harper, 23

Bubble blowing, 65–66

C

Calm app, 86

Catastrophizing, 169

Check-in, Resilience University (RU), 128, 134–135, 140, 145

Child-directed speech, bonding, and playing, 184

Childhood Trauma and Resilience: A Practical Guide, 14

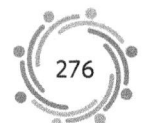

Choices, anticipatory guidance on, 192–193

Chores, anticipatory guidance on, 198

Chronic stress, 15

Clinical scenarios, 213–226

    depression and anxiety, 221–222

    foster care, 224–225

    intellectual or physical disabilities, 214–215

    neurodivergent children, 214

    offsetting clinician stress, 227–228

    oppositional behaviors, aggression, and impulsivity, 222–224

    pain management for psychosomatic symptoms, 226

    self-harm, 216–219

    substance use, 219–221

    suicidality, 215–216

    when a family member is sick, 225–226

Cocreating a plan, 128, 135, 141

Cognitive behavioral therapy, 23

Consequences, 198

Container of love, 170

Coregulation, 35

    meltdowns and, 169

    for teens, 203–204

COVID-19 pandemic, 33, 47, 162

CRAFFT (Car, Relax, Alone, Forget, Family/Friends, Trouble), 199

Curriculum, Resilience University (RU), 124, 125–126t

D

Dakota's 14-year visit, 198–206

Daniel Tiger, 85

Decision-making process, anticipatory guidance on, 204

Deming, W. Edward, 19

Depression

    clinical scenario involving, 221–222

    maternal, 176, 180–181

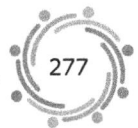
Developmental neuroscience, 17*f*

Dialectical behavior therapy, 23, 108

Discipline, 34–35

    avoiding harsh, 185

    enforcing limits/time-outs, 191

    regarding chores, rules, and consequences, 198

E

"Early Childhood Adversity, Toxic Stress, and the Role of the Pediatrician: Translating Developmental Science Into Lifelong Health," 14

Ecobiodevelopmental (EBD) model of disease and wellness, 14–15, 16*f*, 17*f*, 18, 22

Economic constraints, 164–165, 167

Educational goals, support for, 165–167

Emergencies, 62

Emotional awareness, 68–71, 68*f*, 73

Emotional growth, 79, 80*f*, 82

Emotional regulation, 36–37

    emotional awareness and, 68–70, 68*f*

    by parents, 40

Emotion coaching, 61*t*, 113–115

Endorphins, 65

Engagement, 79, 80*f*, 81

    support system and, 190–191

Environment, 79, 80*f*, 81

Epigenetic regulation, 15, 17*f*

Epistemic trust, 150–151

Evoking, 57–58

F

Family culture, 57

Family feelings chart, 44*f*, 45, 60*t*

Family mealtimes, 182–183

Family structure, 48

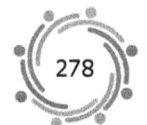

15-month visit, 181–186

Fight, flight, or freeze response, 8, 12, 13, 36, 37–38, 156, 210

Financial constraints, 164–165, 167

"Fire-truck brain," 76, 131, 210

5 Big Deep Breaths, 37, 62–63, 176

5-4-3-2-1, 74, 132

Food and housing insecurity, 176–177

Forkey, Heather, 14, 27

Foster care, 224–225

Framing with strengths, Resilience University (RU), 128, 135, 140, 145

G

Garner, Andrew, 8, 14, 15

General parenting guidance, 210–213

Genetics, 15

Gillespie, R.J., 14, 19

Glitter jar, 67, 129–131, 129*f*

"Good enough" parenting, 33

Gottman, John, 113

Griffin, Jessica, 14, 27

Growth mindset, 152

Guidelines for Adolescent Preventive Services, 199

H

Habit stacking, 177

Handouts, Resilience University (RU), 127–128, 134, 140, 144

Harris, Nadine Burke, 24, 99, 100*f*, 145

Harsh parenting, anticipatory guidance on, 195–196, 204–205

Headspace app, 86

Homelessness, 167

Homework, Resilience University (RU), 133–134, 140, 143

HOPE® (Healthy Outcomes from Positive Experiences), 23, 24*f*, 47, 60*t*, 77, 121, 142, 209

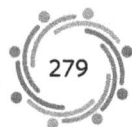
I

Immune response and chronic stress, 15, 17*f*

Impulsivity, 222–224

Institute for Healthcare Improvement, 20

Intellectual or physical disabilities, children with, 214–215

Intergenerational transmission of trauma, 155

Investigating further, 28–29

K

King, Amy, 14, 19

L

Language, 28

Life360, 199

Limits, enforcement of, 191

Lyla's 15-month visit, 181–186

M

Maine Youth Overweight Collaborative (MYOC), 20–21

Masten, Ann, 33

Maternal health, 176, 180–181

McKinney-Vento Homeless Assistance Act, 167

Mealtimes, family, 182–183

Media use and support systems, 186

Medications, 42

Meditation, 60*t*, 66–67

    affirmations, 70–71

    apps for, 86

    emotional awareness, 68–71, 68*f*

    glitter jar for teaching, 67

Meltdown, Anatomy of a, 169

Mental stress, 10

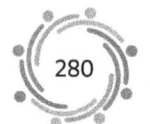

Mindfulness, 60*t*, 65, 71–73, 132
    applied, 76–77
    body scan, 74–76
    5-4-3-2-1, 74
    meditation and, 66
    sensory grounding, 73
Mindfulness-based stress reduction, 23
Mindsight, 76
Mohamed's newborn visit, 175–181, 177*f*
Motivational interviewing (MI), 10, 18, 21, 35, 43, 55–59, 56*f*, 122
    Plan-Do-Study-Act (PDSA) model, 93
    VIVA (Validate, Inform, Validate, Ask) approach, 28, 37, 43, 45, 59, 93, 127
Multigenerational approach, 35–37
My Little Book of Big Feelings, 46, 46*f*, 140, 142–143

N

Neuroception, 37–38, 155
Neurodivergent children, 214
Neuro-endo-immune axis, 17*f*
Neuroplasticity, 155
Newborn visit, 175–181, 177*f*
Ngoc's 7-year visit, 193–198
NICER (Notice, Identify, Connect/coregulate, Explore, Review/repair) parenting, 35, 44, 46, 60*t*, 77, 109–111, 109*b*, 206
    in relationship-based, trauma-informed anticipatory guidance, 152
NICHQ Vanderbilt Assessment Scales, 166
9-5-2-1-0, 84–85, 85*f*
Nonjudgmental responses, 153, 154*f*, 158, 162–163
Nonparent relationships, close, 33
Non-suicidal self-injury (NSSI), 216–218
Nook, self-care, 48–49
Normalizing, 29

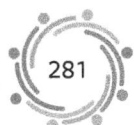

O

Older children, spending time with, 179

Open-ended questions, 58

Oppositional behaviors, 222–224

Ordinary Magic, 33

Overwhelming stress, 13, 156

    anticipatory guidance on responding to, 199–200

Oxytocin, 8, 65

P

Pain management for psychosomatic symptoms, 226

"Parenting hangover," 35

Parenting Kids Who Have Experienced Trauma: Stop, Drop and Stay in Control, 170

Pathologizing, 162–163

Perry, Bruce, 151

PHQ-9 Modified for Adolescents, 166, 198, 199, 216

Physical stress, 10

Physician-caregiver relationship, 38–40

Physicians

    bridging the practice gap for, 40–41

    clinical rotations, 2–3

    expectations about medical training, 1–2, 209

    imposter syndrome in, 2

    offsetting stress in, 227–228

    as parents, 231

    quality improvement for, 18–19

    reasons for choosing to study medicine, 1

    referrals and prescriptions offered by, 42, 62

    self-care for, 1–2

    tiring of the work, 4

    toxic stress in, 18, 232

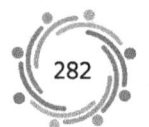
Plan-Do-Study-Act (PDSA) model, 19–22, 20*f*, 21*f*, 26, 35, 41, 53, 149
    motivational interviewing and, 58
    problem-solving using, 91–93, 94*f*
    Resilience University (RU) structure and, 122
    scheduling Resilience University (RU) sessions and, 122
Plan-Do-Study-Check, 19. *See also* Plan-Do-Study-Act (PDSA) model
Polyvagal theory, 22, 37
Porges, Stephen, 22, 37
Positive childhood experiences (PCEs), 5, 6, 8, 23, 54, 118
    anticipatory guidance on promoting, 201–202
    sticker charts and, 104–105, 104–105*f*
    strengths-based approach to begin integrating, 35
Positive stress, 10
Postpartum depression, 176
Poverty, 155–156, 167
"Preventing Childhood Toxic Stress: Partnering With Families and Communities to Promote Relational Health," 13
Proactive integration of healthy coping skills, 103–104
Problem-solving, 27–28, 33, 194–195
    Plan-Do-Study-Act cycles for, 91–93, 94*f*
Psychosomatic symptoms, 226

Q

Quality improvement, 10, 18–26
    HOPE (Healthy Outcomes from Positive Experiences), 23, 24*f*
    as lifelong process, 19
    Maine Youth Overweight Collaborative (MYOC), 20–21
    Plan-Do-Study-Act (PDSA) model for, 19–22, 20*f*, 21*f*, 26
    Resilience University (RU) and, 4, 21, 22
    Roadmap for Resilience, 24, 25*f*
    "See one, do one, teach one" strategy, 24
    Stress-buster wheel, 24, 25*f*

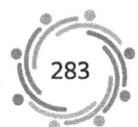

R

Reading, anticipatory guidance on, 192–193

Reassure, Return to Routine, Regulate, 73

Reconnection strategies, 206

Referrals, 42, 62

Reflective listening, 58

Relational health, 79, 80f, 81

    avoiding arguments and, 183–184

    as long-distance event, 196–197

    maternal health and, 176, 180–181

    spending time with older children and, 179

Relational responses to behaviors, 202–203

Relationship-based, trauma-informed anticipatory guidance, 149–150, 150f

    acknowledging trauma in, 151–154, 154f

    avoiding judgment and pathologizing in, 162–163

    being mindful of financial constraints in, 164–165

    bypassing blanket advice in, 164

    cocreating a plan in, 158–167

    diving deeper in, 158–159

    establishing trust in, 150–151

    identifying barriers in, 154–157, 157t

    observing stress in, 160–162

    supporting educational goals, 165–167

    supporting serve and return, 163–164

    tools in, 167–171

Relaxation breathing, 64–65

Resilience. *See also* Quality improvement

    defined, 5

    ecobiodevelopmental (EBD) model of disease and wellness and, 14–15, 16f, 17f, 18

    engineering, 6, 7f

    modifiable factors that enhance, 36

    offsetting adversity with interventions for, 14–15

    offsetting clinician stress, 227–228

    stress and, 8–10, 9f

"Resilience intelligence," 15

Resilience University (RU), 4, 21, 22, 33, 53–54, 117–118

    in action, 41–42

    behavioral health guidance, 34–38

    bridging the practice gap, 40–41

    case scenario, 43–47, 43–47f

    core components of, 122–124, 123–126t

    cultivating a self-care nook, 48–49

    curriculum of, 124, 125–126t

    emotion coaching in, 114

    graduation, 146

    honoring family structure, 48

    integrated for practice enhancement and self-care, 228–229

    launching of, 120–121

    leveraging the physician-caregiver relationship, 38–40

    potential revenue from, 124, 124t

    reflect and celebrate, 145–146

    rooming and scheduling, 127, 134, 144, 144f

    scheduling sessions for, 121–122

    session format, 127–146

    strategies for change, 133

    strengths-based clinical approach in, 27–30

    structure of, 122

    tools for. *See* Tools, Resilience University (RU)

    who can benefit from, 118–120

Revenue from Resilience University (RU), 124, 124t

Review of systems (ROS) approach, 77–82, 83f

Roadmap for Resilience, 24, 25f

Rooming and scheduling, Resilience University (RU), 127, 134, 140, 144, 144f

Rules, anticipatory guidance on, 161, 198

S

Safe, stable, nurturing relationships (SSNRs), 13–14

Safe Environment for Every Kid program, 177

Salzberg, Sharon, 70

Saul, Robert, 8, 14

Saying that trauma/stress may be cause, 27

Scheduling, Resilience University (RU) sessions, 121–122

Screen time, anticipatory guidance on, 165, 191–192

Sege, Robert, 23

Self-actuation, 39

Self-care, 1–2, 18–19

    clinician, 228

    cultivating a nook for, 48–49

    discussions around, 86

    integrating Resilience University for practice enhancement and, 228–229

    for parents, 229

    patient, 228–229

    promoting caregiver, 185

    in relationship-based, trauma-informed anticipatory guidance, 153, 154*f*

    SUNBEAM (See, Unhook, Nurture, Breathe, Emotionally Aware, Mindful, Meditation) tool, 35, 42, 45–47, 60*t*, 77, 111–112, 112–113*b*, 206

    superpowers sticker chart, 45, 45*f*

    for teens, 229

Self-harm, 216–219

Self-regulation skills, 33

Sensory grounding, 73

Sesame Street, 85

Session 1, Resilience University (RU)

    check-in, 128

    cocreating a plan, 128

    frame with strengths, 128

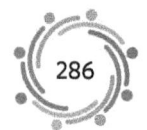
Session 1, Resilience University (RU) (*continued*)
   homework, 133–134

   rooming and scheduling, 127

   strategies for change, 133

   supplies and handouts, 127–128, 129*f*

   tools and skills, 129–133, 129*f*

Session 2, Resilience University (RU)
   check-in, 134–135

   cocreating a plan, 135

   frame with strengths, 135

   homework, 140

   rooming and scheduling, 134

   strategies for change, 137–139, 139*f*

   supplies and handouts, 134

   tools and skills, 135–136, 136*f*

Session 3, Resilience University (RU)
   check-in, 140

   cocreating a plan, 141

   framing with strengths, 140

   homework, 143

   rooming and scheduling, 140

   strategies for change, 141–143

   supplies and handouts, 140

   tools and skills, 141

Session 4, Resilience University (RU)
   check-in, 145

   framing with strengths, 145

   graduation, 146

   reflect and celebrate, 145–146

   review, 145

   rooming and scheduling, 144, 144*f*

   supplies and handouts, 144

Sick family members, 225–226

Siegel, Dan, 76

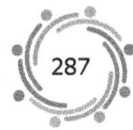
Simple requests, anticipatory guidance on, 192–193

Singing, 65

6 Steps to Connect, 170–171

Smoke exposure, 187–188

Social drivers of health (SDOH), 17, 30, 37, 39, 42, 62, 177

Somatization of emotional pain, 226

Special Supplemental Nutrition Program for Women, Infants, and Children (WIC), 164, 176

SPLINT model, 27–30

"Square" breathing. *See* "Box" breathing

Stepwise change process, 91. *See also* Resilience University (RU)

    defining success in, 94–95

    emotion coaching in, 61*t*, 113–115

    fostering change, 104–105*f*, 104–107

    Plan-Do-Study-Act cycles in, 91–93, 94*f*

    proactively integrating healthy coping skills in, 103–104

    resisting rigidity in, 99–100, 100–101*t*, 100*f*

    retrospectively "backing the bus up" in, 102, 103*f*

    timing is everything in, 97–99

    trauma-informed positive parenting in, 109–111, 109*b*

    validation in, 107–108, 108–109*b*

    when the caregiver(s) is engaged, 95–96

    when the caregiver(s) is temporarily disengaged, 96–97

Sticker charts, 104–105, 104–105*f*, 133–134, 135, 136*f*, 146

Strategies for change, Resilience University (RU), 133, 137–139, 139*f*, 141–143

Strengthening Families approach, 23

Strengths-based approach, 27–30, 35, 177*f*, 211–212, 232

    building block conversations, 83*f*

Stress

    chronic, 15

    emotional regulation strategies for, 36–37

    fight, flight, or freeze response to, 8, 12, 13, 36, 37–38, 156

    mental, 10

    mitigating the response to, 10, 11*f*

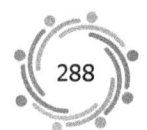

Stress (*continued*)

    neuroception and, 37–38

    offsetting clinician, 227–228

    overwhelming, 13, 156, 199–200

    in parents versus children, 12, 18, 53–54

    physical, 10

    polyvagal theory of, 22, 37

    positive, 10

    preparing families with stepwise problem-solving strategies and tools for, 9–10, 16–17

    previously established methods for lowering, 22–23

    in relationship-based, trauma-informed anticipatory guidance, 160–162

    SPLINT model for, 27–30

    tolerable, 11–12

    toxic, 12, 13, 18, 53, 152–153, 155–156, 231, 232

Stress-buster strategies, 100–101*t*

Stress-buster wheel, 24, 25*f*, 61*t*, 99, 100*f*

Stress reduction plan, 84*f*

Substance use, 35, 200–201, 219–221

Success, defining of, 94–95

Suicidality, 215–216

Summarizing, 58

SUNBEAM (See, Unhook, Nurture, Breathe, Emotionally Aware, Mindful, Meditation) tool, 35, 42, 45–47, 60*t*, 77, 111–112, 112–113*b*, 120, 206

    in relationship-based, trauma-informed anticipatory guidance, 152

Supplies and handouts, Resilience University (RU), 122–124, 123*t*, 134, 140, 144

Support system and engagement, 190–191

    bypassing blanket advice on, 164

Sympathetic nervous system, 8, 9–10, 12

Szilagyi, Moira, 14, 27

T

Talking about feelings, anticipatory guidance on, 197–198

Tantrums, 159

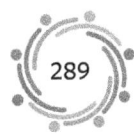
"10 Things I Can Do When I Feel Yucky" list, 46, 47*f*, 60*t*, 134, 140

"Tend and befriend," 9–10

Therapy, treatment, or guidance, 29–30

Thinking Developmentally: Nurturing Wellness in Childhood to Promote Lifelong Health, 8, 14

Three Rs. *See* Reassure, Return to Routine, Regulate

Three Rs: Ways to Support Your Child's Resilience, The, 170

"Tik Tok/YouTube brain," 60*t*, 73

Time-ins, 34–35

Time-outs, 34, 191

Time-versus-emotion curve, 43, 43*f*, 68, 68*f*, 130

Timing of stepwise change, 97–99

Toes-to-nose, 74–76

Tolerable stress, 11–12

Tools, anticipatory guidance, 167–169, 168*t*

    Anatomy of a Meltdown and, 169

    Authentic Apologies, 169–170

    catastrophizing and, 169

    Leveling Up Your Container of Love, 170

    6 Steps to Connect, 170–171

Tools, Resilience University (RU), 53–54

    breathing exercises, 60*t*, 62–66

    check-in, 128, 134–135, 140

    cocreating a plan, 128, 135, 141

    framing with strengths, 128, 135, 140, 145

    general parenting guidance, 210–213

    glitter jar, 67, 129–131, 129*f*

    healthy strategies and the science behind them in, 59, 60–61*t*

    homework, 133–134, 140

    meditation, 60*t*, 66–71, 68*f*

    mindfulness, 60*t*, 65, 71–77

    motivational interviewing (MI), 10, 18, 21, 35, 55–59, 56*f*

    9-5-2-1-0, 84–85, 85*f*

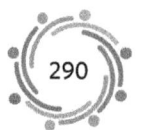
Tools, Resilience University (RU) (*continued*)

 for referrals and emergencies, 62

 in relationship-based, trauma-informed anticipatory guidance, 154

 review of systems (ROS) approach, 77–82, 83*f*

 session 1, 129–133, 129*f*

 session 2, 135–136, 136*f*

 session 3, 141

 sticker charts, 104–105, 104–105*f*, 133–134, 135, 136*f*, 146

 supplies and handouts, 122–124, 123*t*, 127–128, 134, 140, 144

 video resources, 85

Toxic stress, 12, 13, 18, 231, 232

 leading to transactional rather than relational connection, 152–153

 parental yelling and, 53

 poverty and, 155–156

 SPLINT model for, 27–30

Transactional responses to behaviors, 202–203

Trauma

 acknowledging, 151–154, 154*f*

 "big *T*" versus "little *t*," 13

 intergenerational transmission of, 155

Trauma-informed approach, 8, 9*f*, 40, 209–210

 multigenerational, 35–37

 NICER (Notice, Identify, Connect/coregulate, Explore, Review/repair) parenting, 35, 44, 46, 60*t*, 77, 109–111, 109*b*, 206

 in relationship-based, trauma-informed anticipatory guidance. *See* Relationship-based, trauma-informed anticipatory guidance

 Rutgers University behavioral health program core principles for, 153

 universal integration in. *See* Universal integration

Trauma-informed care, SUNBEAM (See, Unhook, Nurture, Breathe, Emotionally Aware, Mindful, Meditation) tool, 35, 42, 45–47, 60*t*, 77, 111–112, 112–113*b*, 206

Trauma-Informed Pediatric Practice: A Resilience-Based Roadmap to Foster Early Relational Health, The, 14, 19

Trust, establishment of, 150–151

2½-year visit, 186–193

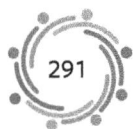

U

Universal integration, 209–210

    examples of clinical scenarios, 213–226

    general parenting guidance, 210–213

    offsetting clinician stress, 227–228

    of Resilience University for practice enhancement and self-care, 228–229

V

Validate, Validate, Validate strategy, 60*t*, 107–108, 108–109*b*

VIVA (Validate, Inform, Validate, Ask) approach, 94*f*, 106, 120

    as abbreviated MI approach, 28, 37, 43, 45, 59, 93, 127

    for addressing barriers, 156–157

    establishing trust and, 151

    for exploring family supports, 164

    in nonjudgmental responses, 158

    in observing stress, 161

    substance use and, 220

Y

Yelling, parental, 53

YouTube, 85, 86, 186

Z

Zachary, Anne, 66

Zero to Three National Parent Survey, 154–155